AF333151

Glare and Contrast Sensitivity for Clinicians

M. Princeton Nadler
David Miller
Daniel J. Nadler

Editors

Glare and Contrast Sensitivity for Clinicians

With 114 Illustrations, 22 in Full Color

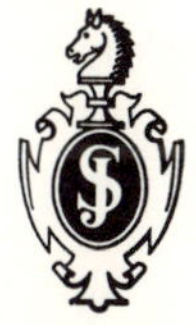

Springer-Verlag
New York Berlin Heidelberg
London Paris Tokyo Hong Kong

M. Princeton Nadler, M.D., Honorary Staff, Sewickley Valley Hospital, Sewickley, PA 15143, USA (*Mailing address:* 406 Edgeworth Lane, Sewickley, PA 15143)

David Miller, M.D., Associate Professor of Ophthalmology, Harvard Medical School; Ophthalmologist-in-Chief, Beth Israel Hospital, Boston, MA 02215, USA

Daniel J. Nadler, M.D., Clinical Assistant Professor of Ophthalmology, University of Pittsburgh, Pittsburgh, PA 15213, Department of Surgery, Sewickley Valley Hospital, Sewickley, PA 15143 USA (*Mailing address:* 409 Broad Street, Sewickley, PA 15143)

Cover: The features in the cover design relating to glare and contrast sensitivity initially were developed by the Art Department of Sewickley Valley Hospital and subsequently were rendered by Sewickley Graphics and Design, both of Sewickley, Pennsylvania. To maintain scientific fidelity, a true sinusoidal grating pattern was used for the background. The bright yellow sunburst pattern with its luminous offshoots symbolizes Nature's most brilliant and intense glare source.

Library of Congress Cataloging in Publication Data
Glare and contrast sensitivity for clinicians / M. Princeton Nadler, David Miller, Daniel J. Nadler, editors.
    p. cm.
  ISBN 0-387-97009-6
  1. Contrast sensitivity (Vision)—Testing. 2. Glare—Testing.
 I. Nadler, M. Princeton. II. Miller, David, 1933–   III. Nadler, Daniel J.
  [DNLM: 1. Contrast Sensitivity. 2. Eye Diseases—diagnosis. 3. Light,
 4. Vision Tests. 5. Visual Acuity. WW 145 G547]
 RE79.C65G53 1990
 617.7—dc20
 DNLM/DLC
 for Library of Congress   89-21882
                                                                    CIP

© 1990 by Springer-Verlag New York, Inc.

All rights reserved. This work may not be translated or copied in whole or in part without the written permission of the publisher (Springer-Verlag, 175 Fifth Avenue, New York, NY 10010, USA), except for brief excerpts in connection with reviews or scholarly analysis. Use in connection with any form of information storage and retrieval, electronic adaptation, computer software, or by similar or dissimilar methodology now known or hereafter developed is forbidden.
The use of general descriptive names, trade names, trademarks, etc. in this publication, even if the former are not especially identified, is not to be taken as a sign that such names, as understood by the Trade Marks and Merchandise Marks Act, may accordingly be used freely by anyone.
While the advice and information in this book are believed to be true and accurate at the date of going to press, neither the authors nor the editors nor the publisher can accept any legal responsibility for any errors or omissions that may be made. The publisher makes no warranty, express or implied, with respect to the material contained herein.

Typeset by Caliber Design Planning, Inc., New York, New York.
Printed and bound by Arcata Graphics/Halliday, West Hanover, Massachusetts.
Printed in the United States of America.

9 8 7 6 5 4 3 2 1

ISBN 0-387-97009-6 Springer-Verlag New York Berlin Heidelberg
ISBN 3-540-97009-6 Springer-Verlag Berlin Heidelberg New York

To Ruth, Renee, and Patty, Our Understanding Wives

Foreword

There have been greater advances in our knowledge of the visual function and its disabilities in the past 50 years than had accumulated in all of the previous years. This applies not only to the basic science of biochemistry, physiology, physiopathology, and cytopathology but also to the diagnosis and treatment of visual dysfunction and ocular disease. These advances have been aided by a proliferation of ingenious instruments.

When I began my residency in ophthalmology at The Wilmer Institute in 1938, one was supposed to learn not only the physiology of vision but also how to diagnose and treat all phases of ophthalmology including disabilities of the orbit, sclera, retina, lens, and cornea. In addition he or she was supposed to understand neuro-ophthalmology, ophthalmic genetics, and so-called uveitis.

It soon became evident that no one could adequately comprehend all of these areas and, therefore, most young trainees today take a year or two of fellowship in a specialized area following their three- to five-year residency training. Following this they join a group of other ophthalmologists and specialize. Thus, they become more expert in the diagnosis and treatment in a limited area in ophthalmology. When I returned to The Wilmer Institute in 1955 as Head of the Department I was the only full-time member of the staff. To date we have some 28 full-time ophthalmologists working in highly specialized areas of our institution.

It is interesting that in spite of the great advances that have occurred in the past 50 years most ophthalmologists still test the patient's visual acuity by the use of a high-contrast letter-based acuity chart devised by Snellen in 1862. We have all known that the vision so taken in a uniformly illuminated room did not explain the patient's complaints of visual perception under a number of different conditions, particularly when attempting to drive a car at night.

I will now quote from one of the authors, David Miller, "We are slowly coming to learn that contrast sensitivity testing and glare testing can explain patient complaints, when Snellen acuity in a darkened examining room is normal. Thus, these tests can help us follow optic neuritis, certain types of cataracts, certain types of corneal disease, etc. It is simply a finer measuring tool, much as the microscope helps us see disease process that gross anatomical studies do not allow us to see."

In explaining the purpose of this text, *Glare and Contrast Sensitivity for Clinicians*, Princeton Nadler has stated, "As you are aware, the subjects of glare disability and contrast sensitivity testing are receiving wide exposure in the field of ophthalmology. There is considerable confusion and misunderstanding in these areas as well as a notable lack of standardization with regard to measurement of these factors. The purpose of our text is to educate clinicians with regard to the subjects of glare and contrast sensitivity by providing them with a comprehensive discussion of these subjects written in language that they can understand."

It is interesting that George Young in 1918 wrote a very interesting paper on "Threshold Tests" in the *British Journal of Ophthalmology*, but ophthalmologists have made little use of this method of examination until recently.

Again I quote David Miller, "Although the world of visual psychologists have worked with and appreciated the importance of contrast sensitivity for about 50 years, clinicians are in general unaware of the data, the importance, the usefulness and vocabulary surrounding this field. Thus, this book is an honest attempt to bring the clinician into that world in language he can understand."

Today we live in an era of extracapsular cataract surgery and posterior chamber intraocular lenses, an era of fewer operative and post-operative complications, an era when the patient is rehabilitated to almost normal vision. Thus, it becomes very important for us to understand the effects of glare and contrast sensitivity both pre-operatively and post-operatively. These tests explain why we are now operating on many patients with cataracts who complain that their vision decreases in bright illumination or who have stopped driving at night although their visual acuity is 20/30 to 20/40 in our examining rooms.

I will now quote Daniel J. Nadler, Princeton's son, "As with any new measurement of visual disability, glare testing and contrast sensitivity testing both have potential for abuse by clinicians. These tests are not intended to provide physicians with another means of boosting their surgical volume but rather should be added to the armamentarium of existing measurements of visual disability and should be applied judiciously. The text of this book is organized in a manner that enables the reader to selectively choose the areas of greatest interest to him. While some of the chapters may not seem immediately clinically relevant they provide the background information that will enable clinicians to better understand future developments that will undoubtedly occur."

Doctors Nadler, Princeton and his son, Daniel, and David Miller have wisely selected some of the most capable basic scientists and clinicians who are doing studies in the field of glare disability and contrast sensitivity to provide chapters for this book. I am certain that reading it will prove helpful to the general eye practitioner, the neuro-ophthalmologist, the glaucoma specialist, the retinal specialist, and lens and corneal specialists. I also believe that as the instruments are perfected, become easier to use, and are produced at a reasonable cost that these tests will become a routine part of the examination of the patient's vision by many ophthalmologists.

A. Edward Maumenee, M.D.
President
The International Council
of Ophthalmology

Preface

During an informal lunch break at the fall 1987 meeting of the American Academy of Ophthalmology, the three of us decided to organize a multi-authored book for clinicians concerning aspects of glare and contrast sensitivity. We had watched the growth in the number of equipment companies producing glare and contrast measuring instruments and we had noted more and more time being devoted to the subject at various clinical meetings. Our objective was to educate clinicians with regard to glare and contrast sensitivity by providing them with a comprehensive discussion *written in language they could understand*. This latter stipulation was stressed to contributing authors, all of whom are experts in their assigned topics. We feel that this goal largely has been attained, although portions of the text will require careful study.

Understandably, each author was most secure and comfortable defining his or her own basic terms and concepts. Despite occasional subtle conceptual differences, there is a strong connecting theme throughout. Repetition of key concepts in different chapters should provide reassuring reinforcement for the reader.

Contemporary clinicians recognize the current evolution and growth of interest in assessing the broad concept of quality of vision, and they are aware that more is involved than simply determining Snellen acuity. Such assessment now is within the realm of standard clinical practice.

We hope that this book will further stimulate your interest in the measuring of glare and contrast sensitivity as a useful and enlightening addition to your clinical diagnostic armamentarium.

M. Princeton Nadler, M.D.
David Miller, M.D.
Daniel J. Nadler, M.D.

Contents

Contents

Contributors

Lloyd M. Aiello, M.D., Director, William P. Beetham Eye Research and Treatment Unit, Joslin Diabetes Center, Boston, Massachusetts; Associate Clinical Professor of Ophthalmology, Harvard Medical School, Boston, Massachusetts 02115, USA

Geoffrey B. Arden, Professor of Neurophysiology, Department of Clinical Ophthalmology, Institute of Ophthalmology, London, United Kingdom

Ivan Bodis-Wollner, M.D., Professor of Neurology and Ophthalmology, Department of Neurology, The Mount Sinai Medical Center, New York, New York 10029-6574, USA

Jerry D. Cavallerano, O.D., Ph.D., Staff Optometrist, William P. Beetham Eye Research Unit, Joslin Diabetes Center, Boston, Massachusetts 02115; Assistant Professor of Optometry, New England College of Optometry, Boston, Massachusetts 02115, USA

Chris A. Johnson, Ph.D., Associate Professor, Department of Ophthalmology, University of California, Davis, Sacramento, California 95816, USA

Philip Lempert, M.D., Lecturer, Department of Applied Engineering and Physics, Cornell University, Ithaca, New York 14850; Research Instructor, Department of Ophthalmology, State University of New York College of Medicine, Syracuse, New York 13210, USA

Mark J. Mannis, M.D., F.A.C.S., Associate Professor, Department of Ophthalmology, University of California, Davis, Sacramento, California 95816, USA

A. Edward Maumenee, M.D., President, The International Council of Ophthalmology, Baltimore, Maryland 21205, USA

David Miller, M.D., Associate Professor of Ophthalmology, Harvard Medical School, Boston, Massachusetts 02115; Ophthalmologist-in-Chief, Beth Israel Hospital, Boston, Massachusetts 02215, USA

Daniel J. Nadler, M.D., Clinical Assistant Professor of Ophthalmology, University of Pittsburgh, Pittsburgh, Pennsylvania 15213, Department of Surgery, Sewickley Valley Hospital, Sewickley, Pennsylvania, 15143, USA (*Mailing address:* 406 Edgeworth Lane, Sewickley, PA 15143)

M. Princeton Nadler, M.D., Honorary Staff, Sewickley Valley Hospital, Sewickley, Pennsylvania 15143, USA (*Mailing address:* 409 Broad Street, Sewickley, PA 15143)

Thomas C. Prager, Ph.D., Clinical Assistant Professor, Department of Ophthalmology, University of Texas Health Science Center–Hermann Eye Center, Houston, Texas 77030, USA

Mark S. Rea, Ph.D., Director, Lighting Research Center, Rensselaer Polytechnic Institute, Troy, New York 12180-3590, USA

Suketu S. Sanghvi, M.D., Department of Ophthalmology, Pacific Presbyterian Medical Center, San Francisco, California 94115, USA

Rita L. Storch, M.D., Research Associate, Department of Ophthalmology, Mount Sinai School of Medicine, New York, New York 10029, USA

Jeremy M. Wolfe, Ph.D., Associate Professor, Massachusetts Institute of Technology, Department of Brain and Cognitive Sciences, Cambridge, Massachusetts 02139, USA

Karla Zadnik, O.D., Assistant Clinical Professor of Optometry, Department of Ophthalmology, School of Medicine, University of California, Davis, Sacramento, California 95816, USA

Daan Zwick, Senior Research Associate (Retired), Research Laboratories, Eastman Kodak Company, Rochester, New York 14650, USA

Terms and Concepts

This glossary of terms and concepts related to glare and contrast sensitivity is intended as a helpful preview, as well as a convenient reference. Many of the definitions were modified from the following sources: *Handbook of Optics*, by the Optical Society of America (McGraw-Hill, New York, N.Y., 1978); *Intraocular Light Scattering*, by D. Miller and G. Benedek (Charles C Thomas, Springfield, Ill., 1973); and the *IES Lighting Handbook, 1984 Reference Volume*, by permission of the Illuminating Engineering Society of North America, New York, N.Y. Readers who desire greater technical detail or precision are referred to the original sources.

A

acuity: see *visual acuity.*

acutance: a measure of the sharpness with which a film can reproduce the edge of an object.

adaptation: the process by which the visual system becomes accustomed to more or less light or light of a different color than it was exposed to during an immediately preceding period; results in a change in the sensitivity of the eye to light. See *scotopic vision, photopic vision.* Adaptation is also used to refer to the final state of the process, as reaching a condition of *dark adaptation* or *light adaptation.*

after image: a visual response that occurs after the stimulus causing it has ceased.

Alzheimers disease: presenile dementia.

ambient lighting: lighting throughout an area that produces general illumination. See *general lighting.*

amblyopia: impaired foveal vision, unilateral or bilateral, in the absence of demonstrable organic disease.

amplitude: the maximum displacement of a particle in harmonic motion or the maximum value of any wave or its harmonic function.

Amsler test: test that involves the use of a grid pattern (Amsler grid) consisting of a 20-cm square subdivided into 5-mm squares. The patient looks at the center of the square so that any defect in the encompassed visual field is projected onto the grid test pattern; sensitive method of assessing abnormalities of the fovea centralis that are so slight as not to be detected by the usual methods of perimetry.

angstrom: unit of wavelength equal to 10^{-10} m (one ten-billionth meter); nanometer (10^{-9} meter) now preferred.

antihalation backing: a coating on the back surface of films to absorb the image light which reaches the rear surface and prevent its reflection back into the emulsion. See *spread function.*

aphakia: the term used to describe the optical condition of the eye when the crystalline lens is absent.

apperceptions: past or learned experiences which are brought to bear to form an integrated impression of a complex optical image. See *Chapter 12, Introduction, Definitions*; see *perception* and *visual perception.*

B

back light: illumination from behind (and usually above) a subject to produce a highlight along its edge and consequent separation between the subject and its background.

band-pass filter: a wave filter that attenuates waves on either side of a specified spatial frequency (Sf) range or band. Signals (waves) within the band are accepted while those outside the specified range are rejected.

The visual system, or any optical system, can be characterized as a filter that selectively passes some spatial frequencies and not others. A filter that selectively passes high spatial frequency gratings but attenuates or blocks low frequency gratings would be called a *high-pass filter*. The optical system of the eye is a *low-pass filter* that attenuates or blocks high frequency gratings. Finally, the *visual system as a whole* attenuates both low and high frequencies. It passes stimuli in a specific range, or band, and is thus referred to as a *band-pass filter*.

black light: the popular term for ultraviolet energy near the visible spectrum.

blinding glare: glare which is so intense that for an appreciable length of time after it has been removed, no object can be seen. As from a flash bulb, direct sun, or an atomic explosion; light intensity beyond physiologic range.

brightness: see *subjective brightness*; see *Chapter 12, Definition*.

brightness contrast threshold: when two patches of color are separated by a brightness contrast the border between the two patches is a brightness contrast border. The contrast which is just detectable is known as the brightness contrast threshold.

C

candela, cd: the International System (SI) unit of luminous intensity. One candela is one lumen per steradian. *Formerly, candle.* Since 1948, the internationally accepted name for the unit of luminous intensity is candela. The difference between the candela and the old international candle is so small that only measurements of high accuracy are affected.

candlepower: luminous intensity expressed in candelas.

cataract: any opacity or cloudiness of the crystalline lens or its capsule. Light, if incident upon the opacity, becomes scattered and superimposed upon the retinal image, degrading it to various degress.

central (foveal) vision: the seeing of objects in the central or foveal part of the visual field, approximately two degrees in diameter. It permits seeing much finer detail than does peripheral vision.

channels: see *spatial frequency channels*. Spatial frequency and/or directionally oriented selective "channels" or "mechanisms" acknowledge that experiments do not directly measure the response of single ganglion cells, but closely related "family groups" of cells. The contrast sensitivity function curve is probably, in aggregate, made up of about six to eight spatial frequency selective contiguous or overlapping channels. See *Chapter 2, Figure 2.13*.

characteristic curve: a curve on a graph which represents the response of specific photographic materials to varying amounts of light. See *Chapter 12, Figure 12.3*.

chroma: the purity of a color, or its saturation and freedom from white or gray.

chromatic adaptation: the process by which the chromatic properties of the visual system are modified by the observation of stimuli of various chromaticities and luminances. See *state of chromatic adaptation*.

chromatic contrast: visual targets that have the same luminance as the background may still be discerned by color information. These equal luminance chromatic contrasts are generally less distinct than achromatic contrasts but under some conditions they can be quite visible. Although significant, chromatic contrast produces maximum visibilities which are generally less than 20 percent of the contrasts that are obtainable from luminance differences. A contrast border can involve both differences in luminance and chromaticity on the two sides of the border.

chromaticity of a color: the dominant or complementary wavelength and purity aspects of the color taken together.

clear sky: a sky that has less than 30 percent cloud cover.

cloudy sky: a sky having more than 70 percent cloud cover.

color: the characteristic of light by which a human observer may distinguish between two structure-free patches of light of the same size and shape. See *object color, hue of a perceived color*.

color comparison, or color grading: the judgment of equality, or of the amount and character of difference, of the color of two objects viewed under identical illumination.

color discrimination: the perception of differences between two or more colors.

color rendering: general expression for the effect of a light source on the color appearance of objects in conscious or subconscious comparison with their color appearance under a reference light source.

conspicuity: the capacity of a signal to stand out in relation to its background so as to be readily discovered by the eye; noticeable, conspicuous.

contrast: the manifestation of differences in luminance or color between objects or areas in space. Usually applied to contiguous areas. See *Chapter 12*. See *luminance contrast, chromatic contrast*.

contrast detection: the basic task from which all other visual behaviors are derived. The simplest visual function is one in which a small change in luminance must be detected in an otherwise uniform surround.

contrast, photographic: a term used to describe the separation of tones in a negative or print. A picture which has only a slight increase in density from tone to tone for a given increase in exposure is termed *low in* *contrast* and one which has a large increase from tone to tone for the same increase in exposure is said to be *high in contrast*.

contrast sensitivity: the ability to detect the presence of minimal luminance differences between objects or areas in space. Quantitatively it is equal to the reciprocal of the contrast threshold. Contrast sensitivity, and spatial frequency, are plotted on logarithmic scales because they better reflect perceptual reality. See *Chapter 2, Methodology of Contrast Sensitivity Testing*.

contrast sensitivity curve: a graphic representation of the patient's vision for a range of spatial frequencies. See *contrast sensitivity function*.

contrast sensitivity function (CSF): a function measured using a range of sinusoidal grating patterns as the visual stimulus. Contrast sensitivity assesses the patient's visual sensitivity to large, intermediate, and small objects (spatial frequencies) under circumstances of varying contrast. The *aggregate* of the patient's visual performance over this range of various target sizes (spatial frequencies) is known as the *contrast sensitivity function*. When plotted in orderly sequence, the curve connecting these threshold measurements is a *graphic* representation of the CSF known as the *Contrast Sensitivity Curve*. It is sometimes also known as the Spatial Modulation Transfer Function (SMTF). See *Chapter 2, Figures 2.3, 2.6, 2.7, 2.13*.

cortical cell tuning: see *tuned cortical cells*.

cut-off frequency: the last point on the spatial contrast sensitivity curve, which represents the finest pattern an observer can detect at a theoretical 100 percent contrast. See *grating acuity*.

D

dark adaptation: the process by which the retina becomes adapted to a luminance less than about 0.034 candela per square meter. See *adaption*.

dazzle glare: or *simultaneous glare*. A form of disability glare; associated with *bright lights* (sun, headlights, street lights, wall lights, unshaded lamps) in the field of view which form images upon peripheral portions of the retina *off the line of sight*. In " . . . one way or another (they) reduce the sensitivity of the eye for seeing objects imaged upon the central . . . region of the retina" (L. L. Holladay, 1926). May be accompanied by *discomfort glare*.

daylight lamp: a lamp producing a spectral distribution approximating that of a photographic image.

density: a numerical measure of the blackening, or light-stopping ability, of a specified daylight.

density range: the measured difference between the maximum and minimum densities of a particular negative or positive. See *Chapter 12*.

density scale: another term for density range.

detection acuity: see *visual acuity*.

deuteranopia: a defect of vision in which the retina fails to respond to green.

diffraction: the bending of a wave around a barrier or in passing through a slit.

diffused lighting: lighting provided on the workplane or on an object, that is not predominantly incident from any particular direction.

diffuse reflection: reflection of light at many different angles by a rough surface; occurs and increases as the smoothness of a surface decreases, thus scattering the incident light in many directions. See *specular reflection*.

direct glare: glare resulting from high luminances or insufficiently shielded light sources in the field of view. It usually is associated with bright areas, such as luminaires, ceilings, and windows which are outside the visual task or region being viewed. It can cause light scatter within the eye, most seriously affecting older people because of age-dependent imperfections in their ocular media. Direct glare is most troublesome when the light source is bright and close to the line of sight to the task. See *veiling glare, entoptic scatter, intraocular light scatter*.

disability glare: glare resulting in reduced visual performance and visibility. It often is accompanied by discomfort. See *light shock, blinding glare, veiling glare, veiling luminance, dazzle glare*.

discomfort glare: glare producing subjective visual discomfort or fatigue. It does not necessarily interfere with visual performance or visibility.

display: a particular visual presentation for analysis or testing in terms of contrast or visibility, such as a disc or figure on a background of different luminance. See *visibility*.

E

electromagnetic spectrum: a continuum of electric and magnetic radiation encompassing all wavelengths; an equivalent statement is that such waves are not intermittent but follow one another without any interval of time between. See *regions of electromagnetic spectrum*.

electromagnetic radiant energy: an energy that provides a physical stimulus that enters the eye and causes the sensation of light and color. See *electromagnetic spectrum*.

electro-oculogram: an electrophysiological measurement of the resting potential of the eye generated by the retinal pigment epithelium. May be used to measure saccadic velocities or to help confirm the diagnosis of Best's disease. See *electrophysiological testing*.

electrophysiological testing: testing applied mostly in research as a more objective approach for obtaining information; examples are electroretinogram testing (ERG), electro-oculogram testing (EOG), and visual evoked potential testing (VEP). Requires no judgment or patient response and only minimal cooperation from patient. Useful in infants and uncooperative patients. See *Chapter 9, Methods of Testing*.

electroretinogram (ERG): an electrophysiological measurement of the integrity of the rods and cones. Can be applied to measure the effects of macular edema, diabetic retinopathy, laser photocoagulation, and other disorders of the photoreceptors. Requires no subjective response from the patient.

emulsion: the light-sensitive coating of a photographic material, mainly silver salts suspended in gelatin; roughly its biologic counterpart is the *retina*.

emulsion speed: the rate of response (sensitivity) of a photographic emulsion to light, determined under standard conditions of exposure and subsequent development; roughly its biologic counterpart is *contrast sensitivity*.

entoptic scatter: a certain amount of light scatter from the refracting surfaces of the eyes, the ocular media, and the fundus. It can lead to a reduction in visibility of objects. See *disability glare*.

exposure: the quantity of light which is allowed to act on a photographic material. The product of the intensity and the duration of the light acting on the emulsion.

F

flare: non-image light which reaches the focal plane of an imaging system. Its source may be any stray light falling directly on or reflected to, from, or within the surfaces of the lens system and its supporting structures. Its general effect is to lower the contrast of the image obtained or to cause unwanted meaningless images, or both, at the focal plane. See *Chapter 12*.

fog: a veil of silver granules of low density on a photographic material; most commonly caused by non-image light striking the material or by incorrect chemical treatment. See *veiling luminance*.

footcandle, fc: the unit of illuminance when the foot is taken as the unit of measurement. It is the illuminance on a surface one square foot in area on which there is a uniformly distributed flux of one lumen, or the illuminance produced on a surface all points of which are at a distance of one foot from a directionally uniform point source of one candela. See *candela*.

footlambert, fl: a unit of luminance equal to $1/\pi$ candela per square foot, or to the uniform luminance of a perfectly diffusing surface emitting or reflecting light at the rate of one lumen per square foot, or to the average luminance of any surface emitting or reflecting light at that rate. The average luminance of any reflecting surface in footlamberts is, therefore, the product of the illumination in footcandles by the luminous reflectance of the surface. The use of this unit is to be deprecated. See *units of luminance*.

Fourier analysis: the mathematical analysis and reduction of any optotype into its sinusoidal component parts.

Fourier's theory: a theory developed by the French physicist, Fourier, showing that it is possible to describe any complex periodic waveform as the sum of a specific series of sine waves. The amplitudes, phases, and frequencies of these waves are a characteristic of the original (fundamental) wave form and constitute a full description of it. See *Chapter 4, Figure 4.3*; see *harmonics*.

fovea: a small region at the center of the retina, subtending about two degrees, containing only cones and forming the site of most distinct vision.

function: a statement or declaration in the form of a data chart, a graph, or an equation, that for any value of one variable, there is a unique value of another.

fundamental frequency (F): the lowest frequency of any free vibration. See *Chapter 4, Figure 4.3*. See *harmonics, harmonic series*.

G

gamma: a numerical designation for the contrast of a photographic material as represented by the slope of the straight-line portion of the *characteristic curve*. The gamma is numerically equal to the tangent of the angle which the straight-line portion makes with the base line. See *Chapter 12, Figure 12.3*.

general lighting: lighting designed to provide a substantially uniform level of illumination throughout an area, exclusive of any provision for special local requirements. See *ambient lighting*.

geniculate body: a way station in the central nervous system for the transmission of most visual impulses (70 percent) from the retina to the visual cortex.

glare: the sensation produced by luminance within the visual field that is sufficiently greater than the luminance to which the eyes are adapted to cause annoyance, discomfort, or loss in visual performance and visibility. The magnitude of the sensation of glare depends upon such factors as the size, position and luminance of a source, the number of sources, and the luminance to which the eyes are adapted. See *Chapter 3, Contrast and Glare for Normal Eyes*. See *blinding glare, direct glare, disability glare, discomfort glare, dazzle, veiling glare*.

grain: minute variations of density in a developed photographic emulsion. Caused by irregular distribution of the silver crystals.

grating acuity: determined by the highest resolvable spatial frequency and represents only the last point on the entire contrast sensitivity curve, the so called *cut-off frequency*. It is roughly equivalent to Snellen acuity. See *visual acuity, contrast sensitivity curve*.

H

halation: a blurring of a photographic image, particularly in highlight areas, caused by light reflected from the back surface of the film emulsion. See *Chapter 12*. See *anti-halation backing*.

halftone: a tone pattern in a photographic reproduction composed of dots of uniform density but varying in size.

harmonics: in general refers to the components of a repetitive waveform having a frequency that is an integral multiple of the fundamental frequency (e.g. a wave with three times the frequency of the fundamental is called the third harmonic). A particular display (waveform) can be made up of the fundamental frequency combined with a number of its harmonics. The sum total of their combined frequencies, amplitudes, and phases will be a complex waveform (e.g. a square wave) rather than a simple sinusoidal one. See *fundamental frequency*; see *Chapter 4, Figure 4.3B*.

harmonic motion (as differentiated from "harmonics"): see *simple harmonic motion*.

harmonic series: a series of numbers, often representing the frequencies of a mixture of waves or vibrations, such that all are integral multiples of the lowest or fundamental frequency. See *fundamental frequency, Fourier's theory*; see *Chapter 4, Figure 4.3*.

hertz, Hz: A unit of temporal frequency equal to one cycle per second; 10 Hz equal 10 cycles per second.

highlight: the lightest portion of a picture. In a negative, the highlights are the areas of highest density, since these correspond to the lightest areas of the original.

high-pass filter: see *band-pass filter*.

hue of a perceived color: the attribute that determines whether the color is red, yellow, green, or blue.

hypertension, ocular (OHT): elevated intraocular pressure without visual field defects or any evidence of ocular nerve damage.

I

illuminance: the density of the luminous flux incident on a surface; it is the quotient of the luminous flux by the area of the surface when the latter is uniformly illuminated. It is measured in lumens per square meter (lm/m^2) or lux.

illumination: the act of illuminating or state of being illuminated. This term has been used for density of luminous flux on a surface (illuminance) and such use is to be deprecated.

image: an optical representation of an object such that each point on the image corresponds to a point on the object.

incandescence: the self-emission of radiant energy in the visible spectrum due to the thermal excitation of atoms or molecules.

indirect lighting: lighting by luminaires distributing 90–100 percent of the emitted light *upward*.

intensity: a shortening of the terms luminous intensity and radiant intensity. Often misused for level of illumination or illuminance.

intraocular light scattering: the optical phenomenon of transmitted light being scattered in a stray unfocused manner by opacities within the ocular media. Superimposed upon the retinal image, it can degrade contrast and image quality depending upon:

1. The amount and intensity of the scattered light.
2. The extent and density of the opacity.
3. The strengths and subleties of contrast within the visual scene being imaged upon the retina.

See *entoptic scatter, veiling luminance, veiling glare, direct glare, glare*.

L

lambert, L: a lambertian unit of luminance equal to $1/\pi$ candela per square centimeter. The use of this term is deprecated.

laser: an acronym for Light Amplification by Stimulated Emission of Radiation. The laser produces a highly monochromatic and coherent (spatial and temporal) beam of radiation. A steady oscillation of nearly a single electromagnetic mode is maintained in a volume of an active material bounded by highly reflecting surfaces, called a resonator. The frequency of oscillation varies according to the material used and by the methods of initially exciting or pumping the material.

lens: a glass or plastic element used in luminaires to change the direction and control the distribution of light rays.

light: radiant energy that is capable of stimulating the retina and producing a visual sensation. The visible portion of the electromagnetic spectrum extends from about 380 to 770 nm. The subjective impression produced by stimulating the retina is sometimes designated as light. Visual sensations are sometimes arbitrarily defined as sensations of light, and in line with this concept it is sometimes said that light cannot exist until an eye has been stimulated. Electrical stimulation of the retina or the visual cortex is described as producing flashes of light. In illuminating engineering, however, light is a physical entity—radiant energy weighted by the luminous efficiency function. It is a physical stimulus which can be applied to the retina.

light adaptation: the process by which the retina becomes adapted to a luminance greater than about 3.4 candelas per square meter. See also *dark adaptation*.

light shock: see *blinding glare*.

local lighting: lighting designed to provide illuminance over a relatively small area or confined space. See *task lighting*.

low-pass filter: see *band-pass filter*.

lumen, lm: SI unit of luminous flux. Photometrically, it is the luminous flux emitted within a unit solid angle (one steradian) by a point source having a uniform luminous intensity of one candela.

luminaire: a complete lighting unit consisting of a lamp or lamps together with the parts designed to distribute the light, to position and protect the lamps, and to connect the lamps to the power supply.

luminance: corresponding to the *formerly photometric brightness* of objects, or areas, and measured in candelas per square meter (cd/m^2) or *nits*. Luminance is used most frequently in specifying the stimulus for vision. See *subjective brightness*.

luminance contrast: defined in several ways. When the contrast of an object is specified one must know which definition is being used. For our purpose, in dealing with *modulation* (contrast) of periodic, or grating patterns, it is defined by

$$\text{Modulation } (contrast) = \frac{L_{max} - L_{min}}{L_{max} + L_{min}}$$

sometimes referred to as the *Michelson contrasts* as opposed to the *Weber contrast*. See *modulation, Weber contrast*.

luminance difference: the difference in luminance between two areas. It usually is applied to contiguous areas, such as the detail of a visual task and its immediate background, in which case it is quantitatively equal to the numerator in the formula for luminance contrast.

luminance threshold: the minimum perceptible difference in luminance for a given state of adaptation of the eye.

lux, lx: the SI unit of illuminance. One lux is one lumen per square meter (lm/m^2).

M

macular photostress test: a sensitive test for detecting patients with macular disturbances such as cystoid macular edema, central serous chorodopathy, and macular degeneration. After time and light-intensity controlled photostress (exposure to a strong light), these conditions are characterized by significantly prolonged recovery of vision. Testing parameters for this test are well standardized in some newer glare testing equipment (Brightness Acuity Tester, BAT).

matte surface: one from which the reflection is predominantly diffuse, with or without a negligible specular component. See *diffuse reflection*.

mesopic vision: vision with fully adapted eyes at luminance conditions between those of photopic and scotopic vision, that is, between about 3.4 and 0.034 candelas per square meter.

metamers: lights composed of different spectral energy distributions but perceived as having the same color (hue); surfaces that appear to retain the same color even though viewed when illuminated by light sources of differing spectral energy distributions.

Michelson contrast: see *luminance contrast*.

middle tones: in general, the tones in a photographic reproduction between the highlights and the shadows.

modulate, modulation: two important terms in the vocabulary surrounding the field of glare and contrast sensitivity. Subtle differences in definition are usually apparent from general context and method of usage.

a. *modulate*, a verb meaning to adjust, change, temper, soften, or tone down; to change the characteristics of a wave form as to frequency or intensity.

b. *modulation*, a noun meaning the state of being modulated, adjusted, changed, tempered, softened, toned down.

For our purposes *modulation*, as a noun, is frequently used interchangeably with *contrast* but is usually and more properly called *modulation*. It applies to periodic patterns, such as gratings, which have one maximum luminance (L_{max}) and one minimum luminance (L_{min}) in each cycle. The equation which defines and quantifies this factor is

$$\text{Modulation } (contrast) = \frac{L_{max} - L_{min}}{L_{max} + L_{min}}$$

modulation, temporal: the term denoting time-dependent contrast. It is the perceived contrast (modulation) of a grating pattern that is dependent upon and varies with the time (temporal) increments or decrements allowed for viewing the grating test pattern.

modulation transfer function (MTF): the MTF applies, by definition, to the imagery of an object or target linear (gratings) pattern whose illuminance can be described by a sinusoidal function or by a combination of sinusoidal functions. It cannot be applied directly to other (nonsinusoidal) patterns.

The modulation (contrast) transfer function, is a measure of the fidelity (in terms of contrast) with which an optical device or system, human or otherwise, transmits images with various spatial frequency components. Because of optical aberrations, or the *spread function*, such transmitted images are less than perfect and therefore this quantity varies from 0 to 1. It can be multiplied by 100 percent to give percent contrast (modulation) of the image as compared to the object contrast (modulation). See *Chapter 2, Stimuli for Measuring Contrast Sensitivity.* MTF can effectively evaluate system imaging performance or that of any of the individual components. See *optical transfer function (OTF); spread function.*

Munsell color system: a system of surface-color specification based on perceptually uniform color scales for the three variables: Munsell hue, Munsell value, and Munsell chroma. For an observer of normal color vision, adapted to daylight, and viewing a specimen when illuminated by daylight and surrounded with a middle gray to white background, the Munsell hue, value, and chroma of the color correlate well with the hue, lightness, and perceived chroma.

N

nanometer: unit of wavelength equal to 10^{-9} *meter* (one-billionth meter). See *angstrom.*

near infrared: the region of the electromagnetic spectrum from 770 to 1400 nanometers.

negative: the image obtained from the original in the conventional photographic process. The tones are the reverse of those in the original subject.

neutral density filter: a filter to reduce uniformly all colors of light.

nit, nt: a unit of luminance equal to one candela per square meter. **NOTE:** Candela per square meter is the International System (SI) unit of luminance.

O

object color: the color of the light reflected or transmitted by the object when illuminated by a standard light source.

optical transfer function (OTF) of an optical system: its modulus is the MTF, also known as the contrast transfer, the frequency response, and sine wave response. See *modulation transfer function.*

optotype: type used on an eye chart.

overcast sky: one that has 100 percent cloud cover; the sun is not visible.

P

panchromatic: a term applied to photographic materials which are sensitive to light of all colors. Their range of color sensitivity approximates that of the human eye.

papilledema: swelling of the optic nerve head.

Pelli-Robson chart: single-size large-letter variable-contrast chart to measure peak threshold contrast sensitivity function (CSF) at spatial frequency (Sf) between 3 and 5 cycles/degree. See *Chapter 9, Meth-*

ods of Testing, psychophysical.

perception: See *visual perception.*

perfect diffusion: that in which light flux is uniformly scattered such that the luminance (radiance) is the same in all directions.

peripheral vision: the seeing of objects displaced from the primary line of sight and outside the central visual field.

peripheral visual field: that portion of the visual field that falls outside the region corresponding to the foveal portion of the retina.

phase: the time relationship of two cyclic, or wave, motions. Two motions are *in phase* if they reach their peaks with the same displacement and direction simultaneously, and *out of phase* if they do otherwise.

photometer: an instrument for measuring photometric quantities such as luminance, luminous intensity, luminous flux, and illuminance.

photopic vision: vision mediated essentially or exclusively by the cones. It is generally associated with adaptation to a luminance of at least 3.4 candelas per square meter. See *scotopic vision.*

photostress test: see *macular photostress test.*

polarization: the act, process, or result of altering the transverse vibrations of light waves so that they are oriented in a specific plane perpendicular to the direction of propagation but are not uniform in amplitude in all directions of that plane; polarization may be obtained by using either transmitting or reflecting media.

polarized: said of an electromagnetic or other transverse wave, having all its vibrations in a single transverse direction.

positive: a photographic image, usually made from a negative, in which the tones are not reversed as in a negative. A positive on paper is usually called a *print,* and one on a transparent base, such as film, is called a positive *transparency.*

protanopia: a defect of vision in which the retina fails to respond to red.

pseudophakia: a term used to describe the optical condition of the eye when the natural crystalline lens has been replaced by an artificial intraocular lens (IOL).

psychophysical testing: based on patient's verbal responses; a subjective way for obtaining a contrast sensitivity function (CSF). Methodology utilizes either printed or electronically generated patterns and permits only threshold data to be obtained. It requires judgment and patient cooperation and is subject to some variabilities in testing conditions and score obtained. See *Chapter 9, Methods of Testing.*

Q

quality of lighting: pertains to the distribution of luminance in a visual environment. The term, used in a positive sense, implies that all luminances contribute favorably to visual performance, visual comfort, ease of seeing, safety, and esthetics for the specific visual tasks involved.

quality of vision: refers to the *holistic* vision or visual experience as compared to a theoretical standard which is characterized by normal visual acuity, light and dark adaption, color vision, full visual field, and contrast sensitivity function, all of which are unimpaired by glare and uncorrected refractive errors or by inadequate ambient and task lighting. See *visual function*.

quartz-iodine lamp: an obsolete term for tungsten-halogen lamp.

R

radiance: radiant brightness or amount of light energy flux emitted or propagated from a source by radiation.

radiation: energy transferred through space as electro-magnetic waves.

recognition acuity: see *visual acuity*.

reflected glare: glare resulting from specular reflections of high luminances in polished or glossy surfaces in the field of view. It usually is associated with reflections from within a visual task or areas in close proximity to the region being viewed. See *veiling reflection*.

reflection: a general term for the process by which the incident flux leaves a surface or medium from the incident side, without change in frequency. Reflection is usually a combination of regular and diffuse reflection. See *regular (specular) reflection, diffuse reflection, and veiling reflection*.

regular reflection: see *specular reflection*.

refraction: the process by which the direction of a ray of light changes as it passes obliquely from one medium to another in which its speed is different.

regions of electromagnetic spectrum: for convenience of reference the electromagnetic spectrum is arbitrarily divided as follows:

Vacuum ultraviolet	
Extreme ultraviolet	10–100 nm
Far ultraviolet	100–200 nm
Middle ultraviolet	200–300 nm
Near ultraviolet	300–380 nm
Visible	380–770 nm
Near (short-wavelength) infrared	770–1400 nm
Intermediate infrared	1400–5000 nm
Far (long-wavelength) infrared	5000–1,000,000 nm

NOTE: The spectral limits indicated above have been chosen as a matter of practical convenience. There is a gradual transition from region to region without sharp delineation. Also, the division of the spectrum is not unique. In various fields of science the classification may differ due to the phenomena of interest.

regular reflection: that process by which incident flux is redirected at the specular angle. See *specular angle, specular reflection*.

regular transmission: that process by which incident flux passes through a surface or medium without scattering.

resolution acuity: see *visual acuity*.

resolving power: the ability of the eye to perceive the individual elements of a grating or any other periodic pattern with parallel elements. It is measured by the number of cycles per degree that can be resolved. The resolution threshold is the period of the pattern that can be just resolved. Visual acuity, in such a case, is the reciprocal of one-half of the period expressed in minutes. The resolution threshold for a pair of points or lines is the distance between them when they can be distinguished as two, not one, expressed in minutes of arc; the ability of a photographic emulsion or lens to record fine detail, usually expressed in lines per millimeter. See *spatial frequency*.

rods: retinal receptors which respond at low levels of luminance below the threshold for cones. At these levels there is no basis for perceiving differences in hue and saturation. No rods are found in the center of the fovea.

S

saccadic movements: fast phase abrupt flick movements of the eyes as obtained in changing fixation from one point to another during reading, following movements, and as the quick phase of nystagmus. See *electro-oculogram*.

scotopic vision: vision mediated essentially or exclusively by the rods. It is generally associated with adaptation to a luminance below about 0.034 candela per square meter. See *photopic vision*.

shadow: the darkest portions of a picture. In a negative, the low-density areas are called the *shadow areas*, because they correspond to the high-density (dark) portions of the original.

sharpness: in photographic materials, the ability to reproduce a sharp edge, of a line, for example. See *acutance*.

shoulder: the portion of a *characteristic curve* above its straight-line section. See *Chapter 12, Figure 12.3*.

simple harmonic motion: harmonic *motion* in which the displacement varies with time in sinusoidal fashion; an equivalent statement is that the acceleration of the particle in harmonic motion is at all times proportional to the negative of the displacement; any back and forth motion around a central point; for our purposes this term is to be distinctly differentiated from *harmonics*.

simultaneous glare: see *dazzle glare.*

sine wave grating: also sinusoidal grating; a pattern of bars whose luminance varies sinusoidally in a direction at right angles to the orientation of the bars. Such a grating looks like a fuzzy set of parallel lines. Because of its simplicity it is the favorite stimulus of researchers studying spatial vision. A specific grating can be characterized by its amplitude, orientation, spatial frequency, and phase. It contains only one fundamental spatial frequency (F). See *harmonics;* see *Chapter 4, Figures 4.2 and 4.3.*

sinusoidal grating: see *sine wave grating.*

size threshold: the minimum perceptible size of an object. It also is defined as the size that can be detected some specific fraction of the times it is presented to an observer, usually 50 percent. It usually is measured in minutes of arc. See *visual acuity.*

sky light: visible radiation from the sun redirected by the atmosphere.

Snellen acuity: visual acuity as determined from testing on a chart designed by Herman Snellen in 1862. It is the most commonly used clinical method for testing sharpness of vision. See text Foreword by A.E. Maumenee, M.D.

solid angle: a measure of that portion of space about a point bounded by a conic surface whose vertex is at the point. It can be measured by the ratio of intercepted surface area of a sphere centered on that point to the square of the sphere's radius. It is expressed in steradians.

spatial frequency: the number of sinusoidal grating cycles (one black bar plus one white bar) per degree of visual space (c/d). Used to specify the "size" or numerical complexity of a particular grating pattern.

spatial frequency channels or mechanisms: experiments on the contrast sensitivity function (CSF) do not directly measure the response of single cells, but of closely related "family" groups of neurons with similar receptive field sizes in human spatial vision. These independent operating mechanisms (channels) are selectively sensitive to a restricted range of spatial frequencies. A limited number of about six to eight of such contiguous or slightly overlapping grouped neurons (channels, mechanisms), in aggregate, underlies the human CSF. See *Chapter 2, Figure 2.13.*

spatial vision: as used here, refers to the ability to see achromatic two dimensional patterns.

specular angle: the angle between the perpendicular to the surface and the reflected ray that is numerically equal to the angle of incidence and that lies in the same plane as the incident ray and the perpendicular but on the opposite side of the perpendicular to the surface.

specular reflection: occurs from a smooth polished surface and has the characteristics of a mirror in which the angle of reflection is equal to the angle of incidence. The incident ray, the normal to the surface, and the reflected ray all lie in the same plane.

specular reflectors: examples of specular reflectors are smooth polished, anodized and electroplated metals, and first-surface silvered glass or plastic mirrors.

speed of light: the speed of radiant energy, including light, is 2.997925×10^8 meters per second in vacuum (approximately 186,000 miles per second). In all material media the speed is less and varies with the material's index of refraction, which itself varies with wavelength.

spread function: in photosensitive materials (film) or its biologic equivalent, the retina, modulation transfer characteristics indicate the effects on the microstructure of the image caused by the diffusion of light within the image. The image of a point or narrow slit is not confined to its nominal borders, but diffuses and spreads out due to turbidity of the emulsion or retinal structural elements. The changed intensity profile of the image is called the *spread function.*

square wave grating: a pattern of alternating parallel black and white bars with clean distinct edges whose luminance changes abruptly at right angles to orientation of the bars.

state of chromatic adaptation: the condition of the eye in equilibrium with the average color of the visual field.

Steradian: see *solid angle.*

Stiles-Crawford effect: manifest by the reduced luminous efficiency of rays entering the peripheral portion of the pupil of the eye.

straight-line portion: that section of a *characteristic curve* which is essentially a straight line. It represents the range of exposures in which the increase in film density is proportional to the increase in the logarithm of the exposure. See *Chapter 12, Figure 12.3.*

stray light (in the eye): light from a source that is scattered onto parts of the retina lying outside the retinal image of the source. See *flare, intraocular light scattering.*

subjective brightness: the subjective attribute of any light sensation giving rise to the percept of luminous magnitude, including the whole scale of qualities of being bright, light, brilliant, dim, or dark. The term brightness often is used when referring to the measurable luminance. While the context usually makes it clear as to which meaning is intended, the preferable term for the photometric quantity is luminance, thus reserving brightness for the subjective sensation. See *luminance.*

sunlight: direct visible radiation from the sun.

T

task lighting: lighting directed to a specific surface or area that provides illumination for visual tasks. See *local lighting.*

temporal modulation: see *modulation, temporal.*

temporal resolution: just as the visual system responds to contrasts in space, it also responds to contrasts in time. Due to movement of target images across the retina (because of eye movements or movements of the object itself) virtually all spatial contrasts can also involve perceptual contrast differences resulting from variations in time of exposure to the target.

threshold: the value of a variable of a physical stimulus (such as size, luminance, contrast, or time) that permits the stimulus to be seen a specific percentage of the time or at a specific accuracy level. In many psychophysical experiments, thresholds are presented in terms of accuracy 50 percent of the time. However, the threshold also is expressed as the value of the physical variable that permits the object to be just barely seen. The threshold may be determined by merely detecting the presence of an object or it may be determined by discriminating certain details of the object. See *brightness contrast threshold, luminance threshold.*

threshold contrast: the contrast at which luminance differences can be detected 50 percent of the time.

time–temperature chart: a chart which indicates the development times necessary at various development temperatures to produce approximately the same degree of contrast as given by the recommended times at 68°F (20°C).

toe: the portion of the *characteristic curve* below the straight-line section of the curve. It represents the area of minimum useful exposure. See *Chapter 12, Figure 12.3.*

transparency: a photographic image intended to be viewed by transmitted light; for example, a 2-by-2-inch Kodachrome slide. See *positive.*

tritanopia: a defect of vision in which the retina fails to respond normally to blue and yellow discrimination.

troland: a unit of retinal illuminance which is based upon the fact that retinal illuminance is proportional to the product of the illuminance of the surface being viewed and the area of entrance pupil. One troland is the retinal illuminance produced when the luminance of the distal stimulus is one candela per square meter and the area of the pupil is one square millimeter. The troland makes no allowance for intraocular attenuation or for the Stiles-Crawford effect.

truncation: the masking or limitation of a grating field by a small, often circular, mask.

tuned cortical cells: receptive fields of many visual cortical cells have a preferred orientation. A CSF measured with horizontal gratings would be the product of the output of a different set of cells from those "tuned" for vertical gratings of the same spatial frequency.

U

units of luminance: the luminance of a surface in a specified direction may be expressed in luminous intensity per unit of projected area of surface or in luminous flux per unit of solid angle and per unit of projected surface area. Typical units are the candela per square meter (lumen per steradian and per square meter) and the candela per square foot (lumen per steradian and per square foot). The luminance of a surface in a specified direction is also expressed (incorrectly) in lambertian units. A typical unit in this system is the footlambert, equal to one lumen per square foot. This method of specifying luminance is not uniform but varies with the angle from which it is viewed. For this reason, this practice is denigrated.

V

veiling brightness: possibly arising from reflection (glossy paper, window glass, wet streets, shiny desk tops, automobile hoods), transmission (print on a thin sheet of paper with light traversing from the underside), diffusion or scattering of light from our surroundings (illuminated fog or dust, soil or dust particles on ones glasses or automobile windshield, etc.).

veiling glare: a type of disability glare due to unwanted stray light from a source *along the line of sight.* When superimposed upon the visual scene, it has a contrast lowering effect that causes decreased visibility and visual performance. See *disability glare, veiling brightness, veiling luminance, dazzle.*

veiling luminance: a luminance superimposed on the retinal image which reduces its contrast. It is this veiling effect produced by bright sources or areas in the visual field that results in decreased visual performance and visibility.

veiling reflection: regular reflections superimposed upon diffuse reflections from an object that partially or totally obscures the details to be seen by reducing the contrast. This sometimes is called reflected glare.

visibility: the quality or state of being perceivable by the eye. In many outdoor applications, visibility is defined in terms of the distance at which an object can be just perceived by the eye. In indoor applications it usually is defined in terms of the contrast or size of a standard test object, observed under standardized view-conditions, having the same thresholds as the given object.

visual acuity: is a measure of the size of the smallest resolvable spatial detail. Can be assessed by testing procedures grouped in three general categories:

1. *Detection acuity* determines the smallest resolvable item, or stimulus element, that the patient can see.
2. *Resolution (Grating) acuity* (GA) determines the highest resolvable spatial frequency of a grating pattern.

3. *Recognition acuity* determines the smallest recognizable item in some set, such as letters or numbers.
See *Chapter 2, Visual Acuity, and Figures 2.1, 2.2, and 2.3*. See also *Snellen acuity*.

visual angle: the angle subtended by an object or detail at the point of observation. It usually is measured in minutes of arc.

visual-evoked potential (VEP): change in the electrical activity of the cerebral cortex that occurs when the retina is stimulated with light. It is recorded from electrodes on the scalp. VEP is a diagnostic tool in assessment of optic nerve abnormalities, transmission of visual impulses through the optic tracts and optic radiation, and cerebral disease.

visual field: the locus of objects or points in space that can be perceived when the head and eyes are kept fixed. The field may be monocular or binocular. See *central visual field, peripheral visual field*.

visual function: broadly defined as the sum total of a person's ability to perform largely or totally visually dependent tasks such as personal grooming, mobility within one's environment, comfortable reading, and identification of people, currency, clocks, and signs. It considers visual acuity, level of contrast sensitivity, light adaptation, color vision, extent of visual field, ambient lighting, tasks being performed, and effects of glare. These components are numerous, varied, interrelated, and not easily or fully measurable in the laboratory or examination room.

visual perception: cognitive process involving direct visual experiences. The interpretation of impressions transmitted from the retina to the brain in terms of information about a physical world displayed before the eye. Visual perception involves any one or more of the following: recognition of the presence of something (object, aperture, or medium), identifying it, locating it in space, noting its relation to other things, identifying its movement, color, brightness, or form. See *apperceptions*.

visual performance: the quantitative assessment of the performance of a visual task, taking into consideration speed and accuracy.

visual surround: all portions of the visual field except the visual task.

visual task: conventionally designates those details and objects that must be seen for the performance of a given activity, and includes the immediate background of the details or objects. The term visual task as used is a misnomer because it refers to the visual display itself and not the task of extracting information from it. The task of extracting information also has to be differentiated from the overall task performed by the observer.

visugram: a term proposed by Bodis-Wollner, analogous to an audiogram and represents the plot of the loss of contrast sensitivity as the difference in logarithmic units (decibels, db) between a patient's CSF and the average normal CSF, which represents the zero level. Thus, a visugram near the zero level implies a normal CSF, while a curve below the zero level indicates the amount of CSF deficit in db. See *Chapter 9, Figure 9.4*.

W

wavelength: the distance between adjacent crests or adjacent troughs of a wave or the distance between two successive points of a periodic wave in the direction of propagation, in which the oscillation has the same phase. The three commonly used units are listed in the following table.

Name	Symbol	Value
Micrometer	μm	$1\ \mu\text{m} = 10^{-6}$ m
Nanometer	nm	$1\ \text{nm} = 10^{-9}$ m
Angstrom*	Å	$1\ \text{Å} = 10^{-10}$ m

*The use of this unit is deprecated.

Weber contrast: for a variable contrast chart or display such as the Pelli-Robson chart; defined as the difference in luminance between the letter and its background divided by the luminance of the background. See *Michelson contrast, luminance contrast*.

work-plane: the plane at which work usually is done, and on which the illuminance is specified and measured. Unless otherwise indicated, this is assumed to be a horizontal plane 0.76 meters (30 inches) above the floor.

1
Contrast Sensitivity: A Viewpoint for Clinicians

Mark J. Mannis, Karla Zadnik, and Chris A. Johnson

Introduction

The chapters that follow will review the physiological, methodological, and theoretical aspects of spatial contrast sensitivity and glare disability in normal observers and in those with ocular and retroocular diseases. In this chapter we will consider the general state of the art and will try to place the utility of contrast sensitivity and glare disability testing in context for the clinician on the basis of both empirical and practical considerations.

The literature available on the subject of such testing is confusing. The clinician is in an understandable quandary when turning to either "trade" magazines or the scientific literature for help in determining how to use contrast sensitivity or glare disability testing for patient management. He or she is faced with a choice of visual psychophysical papers with little or no clinical application or with thinly disguised promotions of contrast sensitivity and glare testing devices occupying ophthalmic tabloids and practice management magazines. Between these two spheres of interest is an area of definable utility for contrast sensitivity and glare disability testing that may help to provide guidelines for patient management.

Measurement of the contrast sensitivity function and of glare disability as a practical clinical tool is an outcome of recognition by vision scientists that there are numerous aspects of visual performance that can be measured above and beyond Snellen visual acuity. Ophthalmic clinicians also realized that visual dysfunction is much more complex than

is described by the Snellen fraction generated in the examining lane. Thus they looked for non-acuity parameters that might help to complete the visual profile of the patient with eye disease. The marriage of these pursuits led to evaluation of contrast sensitivity function in patients with various eye disorders, including glaucoma,[1,2] diseases of the retina and optic nerve,[3-9] lens opacity,[10,11] corneal edema,[12-14] and keratoconus,[13,15-18] in an attempt to better understand the precise nature of the visual deficit. When the contrast sensitivity function was tested in these disease entities, abnormalities were discovered, often in the face of normal Snellen acuity. Unfortunately, such "measureable effects" were obtained using a large variety of testing devices under different conditions. As might be expected, the results often differed.

The situation is even more complex for the measurement of glare disability. Stimulus and response parameters, as well as the type of glare source, exhibit tremendous variations from one investigation to another. The interested clinician, therefore, not only is faced with a lack of consistency in the literature, but must deal with a methodology that has not been standardized and whose clinical implications have not been carefully defined.

Contrast sensitivity and glare disability testing have, nonetheless, been used for diagnosis, vision screening, presurgical and postsurgical evaluation, assessment of the efficacy of medical therapy, and evaluation of contact lenses and intraocular lens implants. The role of these tests in the evaluation of visual function is clearly in evolution.

Potential Clinical Applications

Presurgical Evaluation

The area that has stimulated the greatest interest in clinical contrast sensitivity testing is the evaluation of lens opacities. Clinicians have long been aware that the visual performance of the cataract patient may not be represented accurately by visual acuity measurements in the refracting lane. Clinical visual acuity measurement evaluates the ability to resolve fine detail under conditions of maximum contrast. These conditions are seldom encountered in real life. The patient with a small but dense posterior subcapsular cataract may read the 20/20 optotype in the darkened examination room but may become functionally blind outdoors in the noonday sun. Most ophthalmologists have adapted their routine testing to take this and similar circumstances into consideration by, for example, testing vision in both the darkened and the fully illuminated examining room.

Does the testing of contrast sensitivity and glare disability have a role in expanding our understanding of how vision is affected by lens opacities? Considered by itself, contrast sensitivity testing is probably not a very useful tool for gauging the need for cataract surgery because of its lack of specificity and its undefined relationship to real-world visual function. On the other hand, measurement of glare disability may be helpful in defining the presence of an anterior segment disorder.[19] Glare testing provides an analysis of visual performance under suboptimal or adverse lighting conditions. The effect of glare on Snellen acuity or contrast sensitivity can be readily measured. However, glare disability depends on the distance between the glare source and the visual target, the type of glare source, the ambient lighting conditions, and many other stimulus parameters, as well as on the specific ocular pathology. Unfortunately, careful analysis of glare testing methodology has not accrued at the same rate as the substantial literature on contrast sensitivity testing, so that the available procedures for glare testing are varied and lack universally accepted standards. At this writing, there are at least ten commercially available glare testers, differing from one another primarily in the type of glare source employed. Several use a target surrounded by a broad field of light simulating veiling glare, whereas others utilize point-source glare.

Deranged contrast sensitivity function or glare disability must be understood as a single variable among many in the assessment of the patient with cataract. In our own setting, the primary determinant of suitability for cataract surgery is the ability of the patient to function visually in his or her environment. Adequate visual function is judged by putting together several pieces of a puzzle. These include the patient's subjective assessment of personal visual function, Snellen acuity considered in the context of the patient's visual environment, and nonacuity parameters if the Snellen acuity and the patient's subjective complaints are not internally consistent. In such unusual situations, measurement of the contrast sensitivity function or glare disability may, in contrast to the Snellen test, verify the patient's subjective assessment. What must be avoided at all costs, of course, is the use of deranged contrast sensitivity function or documented glare disability as justification for surgical intervention in the patient in whom Snellen acuity does not fall within the range of surgical potential and whose visual complaints are not significant. There is the unfortunate potential to overinterpret the results of such testing in favor of surgery.[20]

Documentation of the Effects of Corneal Disease

Contrast sensitivity testing may be helpful in clarifying and documenting changes caused by diseases that alter the curvature or clarity of the cornea. We and others have demonstrated a distinct alteration in contrast sensitivity function in patients with keratoconus before Snellen acuity shows any significant decrease.[17,18,21] Complaints of visual distortion often precede a decrement in visual acuity in keratoconus. Altered contrast sensitivity functions may be normalized by optically successful keratoplasty.[17] In cases of keratoconus with reasonably good Snellen acuity, we believe that deranged contrast sensitivity function is a reliable indicator of visual dysfunction that may substantiate the patient's complaints and documents the indications for surgical intervention.[21]

Evaluation of Corneal and Refractive Surgery

An area in which both contrast sensitivity and glare testing may prove to be significant is the realm of corneal and refractive surgery. The population of patients undergoing refractive surgery differs greatly from the traditional surgical patient group in ophthalmology. First, refractive surgery patients are generally in a younger age group. Second, they often go into surgery with excellent corrected Snellen acuity, so that their functional expectations for postsurgical visual performance are very high. They may be quite sensitive to subtle changes in the quality of visual perception. Alterations in glare and contrast sensitivity function have been demonstrated objectively in radial keratotomy[22-25] and epikeratophakia patients.[26,27] Keratoplasty patients may also demonstrate changes in contrast sensitivity function, although the role of the changes engendered by corneal transplantation is not clear.[28,29] Our own data indicate that optically successful keratoplasty in patients with bilateral corneal disease tends to improve contrast sensitivity in the operated eye; nonetheless, the contrast sensitivity curves are not normal when compared with those of normal observers.[29]

Diagnosis of Glaucoma and Optic Nerve Disease

In most instances, optical anomalies and anterior segment disease produce either a generalized depression of the contrast sensitivity function at all spatial frequencies or a selectively greater contrast sensitivity loss for high spatial frequencies. Similar types of contrast sensitivity deficits have been reported for disorders of the neural visual pathways. In a few instances, orientation-specific and/or frequency-specific losses ("notches" in the contrast sensitivity function at a specific spatial frequency) have been reported for optic nerve disease and other neural deficits.[30,31] Such specific losses have been interpreted as reflecting preferential damage to subpopulations of neural elements selectively sensitive to particular spatial frequencies and/or orientations. Unfortunately, recent investigations[32] have reported similar orientation- and spatial frequency-specific contrast sensitivity deficits attributable to optical factors. Thus, the potential differential diagnostic utility of these specific contrast sensitivity losses remains in question.

Contrast sensitivity losses are therefore useful clinically for the early detection of subtle visual disorders. However, contrast sensitivity testing has little or no differential diagnostic value, since the patterns of loss are similar for all types of visual pathology and optical anomalies. The utility of contrast sensitivity testing for medical and/or surgical management of patients and evaluation of the efficacy of therapeutic regimens and related clinical applications will require careful and thorough investigation. At the present time, the primary clinical role for contrast sensitivity testing appears to be as a screening device for detecting early visual abnormalities.

Conclusions

An overview of the clinical literature on contrast sensitivity function and glare testing suggests the following guidelines for clinicians:

1. Both contrast sensitivity and even more so glare disability testing are in a state of evolution from the standpoint of the clinician.
2. Glare testing appears to be more specific for anterior segment pathology than contrast sensitivity testing, but no generalized standards exist for glare testing.
3. When used in the evaluation of a potential surgical patient, nonacuity parameters such as contrast sensitivity and glare disability should provide additional objective data for characterization and quantitation of the patient's complaint. However, these tests should not be the sole deciding factor in a decision to recommend cataract surgery. As always, the visual needs of the patient will dictate the need for surgery.
4. Contrast sensitivity and glare testing may be useful in revealing and documenting subtle corneal disease as well as in assessing vision before and after refractive surgery.

References

1. Arden GB, Jacobson JJ: A simple grating test for contrast sensitivity: Preliminary results indicate value in screening for glaucoma. *Invest Ophthalmol Vis Sci* **17**(1):23–32, 1978.

2. Atkin A, Bodis-Wollner I, Wolkstein M, et al: Abnormalities of central contrast sensitivity in glaucoma. *Am J Ophthalmol* **88**:205–211, 1979.

3. Wolkstein M, Atkin A, Bodis-Wollner I: Contrast sensitivity in retinal disease. *Ophthalmology* **87**:1140–1149, 1980.

4. Marmor MF: Contrast sensitivity and retinal disease. *Ann Ophthalmol* **13**:1069–1071, 1981.

5. Sjostrand J, Frisen L: Contrast sensitivity in macular disease. *Acta Ophthalmol* **55**:507–514, 1977.

6. Kleiner RC, Enger C, Alexander MF, et al: Contrast sensitivity in macular degeneration. *Arch Ophthalmol* **106**:55–57, 1988.

7. Sokol S, Moskowitz A, Skarf B, et al: Contrast sensitivity in diabetics with and without diabetic retinopathy. *Arch Ophthalmol* **103**:51–54, 1985.

8. Regan D, Silver R, Murray TJ: Visual acuity and contrast sensitivity in multiple sclerosis, hidden visual loss; an auxiliary test. *Brain* **100**(3):563–579, 1977.

9. Arden GB, Gucukoglu AG: Grating test of contrast sensitivity in patients with retrobulbar neuritis. *Arch Ophthalmol* **96**:1626–1629, 1978.

10. Hess R, Woo G: Vision through cataracts. *Invest Ophthalmol Vis Sci* **17**:428–435, 1978.

11. Skalka H: Arden grating test in evaluating "early" posterior subcapsular cataracts. *South Med J* **74**(11):1368–1370, 1981.

12. Hess RF, Garner LF: The effect of corneal edema on visual function. *Invest Ophthalmos Vis Sci* **16**:5–13, 1977.

13. Hess RF, Carney LG: Vision through an abnormal cornea: A pilot study of the relationship between visual loss from corneal distortion, corneal edema, keratoconus and some allied corneal pathology. *Invest Ophthalmol Vis Sci* **18**:476–483, 1979.

14. Carney LG, Jacobs RJ: Mechanisms of visual loss in corneal edema. *Arch Ophthamol* **102**:1068–1071, 1984.

15. Carney LG: Visual loss in keratoconus. *Arch Ophthalmol* **100**:1282–1285, 1982.

16. Carney LG: Contact lens correction of visual loss in keratoconus. *Acta Ophthalmol* **60**:795–802, 1982.

17. Mannis MJ, Zadnik K, Johnson CA: The effect of penetrating keratoplasty on contrast sensitivity in keratoconus. *Arch Ophthalmol* **102**:1513–1516, 1984.

18. Zadnik K, Mannis MJ, Johnson CA: An analysis of contrast sensitivity in identical twins with keratoconus. *Cornea* **3**:99–103, 1984.

19. Koch DD: The role of glare testing in managing the cataract patient, in *Focal Points 1988: Clinical Modules for Ophthalmologists.* American Academy of Ophthalmology, Vol VI, Mod 4, 1988.

20. Sweeney CC, Steen WH: Contrast sensitivity as a cataract practice builder. *Ophthalmol Manage,* May 1987, pp 32–36.

21. Zadnik K, Mannis MJ, Johnson CA, et al: Rapid contrast sensitivity assessment in keratoconus. *Am J Optom Physiol Opt* **64**:693–697, 1987.

22. Miller D, Miller R: Glare sensitivity in simulated radial keratotomy. *Arch Ophthalmol* **99**:1961–1962, 1981.

23. Applegate RA, Trick LR, Meade DL, et al: Radial keratotomy increases the effects of disability glare: Initial results. *Arch Ophthalmol* **19**:293–297, 1987.

24. Krasnov MM, Avetisov SE, Makashova NV, et al: The effect of radial keratotomy on contrast sensitivity. *Am J Ophthalmol* **105**:651–654, 1988.

25. Tomlinson A, Caroline P: Effect of radial keratotomy on the contrast sensitivity function. *Am J Optom Physiol Opt* **65**:803–808, 1988.

26. Justin N, Asbell PA, Friedman A: Glare and contrast sensitivity testing in epikeratoplasty. *Invest Ophthalmol Vis Sci* **28**(suppl):225, 1987.

27. Mannis MJ, Zadnik K, Johnson CA, et al: Contrast sensitivity after epikeratophakia. *Cornea* **7**(4):280–284, 1988.

28. Carney LG: Visual deficits remaining after penetrating keratoplasty. *Invest Ophthalmol Vis Sci* **26**(suppl):148, 1985.

29. Mannis MJ, Zadnik K, Johnson CA, et al: Contrast sensitivity after penetrating keratoplasty. *Arch Ophthalmol* **105**:1220–1223, 1987.

30. Apkarian P, Tijsson R, Spekreijse H, et al: Origin of notches in CSF: Optical or neural? *Invest Ophthalmol Vis Sci* **28**:607–612, 1987.

31. Regan D, Whitlock JA, Murray TJ, et al: Orientation-specific losses of contrast sensitivity in multiple sclerosis. *Invest Ophthalmol Vis Sci* **19**:324–328, 1980.

32. Applegate RA, Johnson CA, Howland HC, et al: Optical aberrations of the eye following radial keratotomy—initial results. *Invest Ophthalmol Vis Sci* **29**(suppl):280, 1988.

2
An Introduction to Contrast Sensitivity Testing

Jeremy M. Wolfe

Introduction

In the treatment of visual disorders and eye disease, it is obviously useful to assess the patient's visual abilities. In principle, a great number of abilities could be tested (e.g., perception of motion, depth, color, faces, etc.). In practice, however, the first and often the only aspect of vision to be tested is spatial vision in or near the fovea. As used here, the term *spatial vision* refers to the ability to see achromatic, two-dimensional patterns. The most common clinical measures of spatial vision are visual acuity measures. In recent years there has been increasing awareness of the limitations of acuity measures and a corresponding rise in interest in other measures of visual function, in particular, contrast sensitivity.

This chapter briefly discusses acuity measures and then turns to contrast sensitivity. It covers the basic rationale for contrast sensitivity testing, methodological factors that influence the results of such testing, the underlying psychophysics and physiology, the clinical uses of contrast sensitivity testing, and clinical constraints on methodology.

Visual Acuity

When patients read an eye chart, be it a 19th century standard such as the Snellen letters, Landolt *C*'s, tumbling *E*'s, or a newer chart such as the *ETDRS* chart, their visual acuity is being measured. Visual acuity is a measure of the size of the smallest resolvable spatial detail. Ways to assess acuity can generally be grouped into three large categories: detection, resolution, and recognition.

In tests of detection, one might determine the smallest stimulus element that the patient can see (Fig. 2.1).* Certain pitfalls have to be avoided. For example, assuming that it is bright enough, a white spot on a dark background can be seen no matter how small the spot. A point light source forms a disk of light on the retina. The optics of the eye ensure that the disk always illuminates several cones. Detection of a white spot, therefore, becomes a matter of absolute visual sensitivity and not of visual acuity. (A star is a good example of a bright spot that is visible even though it subtends a very small angle.) Detection of dark disks on a light background would be a better acuity test (Fig. 2.1). In such a test, 30 seconds of arc is a good estimate of the limits of resolution.[1,2]

Rather than detect a single item, it is possible to measure visual acuity by having patients look for separation between elements in a stimulus. For example, rather than measure the smallest visible disk, we could measure the smallest gap that can be seen between two disks. A particularly useful version of such a resolution test is shown in Figure 2.2. Here acuity would be measured by the finest resolvable grating. Typically, the bar width at the

---

*To correct for viewing distance, the size of visual stimuli is generally given in degrees of visual angle. The visual angle of any small target may be approximated by the equation:

$$\text{Visual angle} = \arctan\left(\frac{\text{size}}{\text{viewing distance}}\right)$$

Thus a 1.25-cm thumbnail held at a 70-cm arm's length from the eye subtends $\arctan(1.25/70) = 1.02$ degrees of visual angle.

FIGURE 2.1. Detection acuity determines the smallest resolvable item.

limits of acuity is between 40 and 60 seconds.[2,3] Gratings may also be described in terms of the number of cycles per degree of visual angle. If the acuity limit is 60 seconds for a single bar, then a cycle (one white and one black bar) would be 120 seconds (2 minutes). This corresponds to an acuity limit of 30 cycles per degree (cpd).

In conditions such as astigmatism, grating acuity will be dependent on the orientation of the grating, because different gratings of one orientation will be in better focus than gratings of other orientations. However, the impact of the same clinical condition on other measures of acuity is less clear, because those measures (e.g., Snellen) involve stimuli containing a variety of orientations.

Tests like the Snellen letters are examples of recognition measures of acuity; they are the most common measures (see Fig. 2.3). Here the task of the patient is to name the target (a letter or number) or to name the location of some particular element of the target (the gap in a Landolt *C*, the direction of an *E*, etc.). Acuity is determined by the size of the elements making up the target (line width of letters, size of the gap) and is often rendered as a fraction: 20/20 designates an ability to recognize a target whose critical elements subtend 1 minute of arc at 20 feet. Various other systems use 6 meters or 10 feet, or some other standard, yielding 6/6 or 10/10 as "normal acuity." An acuity of 20/40 corresponds to an element size of 2 minutes, 20/80 to 4 minutes, and so on. It is certainly possible to resolve elements of under 1 minute, and 20/20 does not represent a limit on acuity nor, in any real sense, on "normal" acuity. A large portion of the healthy young population ($>50\%$ under age 40[4]) can resolve letters at 20/15.

HTOVAKE
OVKZENH
KEFVTOH
XZTVONF
HVENZO
ZHKOEVK

FIGURE 2.3. Recognition acuity determines the smallest recognizable item in some set, here letters.

Methodological Issues in Acuity Measures

Acuity measures vary systematically with factors such as pupil size,[5] luminance,[6] and contrast.[7] Further, the style of testing can have a strong impact on the acuity measures. A tester who simply asks the patient to read as many letters as possible will get a quite different result from one who asks the same patient to "guess" at hard-to-see letters. Similar methodological issues affect contrast sensitivity testing and will be discussed in greater detail later in this chapter. For any measure of this sort, consistency is vitally important if measures are to be compared with each other. If the testing method is changed between a patient's visits, changes in the measured acuity are more difficult to interpret. For similar reasons, it may be difficult to evaluate changes in acuity measures for a patient if those measures come from different doctors or hospitals.

Contrast Sensitivity

The most important limitation on the usefulness of acuity measures is not methodological. Even if the methodology were flawless, acuity measures could not contain all the information needed to describe spatial vision. The heart of the matter is that acuity is a one-dimensional answer to a two-dimensional

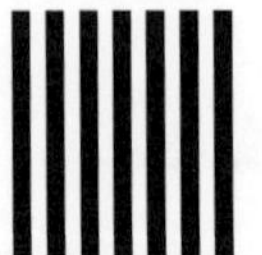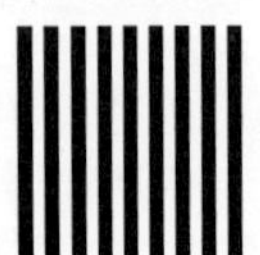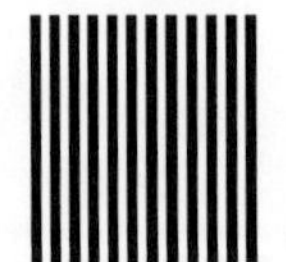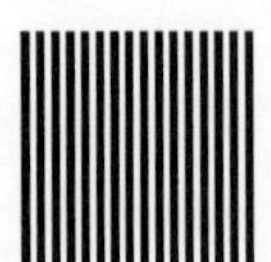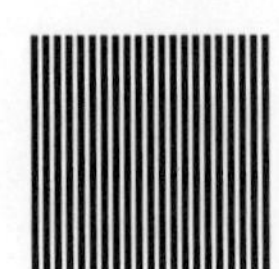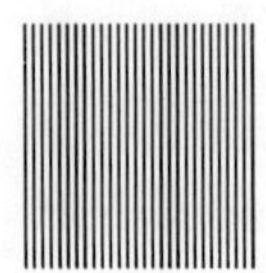

FIGURE 2.2. Grating acuity determines the highest resolvable spatial frequency.

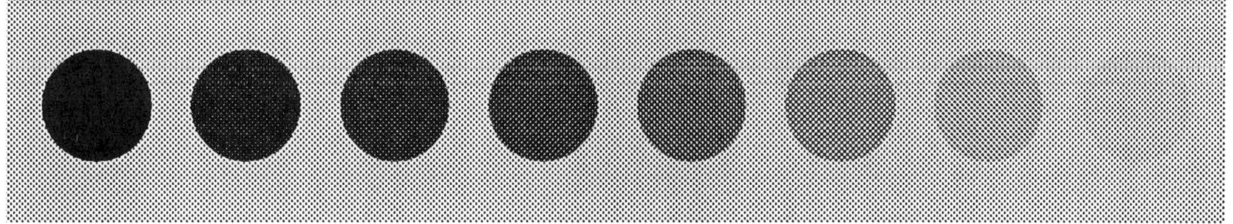

FIGURE 2.4. Contrast sensitivity determines the lowest detectable contrast for stimuli of a fixed size.

problem.* Let us consider one of the black spots in Figure 2.1. It has two salient attributes: size and contrast. In this figure all of the spots are of high contrast (black on white) and visibility is reduced by reducing the size of the spots. Instead of manipulating size, visibility could be reduced by reducing the contrast of a series of spots of equal size (Fig. 2.4). Spatial patterns varying in size and contrast occupy a two-dimensional (size × contrast) space (Fig. 2.5). Acuity tests locate the upper limit in the size dimension: the size below which an item cannot be resolved regardless of its contrast. There must be a similar limit in the contrast dimension: a contrast below which an item cannot be detected regardless of its size (Fig. 2.6). A car looming up in the fog might be an example of an important low-

contrast stimulus. Cataract is an example of a clinical disorder that could lower a contrast limit as well as the acuity limit. Figure 2.6 makes the unrealistic assumption that contrast and size limits are independent of each other. In fact, they are not. The minimum visible contrast varies as a function of the size of the item, and so we get a "contrast sensitivity function," or CSF (Fig. 2.7), that partitions the size × contrast space into visible and invisible stimuli. As will be discussed later in this chapter, the normal CSF shows greatest sensitivity to test patterns of intermediate size. Sensitivity decreases gradually as the patterns become smaller, approaching the acuity limit. Sensitivity also decreases as the patterns enlarge. This can be thought of as a relative insensitivity to gradual changes in illumination (e.g., indistinct shadows on the wall). It follows that unless one makes a number of strong assumptions, knowledge of the acuity limit alone is insufficient to specify the

___

*Three dimensional, if we include luminance as a variable.

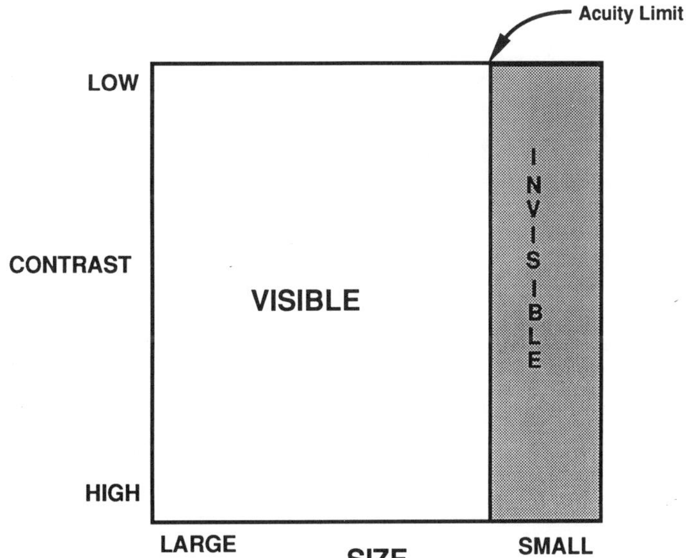

FIGURE 2.5. Alone, acuity determines a size limit on visibility but ignores the dimension of contrast.

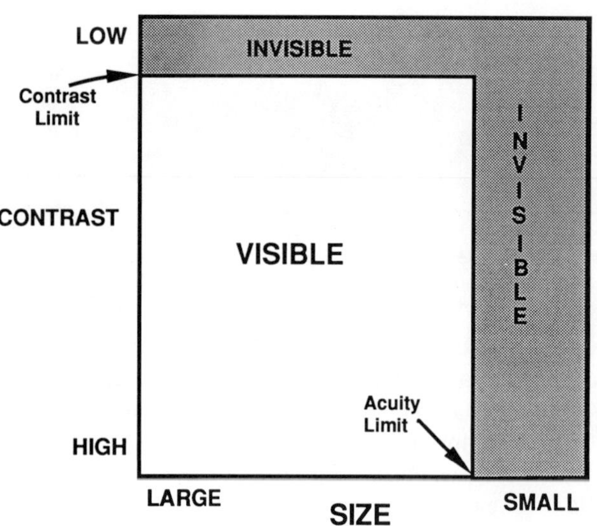

FIGURE 2.6. There must be some contrast below which stimuli are not visible.

entire CSF. It is certainly possible to have "normal" acuity and significantly reduced contrast sensitivity with serious visual consequences.

Stimuli for Measuring Contrast Sensitivity

Just as a variety of stimuli can be used to measure the acuity limit, a variety of stimuli can be used to measure contrast sensitivity. In practice, however, most work in the last 20 years has involved sinusoidal or "sine wave" gratings. A sine wave grating is a pattern of bars whose luminance varies sinusoidally in the direction orthogonal to the orientation of the bars. Such a grating looks like a fuzzy set of parallel lines. The size of a grating is specified in terms of its spatial frequency: the number of sinusoidal cycles per degree of visual space. Contrast of a grating (or, indeed, of any other pattern) is generally given as

$$\frac{\text{Maximum intensity} - \text{minimum intensity}}{\text{Maximum intensity} + \text{minimum intensity}}$$

This quantity varies from 0 to 1 and can be multiplied by 100 to give percent contrast. With sinusoi-

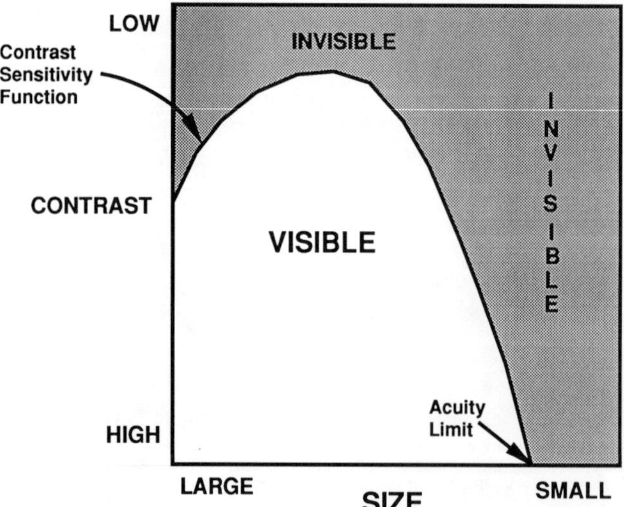

FIGURE 2.7. A more realistic figure shows that visibility depends on both the size (more precisely, the spatial frequency) and the contrast of the stimulus.

dal gratings, acuity is the highest frequency that can be seen at 100% contrast. As with black and white (or "square wave") gratings, the limit of normal resolution is 30 to 45 cpd. The lower figure, 30 cpd, is equivalent to 20/20 Snellen acuity.*

Sine waves have properties that make them attractive stimuli for measuring contrast sensitivity. First, Fourier's theorem holds that any complex waveform can be decomposed into a set of sine waves. For example, a black and white square wave (e.g., Fig. 2.2) can be created by taking a sine wave of the same spatial frequency (the "fundamental frequency") and adding to it a sine wave of three times the fundamental frequency at one third the amplitude of the fundamental plus a sine wave of five times the frequency at one fifth the amplitude, and so on for all of the odd harmonics of the fundamental. These gratings must be added in the correct relationship to each other. In this case, for example, the minima of harmonics must be aligned with the maxima of the fundamental so that the harmonics subtract light from the peak of the fundamental, flattening the sinusoid into a square wave. This positional relationship is known as *phase*. If we allow for gratings of different orientation, we can in principle generate any two-dimensional pattern by combining a set of sine waves having the correct frequency, amplitude, phase, and orientation.

For some purposes, the visual system can be treated as a device that adds up sine waves in a linear fashion. Then the system's sensitivity to any arbitrary two-dimensional pattern can be estimated by knowing its sensitivity to sine waves. Moreover, since contrast sensitivity is a smooth, continuous function, it is not necessary to measure the system's response to every spatial frequency. A properly selected set of frequencies allows the overall function to be estimated. For example, we have described how a square wave grating can be created by adding together a series of sinusoidal gratings. Going in reverse, a square wave of 30 cpd can be decomposed into a series of sinusoids — in this case

a fundamental sine wave of 30 cpd, a third harmonic of 90 cpd at one third the amplitude of the fundamental, a fifth harmonic at 150 cpd and one fifth the amplitude, and so on through all the odd harmonics of the 30-cpd fundamental. However, we have already noted that the visual system does not respond to sine waves above about 45 cpd. Therefore, all of the harmonics are invisible and the 30-cpd square wave should be and is indistinguishable from a 30-cpd sine wave. More on this "linear systems" or Fourier approach to spatial vision can be found in Cornsweet[9] and Ginsburg.[10]

Sine waves have a second property that is useful in a clinical setting. Defocus reduces the contrast of a sine wave but does not alter its form. A blurred sine wave is still a sine wave, albeit a fainter one, while a blurred *E* on a Snellen chart, for example, changes its appearance as well as its contrast. Other sets of stimuli have the attractive properties of sine wave gratings, but sine waves have become the standard.

Methodology of Contrast Sensitivity Testing

Thresholds and Guessing

In principle, measurement of a contrast sensitivity function is straightforward. For a variety of spatial frequencies, one determines the minimum detectable contrast. Sensitivity is defined as the inverse of the minimum contrast (hence the apparently inverted y axis in Figs. 2.5, and 2.6). Sensitivity plotted as a function of spatial frequency gives the contrast sensitivity function.

In practice, a number of methodological issues complicate matters. First is the definition of "minimally detectable." It is incorrect to assume that there is some contrast above which a particular stimulus is visible and below which it is not. Figure 2.8 shows hypothetical results from an experiment where contrast is varied from 0 to 100% and the observer is asked to respond if the stimulus is seen. If, after many repetitions at each contrast level, percent stimuli detected is plotted as a function of contrast, results from almost any experiment of this sort will have the characteristic sigmoid shape shown in Figure 2.8.

There are a number of ways to understand this lack of a sharp criterion. Perhaps the most straight-

---

*In general, acuity measured in cycles per degree can be converted to Snellen notation by dividing the acuity by 30 cpd and then multiplying by 20/20 or 6/6. Because Snellen and grating acuity may not measure exactly the same thing, there is some doubt about the validity of this transformation (e.g., Thorn and Schwartz[8]).

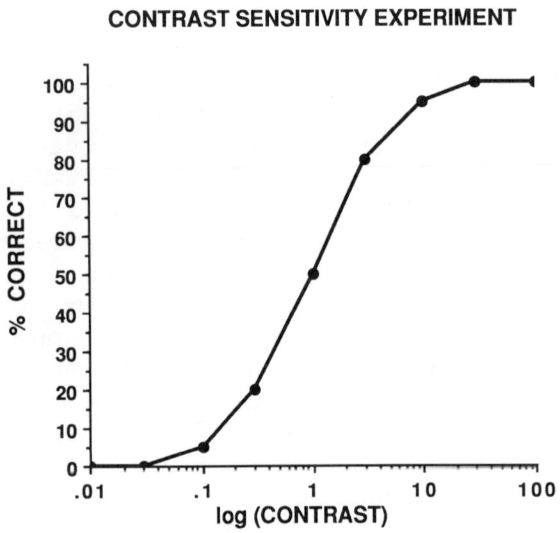

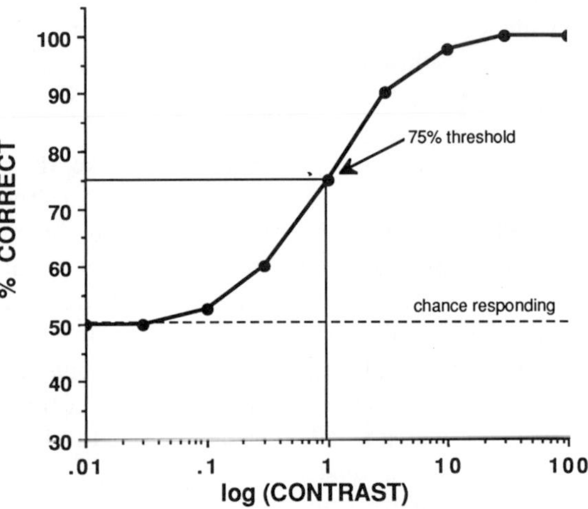

FIGURE 2.8. Contrast sensitivity experiment. As contrast is increased, observers will detect the stimulus with greater and greater accuracy. "Contrast threshold" is an arbitrary point on this smoothly increasing function. There is no sharp division between visible and invisible.

FIGURE 2.9. Two-alternative, forced-choice method to correct for guessing in threshold determination tasks, observers are asked to locate the stimulus in one of two locations in space or time. The contrast threshold is a point (e.g., 75%) on a function that increases from a 50% chance responding level to 100% correct.

forward is to realize that detection of a faint stimulus requires detection of a weak neural event in a system subject to random fluctuations in the background response rate of neurons. Near threshold some signals will be lost in this neural "noise."

This raises a second problem. Some fluctuations in internal noise might be mistaken for the presence of the stimulus by an observer straining to detect a barely visible stimulus. That observer might incorrectly state that the stimulus is visible. In fact, in the experiment just described, the observer could get 100% correct simply by stating that the stimulus was present on each trial. Such a result would be meaningless. Thus, reliable tests of contrast sensitivity (or any other measurement of threshold) require a method to counteract the effects of guessing. More extensive discussion of issues of this sort can be found in Falmagne[11] and in Snodgrass, Levy-Berger, and Haydon.[12]

The experiment just described could be conducted in a slightly different manner. The observer could be presented with two possible stimulus locations and be asked to state which of the two contains the stimulus. On each trial one location would contain a grating of some contrast and the

other would contain a blank gray field of the same average luminance. The two locations could be separated in space or in time. The vital aspects of this "two-alternative, forced-choice" (2AFC) method are that the observer (or patient) is forced to make a response and that guessing, which is perfectly permissible in this case, will yield correct answers a predictable 50% of the time. Hypothetical results are shown in Figure 2.9. Again, there is no sharp threshold. However, a fixed criterion level can be picked (e.g., 75%). Since this method incorporates a correction for guessing, more reliable comparisons can be made between observers and between sessions for a single observer.

The problem of guessing can be dealt with in other ways as well. For example, a Snellen chart is, to a first approximation, a 26-alternative test. In this case the effects of guessing are minimal, because the chance of guessing correctly is under 4%. In reality, guessing effects in letter tests are somewhat more complicated because a patient may be able to narrow the field of possible letters by noting the overall shape even if he or she cannot resolve the details (i.e., G might be mistaken for C or Q, not A or L).

Speed Versus Accuracy

In the 2AFC experiment just described, observers would be tested at several spatial frequencies and at a range of contrasts for each frequency. Curves of the sort shown in Figure 2.9 would be generated for each frequency, the 75% point would be estimated, and the set of 75% points would serve as the CSF. While this test should produce a reliable CSF, it can take a very long time. Suppose ten contrast levels are chosen for each of six frequencies. Further, suppose that 100 trials are run at each contrast level, giving "percent correct" results in 1% steps. This test, for one eye at one orientation, requires $10 \times 6 \times 100$ or 6000 trials. At one trial every 3 seconds (unlikely), the test would take 5 hours. To scientifically establish the existence of the CSF this might be acceptable. However, the test is obviously too arduous for clinical use or, indeed, for most laboratory use.

More efficient methods exist. In general there is a trade-off between accuracy and efficiency, but some small or at least tolerable sacrifices in accuracy can yield substantial savings in time. For example, many of the trials in the 2AFC experiment contain very little information. One-hundred trials at a contrast that can be seen all the time are more than are necessary. If contrast threshold is defined as one point on a function of the sort shown in Figure 2.9, then time and effort should be concentrated at that threshold. Since the threshold is not known in advance, particularly in clinical cases, methods are required to guide the test to the correct contrast levels.

Staircase Methods

One such method was brought into the realm of experimental psychology from work with munitions. One way to determine the amount of force required to explode a bombshell was to carry the shell up, say, ten steps of a ladder and drop it. If it exploded, the next shell was carried up only nine steps. If the first shell did not explode, the next one was carried up 11 steps. This procedure, if repeated many times, will oscillate around the height that causes explosions 50% of the time.

The staircase method can be imported to vision testing very easily. If an observer reports seeing the stimulus in a contrast sensitivity experiment, the contrast is lowered one step. If the observer does not see the stimulus, the contrast is raised one step. This staircase will locate the 50% point on a function such as the one shown in Figure 2.8. This version of a staircase experiment is subject to errors due to guessing. A 2AFC version requires a modification of the staircase rule. The 50% point is the chance response level and is not useful. For the 2AFC case, a better rule is: Decrease contrast if the observer makes *two* correct responses at a given contrast level.[13] Increase contrast if the observer makes *one* incorrect response.

An example of the workings of such a two-down, one-up rule is shown in Figure 2.10. Contrast starts at 100%. It is decreased to 30% after two correct responses, to 10% after two more, and to 3% after two more. At 3% the observer makes an incorrect choice and so the staircase goes back up to 10%, and so on. It can be shown that this staircase estimates the 70.7% point on a 2AFC function such as is shown in Figure 2.9.[14]

The threshold estimate is obtained by averaging the peaks and troughs of the function shown in Figure 2.10. Starting from the right side of the figure, the first trough is at 0.3%; the first peak at 3%, then at 1%, 3%, 0.3%, 3%, and so on. It is important to average an equal number of peaks and troughs to avoid biasing the estimate. It is also important that the contrast steps be equal. Here they are roughly equal on a logarithmic scale. If we take the six values listed here and average their logarithms, we get an estimate of 1.2% for the contrast that is detectable 70.7% of the time.

Figure 2.10 shows an estimate of threshold obtained in 60 trials. That is a great savings over the 900 trials (100 trials at nine contrasts) required to obtain the data in Figure 2.9. These 60 trials can be further reduced. A staircase is usually run for a fixed number of peaks and troughs (reversals). The accuracy of the threshold estimate improves with the number of reversals, but the 18 reversals shown in Figure 2.10 are probably more than are needed. Using ten reversals would require 33 trials in this example. The number of trials required for a fixed number of reversals will vary with the reliability of the observer, fewer trials being required for a careful, reliable observer. Figure 2.10 would represent data from a "good" observer.

The 2AFC staircase procedure is by no means the only reliable method of obtaining a contrast sensitivity function (e.g., Tyrell and Owens[15]). However, the issues addressed by this method

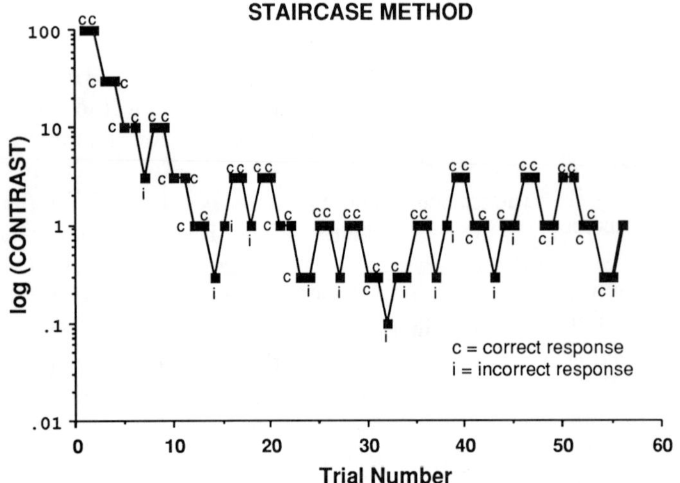

Figure 2.10. "Staircase" method. The time required to determine a contrast threshold may be shortened by using a "staircase" method. If the observer can see the stimulus, contrast is decreased; if not, it is increased. The staircase comes to oscillate around the threshold. See text for details.

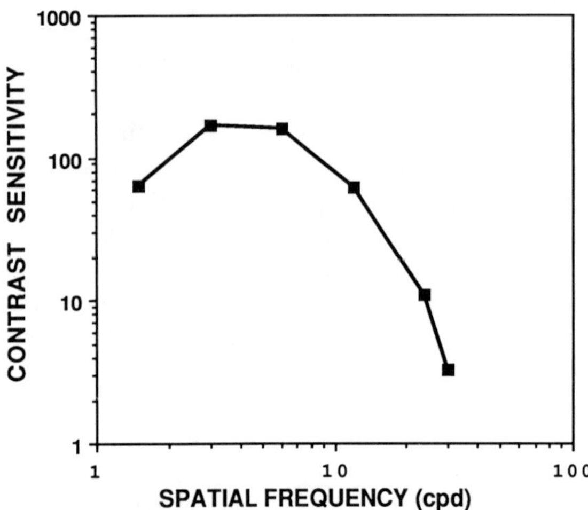

Figure 2.11. Average contrast sensitivity for eight young, healthy observers. Sensitivity is the reciprocal of threshold contrast. Both spatial frequency (cycles per degree, cpd) and sensitivity are plotted on logarithmic scales.

Figure 2.11 shows actual data from an experiment of this sort. Average monocular sensitivity for eight young subjects is plotted as a function of spatial frequency on logarithmic axes.* These data were obtained with a three-alternative, forced-choice method (stimuli could be vertical, tilted 15 degrees left, or tilted right). Fourteen reversals of the two-down, one-up staircase were used. Mean luminance was 85 candela (cd)/m² and the stimuli subtended 1.9 × 1.7 degrees at the 10-foot viewing distance. Stimuli appeared gradually over the course of 0.5 second, remained at full contrast for 1 second, and faded over 0.5 second. Under these conditions, sensitivity was maximal at 3 to 6 cpd, corresponding to correct identification of gratings of less than 1% contrast. Acuity can be estimated by extending the high-frequency limb of the function to the x axis. This yields an estimate of between 30 and 40 cpd (20/20–20/15). These results with a peak at 3 to 6 cpd and sensitivity falling off at both high and low frequencies are a fair representation of a normal CSF.

Stimulus Variables

Virtually all of the variables that might affect contrast sensitivity do affect contrast sensitivity. If

(e.g., the probabilistic nature of "thresholds," guessing, speed–accuracy trade-offs, etc.) are issues that any method should address. At a minimum, those using a method should understand the effects of these factors. In some cases, particularly in some clinical settings, further methodological shortcuts may be justified. This point will be discussed later in this chapter.

---

*Logarithmic axes are used here because they better reflect perceptual reality. For example, the difference between 3 and 6 cpd is much more salient than the difference between 33 and 36 cpd.

measurements are to be comparable one to another it is important that these stimulus variables be held constant. Contrast sensitivity improves as mean luminance increases[16] and as the size of the stimulus increases.[17,18] Thus, if grating stimuli are used, it will be easier to detect six cycles of a 3-cpd grating than to detect two cycles of that grating. Retinal location is important, since acuity and contrast sensitivity for medium and high frequencies decline rapidly from the fovea to the periphery.[19] Acuity and contrast sensitivity vary with the orientation of stimuli even in nonastigmatic observers.[20,21] In general, Caucasians show decreased sensitivity to oblique orientations (oblique effect). This effect may be reduced or absent in other groups[22,23] and may be altered by extensive practice.[24]

Temporal factors may also influence the CSF.[25] Of particular interest in clinical settings, contrast sensitivity at low frequency is likely to be enhanced by abrupt stimulus onset. If desired, this effect can be minimized by having the stimuli appear and disappear slowly (e.g., contrast increases for 0.5 second, is steady for 1 second, and fades over 0.5 second). In general, comparisons between observers or between multiple tests of a single observer will be valid only if these stimulus factors are held constant or if the stimulus variations are taken into consideration in the comparison. More detailed discussion of these factors can be found in Olzak and Thomas.[26]

Refractive state and pupil size affect the quality of the retinal image and therefore affect contrast sensitivity. Defocus has predictable effects on all frequencies, not merely on visual acuity.[27-29] It is important to consider changes in refractive state as possible causes for changes in the shape of the CSF. Refractive error can even produce "notches" in the CSF.[30] Pupil size has two primary effects. Retinal light level varies with pupil size and large pupils introduce larger optical aberrations. Intermediate pupil size (2–5 mm) provides the best acuity and contrast sensitivity.[5,31]

Observer/Procedural Variables

Differences in testing protocol can make surprisingly large differences in results of acuity and contrast sensitivity measures. Naive observers (by which we mean individuals who do not know the purpose of a test and do not have extensive experience with it; e.g., patients) tend to be unwilling to

be conservative when reporting on faint, near-threshold stimuli. That is, returning to Figure 2.8, they might claim to be unable to see stimuli that fall below the 90% point on their underlying sensitivity function. Just as they correct for guessing, 2AFC procedures can correct for this conservative tendency. However, the forced-choice must be a true-false choice. Observers cannot be allowed to use the third choice of "I don't know." This need for true forced-choice holds in others tests. For example, an observer who is asked to locate the smallest visible line on a Snellen chart is likely to yield a poorer acuity measure than an observer who is asked to make a real 26-alternative, forced-choice "guess" at the letters on subsequent lines.

Consistent use of forced-choice methods also makes comparison between observers more trustworthy. Without forced choice, a difference in sensitivity or acuity measures could be attributed either to a "real" difference in vision or to a difference in response criteria. (Forced-choice measures are often called *criterion-free methods*). Further, some observers are less reliable than others and will make careless errors. The results obtained by criterion-free methods are less vulnerable to distortion by errors.

Underlying Mechanisms of Contrast Sensitivity Testing

The shape of the CSF is a product of optical, retinal, and neural factors. There is a basic scientific interest in explaining the CSF. Moreover, our interpretation of deviations from the "normal" CSF are based on our understanding of the processes that give rise to that normal function.

Optics and Photoreceptors

Over the past 20 years, a host of psychophysical and physiological experiments have provided a fairly clear picture of the underlying mechanisms that give the normal contrast sensitivity function its characteristic shape. Optical and photoreceptor characteristics provide the primary limitations for visual acuity (and thus for high spatial frequencies). The optics of the eye act to reduce the contrast of spatial frequencies above about 5 cpd. The reduction increases with spatial frequency and becomes complete at about 60 cpd.[9,19,27] Under

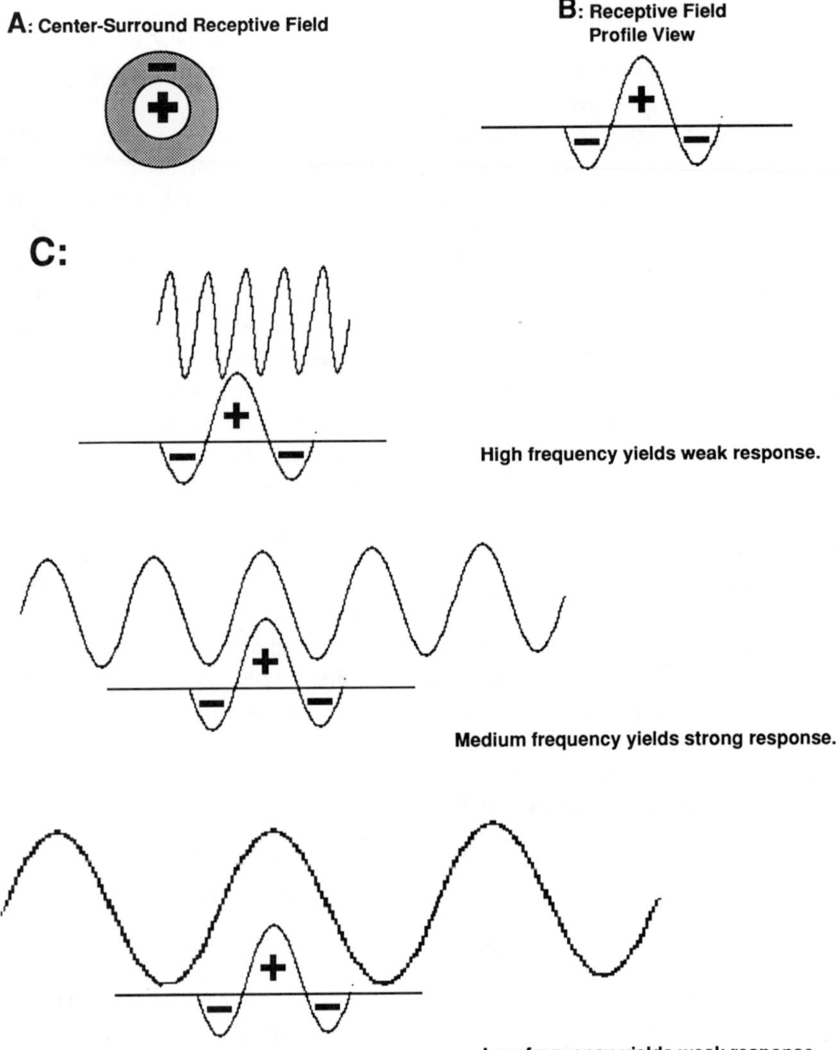

FIGURE 2.12. Individual cells in the retina and central visual pathways have receptive fields that render them more responsive to some spatial frequencies than to others.

normal viewing conditions, spatial frequencies above 60 cpd are not imaged on the retina, so it is no surprise that they are not detected. It is possible, using interference patterns, to form higher frequency gratings directly on the retinal surface. However, even when the optics of the eye are bypassed in this manner, acuity does not improve.[31] Given an image on the retina, the limitation becomes the density of the foveal photoreceptors. Roughly speaking, to see a grating an observer needs photoreceptors packed so that at least one photoreceptor is stimulated by each light bar and one by each dark bar. Not surprisingly, the density of photoreceptors roughly matches the optical limits of the eye.*

*With interference patterns it is possible to see higher spatial frequencies. Imagine that the light from three bright bars and two dark bars of a very fine grating stimulates one photoreceptor while the light from two bright bars and three dark bars stimulates a neighboring photoreceptor. Under these circumstances a pattern might be detected, though it would have an apparent spatial frequency lower than its physical frequency. This interesting phenomenon, known as *aliasing*,[32] does not have important consequences for normal contrast sensitivity or acuity measures.

FIGURE 2.13. Individual cells measured physiologically, or "channels" measured psychophysically, will have contrast sensitivity functions that, when summed together, yield the contrast sensitivity function (CSF) for the organism as a whole. Here, for illustrative purposes, four hypothetical channels are shown underlying the CSF.

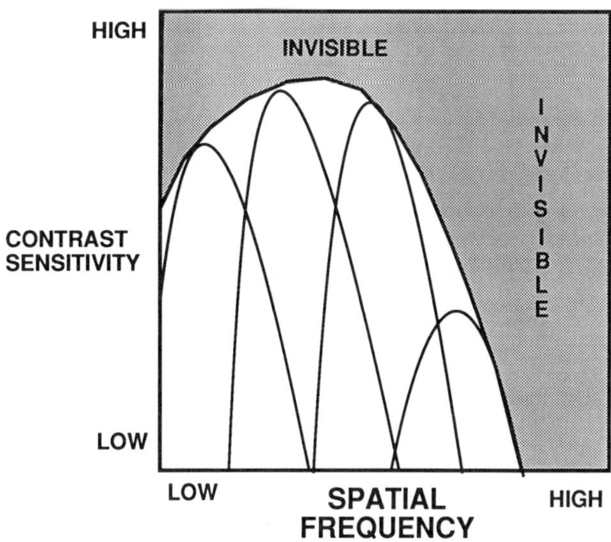

Ganglion Cells

The axons of the retinal ganglion cells form the optic nerve. By means of quite complicated neuronal circuitry in the retina,[33,34] these ganglion cells act to pool responses from a patch of photoreceptors. That patch of retina or, equivalently, the portion of visual space that forms an image over that set of photoreceptors, is known as the *receptive field of the cell.* Ganglion cell receptive fields have a characteristic "center-surround" organization, as shown in Figure 2.12A. Stimulation of the photoreceptors in the center causes an increase in the cell's response. Stimulation of the surround causes a decrease. Another useful representation of the receptive field's response properties is shown in Figure 2.12B. Here the response of the cell is shown for a one-dimensional slice through the receptive field center. Again, stimulation of the center excites the cell. Stimulation of the surround inhibits the cell. It is possible to have the arrangement reversed so that the cell is activated by an absence of light in the center. More information about ganglion cell receptive field properties can be found in Dowling[33] and Bishop.[35] Stimulation by a large patch of light will activate both center and surround and, because of the inhibitory action of the surround, will produce relatively little activation of the ganglion cell.

A ganglion cell with the response profile shown in Figure 2.12B will have a contrast sensitivity function associated with it. This can be understood by comparing the response profile of the cell with the luminance profile of a grating stimulus (Fig. 2.12C). The response of the ganglion cell will be greatest when the response profile matches the periodicity of the luminance profile. Put another way, the response of the cell will be greatest when a bright bar falls on the center of the receptive field while flanking dark bars fall on the inhibitory surround regions. Thus, for the receptive field shown in Figure 2.12B, there will be an optimal spatial frequency with response falling off as the frequency becomes higher or lower than the optimal.

Ganglion cells can have receptive fields of different sizes. As Figure 2.13 indicates, a set of such cells with their associated contrast sensitivity functions could, in aggregate, give rise to the contrast sensitivity function of the observer as a whole.

Spatial Frequency Channels

The preceding assertion is somewhat of an oversimplification. The CSF is not determined completely at the level of retinal output. The output goes to the lateral geniculate nucleus of the thalamus and from there to the visual cortex. Rather than being circularly symmetric, the receptive fields of many visual cortical cells have a preferred orientation. Thus, a CSF measured with horizontal gratings would be the product of the output of cortical cells "tuned" for horizontal orientations, whereas a CSF measured with vertical gratings would involve a different set of cortical cells, those tuned for vertical orientations. Presumably, this orientational selectivity is responsible for the oblique effect already mentioned.[36,37] The matter is not completely clear, however.

We generally assume that the physiology underlying the human CSF is similar to the physiology discussed here, though our data come primarily from monkey and cat. The properties of the human system can be probed only indirectly using psychophysical methods. When discussing human vision, we tend to talk about spatial frequency and/or orientation selective "channels" or "mechanisms," to acknowledge that the experiments do not directly measure the responses of single cells.

Human psychophysical studies of these underlying mechanisms attempt to specify their number, shape, and size. In Figure 2.13, the number of mechanisms would be four. Their shape would be roughly parabolic. Of course, "shape" is used here in a graphic sense and is dependent on the axes used. Normally CSFs are plotted as log sensitivity as a function of log spatial frequency. Finally, the "width" of the mechanism gives an estimate of the range of spatial frequencies to which the mechanism responds. Width is usually defined as the width at half the height of the channel. Thus, if the maximum sensitivity of a channel were 2 log units ($=100=1\%$ contrast), width would be defined as the range of spatial frequencies that stimulate the channel at 1 log unit ($=10=10\%$ contrast).

Several experimental paradigms provide converging evidence that there are a limited number (perhaps six to eight) of spatial frequency selective channels underlying the human CSF. Four of these methods will be described here: adaptation, discrimination at detection thresholds, subthreshold summation, and masking. The existence of multiple spatial frequency channels is of more than purely scientific interest. Given that multiple mechanisms underly human spatial vision, a simple acuity measure may be inadequate, since it will reflect only activity in the high-frequency channels.

Adaptation

Stimulation of a channel renders that channel less sensitive to subsequent stimulation for some period of time. This is known as adaptation. Adaptation of a psychophysical channel is directly analogous to adaptation of photoreceptors to light. Exposure to light reduces the photoreceptor's ability to respond to light. Sensitivity is reduced until the photoreceptor returns to its unadapted state. In adaptation to spatial frequency, it is assumed that exposure to a spatial pattern either depletes some limited resource (perhaps neurotransmitter) or produces some prolonged inhibition. This is made manifest as a reduction in the observer's sensitivity to the adapting stimulus. Sensitivity recovers as the limited resource is replenished or the inhibition dissipates.

Given that adaptation to a grating reduces sensitivity to that grating, information about the nature of underlying spatial frequency channels can be obtained by adapting to a grating of one spatial frequency and looking for effects of that adaptation at other frequencies. If the CSF reflected the sensitivity of a single underlying channel, then adaptation at one spatial frequency should reduce sensitivity at all visible frequencies. The analogous example from light adaptation would be adaptation of the rod photoreceptors. There is a single type of rod with a single spectral sensitivity function. Adaptation to any wavelength of light decreases sensitivity to all other wavelengths. At the opposite extreme, there could be a distinct, narrowly tuned channel for each spatial frequency such that a single frequency would stimulate one and only one channel while a neighboring frequency would stimulate a different channel. In this case, adaptation at one frequency would reduce sensitivity only to that frequency.

Reality lies between the extremes. Adaptation to a single frequency reduces sensitivity to a range of spatial frequencies surrounding the adapting frequency[38] (see Fig. 2.14). These results provide evidence for multiple spatial frequency selective channels and give an estimate of their tuning (the degree of their selectivity). For a number of reasons, it is not simple to infer the precise tuning of the underlying channels from the results of adaptation studies. For instance, adaptation at one frequency may influence several underlying channels. Therefore, the spread of the elevation in threshold cannot be used to estimate directly the shape of any single channel.

Discrimination at Detection Thresholds

No simple, one-channel model of the CSF could be correct, because a single channel could not provide information about spatial frequency. Two spatial frequencies could produce identical outputs from a

FIGURE 2.14. Spatial frequency adaptation. If an observer views a sinusoidal grating of a particular spatial frequency, sensitivity at that frequency and at its near neighbors will be reduced. Remote frequencies will show no reduction.

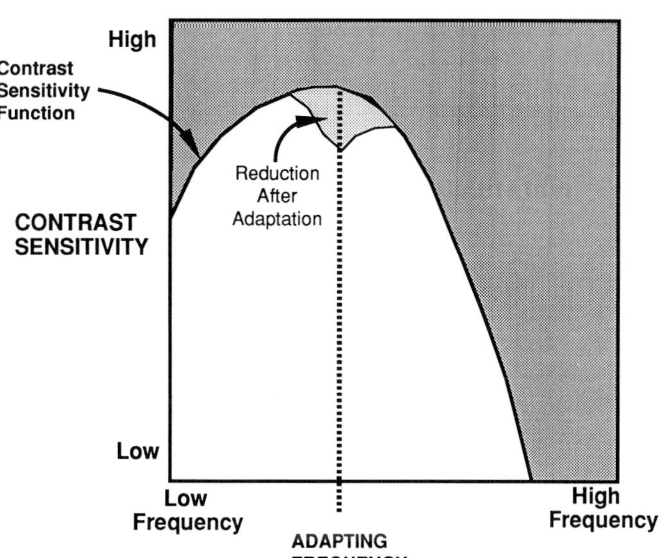

single channel and the stimuli would be indiscriminable. This observation can be turned into a method for studying spatial frequency channels. At the detection threshold, a grating is presumed to be detected exclusively by the channel most sensitive to that spatial frequency. If a grating of a neighboring frequency stimulated the same channel at threshold, the two frequencies should be indistinguishable. Each is producing a minimal activation of the same channel. If, however, the second grating is detected by a second channel, the two gratings should be discriminable at threshold. By examining the discriminability of numerous pairs of spatial frequencies it is possible to estimate the number and shape of the underlying spatial frequency selective mechanisms. For example, Watson and Robson[39] used this method to obtain an estimate of seven selective mechanisms (see also Nachmias and Weber,[40] Thomas and Gille,[41] and Thomas, Gille, and Barker[42]).

Subthreshold Summation

Two other methods, subthreshold summation and masking, emerge from the idea that gratings should interact if their spatial frequencies are similar enough to stimulate the same mechanisms. Subthreshold summation is best understood if we consider detection of a simple spot of light. Sup-

pose that 100 units of light are required for detection and suppose that the available stimuli are two 75-unit light sources. Each of these is "subthreshold," but if both shine on the same patch of retina the energy will summate and the resulting 150 units will be detectable. If the two sources shine on separated patches of retina, no summation will occur and no light will be detected.

Similarly, if two sinusoidal gratings are presented to the same patch of retina at subthreshold contrast, they may summate and produce a detectable stimulus if they stimulate the same underlying spatial frequency channel. However, if the two gratings are far enough apart in spatial frequency that they stimulate entirely different channels, no summation and no detection will occur. Experiments of this sort indicate that gratings can show summation if their spatial frequencies differ by less than a 2:1 ratio.[43] Interestingly, frequencies that are much farther apart may inhibit each other.[44]

Masking

The use of masking in the study of spatial frequency channels can also be understood by analogy to detection of a spot of light. We again assume that, in the absence of other light, the threshold for detection is 100 units of light. It is intuitively clear and factually correct that those 100 units of light will not be detected if they are presented in a location already illuminated by 1000 units of light. The 1000 units *mask* the 100 units. If the 1000 units are presented elsewhere in the visual field, the masking effect will be reduced or eliminated. Switching to spatial frequency, the threshold for a test grating of one spatial frequency will be raised by the presence of a second masking frequency if that masking frequency stimulates the same channels as the test frequency. In masking experiments, gratings mask each other when their spatial frequencies differ by less than a factor of 2. Estimates of the number of underlying mechanisms are similar to those obtained by other methods (e.g., six channels[45]).

While different studies do yield different estimates of the number and shape of spatial frequency channels, an estimate of six to eight channels seems reasonable. The shape of the CSFs for these channels appears to be roughly parabolic plotted on logarithmic coordinates. The width of these channels at half height appears to be about 1 octave (a factor of 2; i.e., a channel that responds maximally to, say, 8 cpd would respond with roughly half that enthusiasm to 6 or 12 cpd). These estimates change as other properties of the stimulus change. For example, if the stimuli are flickering on and off, estimates of the number of channels drop (e.g., from seven to three in Watson and Robson's 1981 study[39]). Spatial frequency channels are tuned for orientation as well as spatial frequency. This means that the channel that detects a vertical 3-cpd grating will be quite insensitive to horizontal gratings of the same frequency. Estimates for the width of the tuning for orientation generally fall in the range of 5 to 20 degrees (see Olzak and Thomas[26]). Methods for determining orientation tuning are similar to those for spatial frequency tuning. For example, detection of a vertical grating would be masked by the presence of another grating oriented near vertical but not masked by a grating oriented at 45 degrees.

As noted previously, a two-dimensional spatial pattern can be decomposed into a set of sinusoids of varying amplitude, phase, frequency, and orientation. The set of spatial frequency channels can be thought of as filters that can selectively attenuate the components of specific frequencies (or orientations). The CSF is the sum of all of those filters. When it is "normal," the world looks normal. Deviations from the normal CSF produce deviations from normal vision that are the natural consequence of a different filter being used to modify visual input. For example, in a reasonably close encounter with a zebra, the highest frequency channels will be activated by the small details: hairs, a small spot, and so on. A loss in the high-frequency end of the CSF would cause a loss in the ability to resolve those fine details. Let us suppose that the stripes on the zebra are of medium spatial frequency. Because they are black and white "square-wave" stripes, they stimulate the medium spatial frequency channels *and* the high-frequency channels. The high-frequency channels are being stimulated by the sharp edge; they would not be stimulated by a sinusoidally striped zebra. If the CSF were depressed in the medium-frequency range, the high-frequency channels might note the edges of the stripes but the stripes would look "washed out" due to a lack of the normal response from the medium-frequency channels. The lowest frequency channels would respond to more substantial chunks of the whole animal: head, limbs, and so forth. A low-frequency loss might cause the animal to appear somehow indistinct while small details remain visible.

Clinical Uses of Contrast Sensitivity Testing

As already noted, the evidence for multiple spatial frequency channels is a strong argument against the use of a single visual acuity test as a measure of spatial vision. A condition that disrupts low-frequency channels may have no influence on acuity. There are numerous reports in the clinical literature of just this situation: clear disruption of spatial vision in spite of Snellen acuity of about 20/20 (e.g., cataract, Hess and Woo[46]; glaucoma, Ross[47]; macular degeneration, Loshin and White[48]; optic neuritis, Fleishman et al.[49]; anterior pathway compressive lesions, Kupersmith, Siegel, and Carr[50,51]). As described in the zebra example, low- or mid-frequency loss with normal acuity can lead to complaints that the visual scene looks washed out or indistinct even though the patient can read small print. These reports are easy enough to understand. Consider a 20/400 *E* on a Snellen chart. The edges of this letter stimulate high spatial frequency channels. The broad areas of black stimulate medium- and low-frequency channels, while the sharp edges stimulate the high-frequency channels. If the medium- and low-frequency channels are not functioning properly, the edges will be seen normally while the bulk of the letter will provide a weaker than normal signal. A weaker signal is interpreted as reduced contrast, and the letter appears washed out.

There are at least four general uses for contrast sensitivity testing: screening, diagnosis, documentation, and tracking. At the present time, for each category, honest investigators may differ about the value of contrast sensitivity testing.

Screening

Contrast sensitivity testing could be made a part of many routine examinations, replacing or augmenting current acuity measures. For example, early cataract may have significant effects at medium and low spatial frequencies and might not be detected by an acuity measure.[10,46] Like most visual tasks, driving involves use of low and medium frequencies. Therefore, it has been argued that state driver's exams could use CSF and not acuity alone.[52] Screening tests need not be as accurate as tests done under laboratory conditions. Clinical constraints on testing will be discussed below.

Diagnosis

Many of the subsequent chapters in this book will deal with the effects of specific disorders on the CSF. While it is clear that a large number of disorders cause changes in the CSF, it is substantially less clear that the nature of that change is diagnostic of the disorder. Cataract, for example, produces a reduction in contrast sensitivity but the nature of that reduction may not be distinguishable from reductions due to other causes (e.g., diabetic retinopathy, Howes, Caelli, and Mitchell[53]; see discussion in Rubin*).

There are reports that some disorders produce specific "notches" in the CSF resembling those seen after adaptation to a specific spatial frequency (see Fig. 2.14) (e.g., multiple sclerosis, Regan, Silver, and Murray[54]). However, notches do not

appear in all cases,[55] and some notches may be due to purely optical causes.[30] That said, CSFs are of some use in locating the source of a visual problem. For example, a loss that is restricted to medium and low spatial frequencies is unlikely to be optical in origin. As a different example, it might be possible to use contrast sensitivity testing in conjunction with acuity testing to detect psychogenic visual defects and/or malingering. An abnormal relationship between the two measures (e.g., 20/200 Snellen acuity with 20-cpd grating resolution) could be an indication of a problem without an organic cause.

Documentation

Cataract is a good example of a disorder that is easily diagnosed without the aid of contrast sensitivity testing. However, measurement of the CSF can serve to document the visual loss that accompanies the cataract. The degree of visual impairment can then be used as a guide to treatment. Similarly for other disorders, reduction in spatial vision can be quantified by comparing the patient's CSF with a standard (e.g., Vistech provides standard ranges for "normal" contrast sensitivity with its equipment). The ability to document loss has led to a desire for criteria for treatment. When is a loss in contrast sensitivity sufficient to warrant, for example, the removal of a cataract? Unfortunately, there is inadequate data on the impact of contrast sensitivity losses on normal visually guided behavior. With an acuity loss, it is possible to state the behavioral consequences fairly precisely. The patient might be unable to read standard newsprint or traffic signs. The behavioral impact of, for example, a 25% loss in overall contrast sensitivity is less clear. For CSFs the situation is further complicated because losses can be restricted to a range of frequencies.

A sensible approach might be to look at the area under the CSF. One can imagine a criterion that recommends removal of a cataract if the area under the CSF has been reduced by X% regardless of the spatial frequency specificity of the loss. At the present time, however, there does not appear to be firm scientific evidence to back any particular criterion.

That said, documentation remains an important use for the CSF. If a patient complains of problems with spatial vision in spite of 20/20 acuity, a CSF

---

*Rubin GS: Contrast sensitivity and glare testing in the evaluation of anterior segment disease. In press.

can document the presence (or absence) of a visual deficit and can be an argument for treatment or nontreatment, even if firm numerical criteria for treatment do not exist at the time.

Tracking

Tracking (longitudinal testing) is a logical extension of documentation. If a disorder causes a CSF change, the course of the disease and/or the effect of treatment may be tracked by repeated CSF measures. Cataract can be used again as an obvious example. Prior to treatment, the CSF may be tracked to determine when the visual loss warrants lens extraction. After removal of the cataract, recovery can be measured by longitudinal testing of the return of the CSF to normal. In cases of degenerative disease, CSF longitudinal testing can be used to monitor the rate of decline and, of course, the efficacy of treatment. In some cases, longitudinal testing of the CSF can reveal the presence of subtle residual deficits even after an acute condition has resolved (e.g., optic neuritis[49]).

In summary, in conjunction with acuity testing, contrast sensitivity testing provides a more accurate assessment of a patient's spatial vision than does acuity alone. At the present time it appears to be of more use in the quantification of visual loss than in the diagnosis of disorders. A clinician with some familiarity with the test should be able to use it to monitor the visual consequences of disease and of treatment.

Clinical Constraints on Psychophysical Methods

As discussed, there are psychophysically "correct" methods for obtaining CSFs. Two major factors act to undermine the use of these methods in clinical settings: the fact that patients are not trained, highly motivated psychophysical observers, and lack of time.

Patients as Psychophysical Observers

Two-alternative, forced-choice (2AFC) methods guard against blind guessing and, to some extent, against the unwillingness of observers to report the presence of near-threshold stimuli. These concerns remain important in a clinical setting. Patients may have very different motivations from those of a volunteer observer in a laboratory. They may wish to prove the existence of a problem, or its absence. They may be relatively uncooperative. Forced-choice methods can help to overcome these impediments to accurate measurement. The central elements of any such method should be a true forced choice. For example, is the stimulus in location 1 or 2? Is the grating tilted left or right or is it vertical? (Note: A three-alternative, forced-choice method as is used in many clinical contrast sensitivity devices is a perfectly valid method with properties only slightly different from those of the 2AFC.) Just as important, the patient should be "forced" (or cajoled or whatever) into making a response. If all tests are administered with consistent, firm instructions to make one of the designated choices, the effects of the patients' response criteria and biases will be reduced.

Clinical Shortcuts

The 2AFC staircase method outlined earlier in this chapter is reasonably efficient by laboratory standards but may still take too long for routine clinical use. Several shortcuts are possible based on the demands of the particular clinical situation and on some simplifying assumptions. The existence of six to eight spatial frequency channels suggests that no more than six to eight spatial frequencies need be chosen to obtain an estimate of the overall shape of the CSF. Great savings may be obtained with the further assumption that the CSF is roughly parabolic. If that is so, as a quadratic function the CSF could be completely specified by two free parameters. In practice, these numbers could be an acuity measure and a single contrast sensitivity measure designed to give the height of the peak of the CSF. Pelli, Legge, and Rubin[56] have proposed such a test and have presented data showing that abnormal CSFs can be treated as if they are normal CSFs (see Fig. 2.11) that are shifted either to the left (reduced acuity) or down (reduced sensitivity), or both. The two numbers required for their method can be obtained with two letter charts: one a version of a Snellen chart and the other a chart with letters of fixed, large size but decreasing contrast.[57] This method, appealing as it is, relies on the assumption that notches and other departures from the parabolic shape of the CSF are either nonexistent or at least of no clinical significance. As indicated previously, this assumption is controversial.

Without a strong assumption about the shape of the CSF, it is necessary to measure more than two points. However, particularly in screening tests where the clinical task is to simply distinguish between normal and abnormal findings, a high level of precision is not needed. Substantial savings in time may be effected by reducing the theoretical accuracy of the estimate of a point on the psychometric function that underlies threshold measures. An example is the Vistech contrast sensitivity (VCTS) wall chart that has been incorporated into a number of testing devices. In this test, patients do what amounts to a one-reversal staircase. For each of five spatial frequencies the patient is asked to identify the orientations of a succession of grating patches of decreasing contrast. There are three possible orientations, so this is a three-alternative, forced-choice situation (always assuming that the patient is required to respond, an assumption at variance with the test's published instructions). The estimate of threshold is taken as the contrast step higher than the first incorrect response. (This can also be considered a one-trial version of a "descending method of limits.")

Obviously, observer errors and guessing can adversely affect this measure.[57] However, with fairly widely spaced contrast steps, the chance of error is reduced, and tests of this sort do appear to provide a rapid estimate of the CSF that is comparable to the estimates obtained with other methods.[58] This type of test would be expected to identify individuals with abnormal CSFs and could give a reasonable estimate of the magnitude of the departure from normal. However, for more fine-grained use of CSF testing (e.g., detailed longitudinal testing of the CSF), it seems likely that more precise and thus more laborious methods will be needed.

A Note About Glare Testing

In a book entitled *Glare and Contrast Sensitivity for Clinicians*, a chapter on the basics of contrast sensitivity testing needs to say something about glare testing, if only that the two topics are logically separable. Glare testing refers to the measurement of visual function in the presence of a glare source. One could measure the CSF in the presence of a glare source. In fact, this is probably an excellent idea in early cataract (e.g., Rubin*). However, one could also measure acuity or color vision or motion detection or any other visual function in presence of the same glare source. From the point of view of contrast sensitivity testing, the glare source acts to degrade the stimulus by reducing the contrast of the stimulus image on the retina. The reduction will be a function of the position and intensity of the source and the light-scattering properties of the visual optics (see Chap. 4). If the glare reduces the retinal contrast below the detection threshold, the grating will not be seen, regardless of its physical contrast. This could be considered as a version of a masking paradigm (see previous discussion). Because of the possibility that light scatter of the glare source may have different effects at different frequencies, glare testing with the contrast sensitivity as the underlying measure is no doubt a good idea. Nevertheless, glare testing does not require a CSF, nor does measurement of the CSF require a glare source.

General Conclusions

Contrast sensitivity testing provides more information about spatial vision than do simple acuity measures. It tests optical and neural properties of the visual system that acuity measures cannot test. Accurate assessment of the CSF can be fairly time consuming but is possible within a clinical setting. Moreover, radically shortened methods can provide useful information. Firm criteria for basing treatment options on specific CSF test results await further research. It is clear, however, that CSF testing can document and quantify visual loss that other visual tests cannot measure.

Acknowledgments. I thank Gary Rubin, Nancy Newman, David Miller, and Marian Stewart for useful comments on earlier drafts of this chapter. Writing of this chapter was supported by Massachusetts Eye and Ear Infirmary, the MIT Class of 1922, and by grants from the National Eye Institute (RO1-EY05087) and the Educational Foundation of America.

---

*Rubin GS: Contrast sensitivity and glare testing in the evaluation of anterior segment disease. In press.

References

1. Pickering WH: Report on Mars, No. 11. *Pop Astron* **23**:569–588, 1915.
2. Riggs LA: Visual acuity, in Graham CH, Bartlett NR, Hsia Y, et al., *Vision and Visual Perception.* New York/London/Sydney, John Wiley, 1965.
3. Keesey UT: Effects of involuntary eye movements on visual acuity. *J Opt Soc Am* **50**:769–774, 1960.
4. Frisen L, Frisen M: How good is normal visual acuity? A study of letter acuity thresholds as a function of age. *Gr Arch Clin Exper Ophthalmol* **215**:149–157, 1981.
5. Leibowitz H: The effect of pupil size on visual acuity for photometrically equated test fields at various levels of luminance. *J Opt Soc Am* **42**:416–422, 1952.
6. Craik KJW: The effect of adaptation upon visual acuity. *Br J Psychol* **29**:252–266, 1939.
7. Byram GM: The physical and photochemical basis of visual resolving power. I. The distribution of illumination in retinal images. *J Opt Soc Am* **34**:571–591, 1944.
8. Thorn F, Scwartz F: Effects of dioptric blur on Snellen and grating acuity. *Am J Optom Physiol Opt*, in press.
9. Cornsweet TN: *Visual Perception.* New York/London, Academic Press, 1970.
10. Ginsburg AP: Spatial filtering and visual form perception, in Boff K, Kaufman L, Thomas J (eds), *Handbook of Perception and Human Performance.* New York, John Wiley, 1986.
11. Falmagne JC: Psychophysical measurement and theory, in Boff K, Kaufman L, Thomas J (eds), *Handbook of Perception and Human Performance.* New York, John Wiley, 1986.
12. Snodgrass JG, Levy-Berger G, Haydon M: *Human Experimental Psychology.* New York/Oxford, Oxford University Press, 1985.
13. Heinemann EG: The relation of apparent brightness to threshold for differences in luminance. *J Exper Psychol* **61**:389–399, 1961.
14. Levitt H: Transformed up-down methods in psychoacoustics. *J Acoust Soc Am* **49**:467–477, 1971.
15. Tyrell RA, Owens DA: A rapid method to assess the resting state of the eyes and other threshold phenomenon: A modified BIN search (MOSS). *Behav Res Meth Comp* **20**:137–141, 1988.
16. Van Nes FL, Bouman MA: Spatial modulation transfer in the human eye. *J Opt Soc Am* **57**:401–406, 1967.
17. Hoekstra J, Van der Goot DPA, Van den Brink G, et al: The influence of the number of cycles upon the visual contrast threshold for spatial sine wave patterns. *Vis Res* **14**:365–368, 1974.
18. Savoy RL, McCann JJ: Visibility of low-spatial-frequency sine wave targets: Dependence on number of cycles. *J Opt Soc Am* **65**:343–350, 1975.
19. Westheimer G: The spatial sense of the eye. *Invest Ophthalmol Vis Sci* **18**:893–912, 1979.
20. Appelle S: Perception and discrimination as a function of stimulus orientation: The "oblique effect" in man and animals. *Psych Bull* **78**:266–278, 1972.
21. Zemon V, Gutowski W, Horton T: Orientational anisotropy in the human visual system: an evoked potential and psychophysical study. *Int J Neurosci* **19**:259–286, 1983.
22. Timney BN, Muir DW: Orientation anisotropy: Incidence and magnitude in Caucasian and Chinese subjects. *Science* **193**:699–701, 1976.
23. Bauer JA, Fang L, Gwiazda J, et al: Meridional anisotropies in Chinese and Caucasian infants and adults. *Invest Ophthalmol Vis Sci (suppl)* (ARVO) **26**:136, 1985.
24. Mayer MJ: Practice improves adults' sensitivity to diagonals. *Vis Res* **23**:547–550, 1983.
25. Henning GB: Spatial-frequency tuning as a function of temporal frequency and stimulus motion. *J Opt Soc Am-A* **5**:1362–1373, 1988.
26. Olzak LA, Thomas JP: Seeing spatial patterns, in Boff K, Kaufman L, Thomas J (eds), *Handbook of Perception and Human Performance.* New York, John Wiley, 1986.
27. Westheimer G: Pupil size and visual resolution. *Vis Res* **4**:39–45, 1964.
28. Mitchell DE, Wilkinson F: The effect of early astigmatism on the visual resolution of gratings. *J Physiol* **243**:739–756, 1974.
29. Legge GE, Mullen KT, Woo GC, et al: Tolerance to visual defocus. *J Opt Soc Am-A* **4**:851–863, 1987.
30. Apkarian P, Tijssen R, Spekreijse H, et al: Origin of notches in CSF: Optical or neural. *Invest Ophthalmol Vis Sci* **28**:607–612, 1987.
31. Campbell FW, Green DG: Optical and retinal factors affecting visual resolution. *J Physiol* **181**:576–593, 1965.
32. Williams DR: Aliasing in human foveal vision. *Vis Res* **25**:195–205, 1985.
33. Dowling JE, Dubin MW: The vertebrate retina, in Darian-Smith I (ed), *Handbook of Physiology.* Baltimore, American Physiological Society, 1984.
34. Masland RH: The functional architecture of the retina. *Scient Am* **254**(12):102–111, 1986.
35. Bishop PO: Processing of visual information within the retinostriate system, in Darian-Smith I (ed), *Handbook of Physiology.* Baltimore, American Psychological Society, 1984.
36. Mansfield RJW: Neural basis of orientation perception. *Science* **186**:1133–1135, 1974.
37. Mansfield RJW, Ronner SF: Orientation aniso-

tropy in monkey vision. *Brain Res* **149**:229–231, 1978.

38. Blakemore C, Campbell FW: On the existence of neurons in the human visual system selectively sensitive to the orientation and size of retinal images. *J Physiol* **203**:237–260, 1969.

39. Watson AB, Robson JG: Discrimination at threshold: Labelled detectors in human vision. *Vis Res* **21**:1115–1122, 1981.

40. Nachmias J, Weber A: Discrimination of simple and complex gratings. *Vis Res* **15**:217–223, 1975.

41. Thomas JP, Gille J: Bandwidths of orientation channels in human vision. *J Opt Soc Am* **69**:652–660, 1979.

42. Thomas JP, Gille J, Barker RA: Simultaneous detection and identification: Theory and data. *J Opt Soc Am* **72**:1642–1651, 1982.

43. Graham N, Nachmias J; Detection of grating patterns containing two spatial frequencies: A comparison of single-channel and multiple-channel models. *Vis Res* **11**:251–259, 1971.

44. Olzak L, Thomas JP: Why frequency discrimination is sometimes better than detection. *J Opt Soc Am* **71**:64–70, 1981.

45. Wilson HR, McFarlane DK, Phillips GC: Spatial frequency tuning of orientation selective units estimated by oblique masking. *Vis Res* **23**:873–882, 1983.

46. Hess R, Woo G: Vision through cataracts. *Invest Ophthalmol Vis Sci* **17**:428–435, 1978.

47. Ross JE: Clinical detection of abnormalities in central vision in chronic simple glaucoma using contrast sensitivity. *Int Ophthalmol* **8**:167–177, 1985.

48. Loshin DS, White J: Contrast sensitivity: The visual rehabilitation of the patient with macular degeneration. *Arch Ophthalmol* **102**:1303–1306, 1984.

49. Fleishman JA, Beck RW, Linares OA, et al: Deficits in visual function after recovery from optic neuritis. *Ophthalmology* **94**:1029–1035, 1987.

50. Kupersmith MJ, Siegel IM, Carr RE: Reduced contrast sensitivity in compressive lesions of the anterior visual pathway. *Neurology* **31**:550–554, 1981.

51. Kupersmith MJ, Siegel IM, Carr RE: Subtle disturbances of vision with compressive lesions of the anterior visual pathway measured by contrast sensitivity. *Ophthalmology* **89**:68–72, 1982.

52. Evans D, Ginsburg A: Contrast sensitivity predicts age-related differences in highway sign discriminability. *Hum Fact* **27**:637, 1985.

53. Howes SC, Caelli T, Mitchell P: Contrast sensitivity in diabetics with retinopathy and cataract. *Aust J Ophthalmol* **10**:173–178, 1982.

54. Regan D, Silver R, Murray TJ: Visual acuity and contrast sensitivity in multiple sclerosis—hidden visual loss: An auxiliary diagnostic test. *Brain* **100**:563–579, 1977.

55. Hess RF, Plant GT: The psychophysical loss in optic neuritis: Spatial and temporal aspects, in Hess RF, Plant GT (eds), *Optic Neuritis*. Cambridge, England, University of Cambridge, 1986.

56. Pelli DG, Rubin GS, Legge GE: Predicting the contrast sensitivity of low vision observers. *J Opt Soc Am-A* **3**:56, 1986.

57. Pelli DG, Robson JG, Wilkins AJ: The design of a new letter chart for measuring contrast sensitivity. *Clin Vis Sci* **2**:187–199, 1988.

58. Corwin TR, Richman JE: Three clinical tests of the spatial contrast sensitivity function: A comparison. *Am J Optom Physiol Opt* **63**:413–418, 1986.

3
Light Scattering: Its Relationship to Glare and Contrast in Patients and Normal Subjects

David Miller and M. Princeton Nadler

Introduction

In the body, collagen bundles, interstitial fluids, and cellular elements all combine to make tendons white, dura opaque, and epidermis translucent.

Yet the same ingredients combined in the eye produce transparent cornea, lenses, vitreous. Theoretically, the cornea in particular should not be transparent. In this structure clear delicate collagen fibrils of index refraction 1.47 (close to that of glass) are surrounded by a mucopolysaccharide matrix with an index of refraction of about 1.33 (similar to that of water). David Maurice[1] of Stanford studied the organization of the corneal stromal fibers and noted that the collagen fibers are about 200 Å in diameter and are separated from each other by about 600 Å. He felt the arrangement resembled a uniform lattice pattern. Such a pattern would produce destructive interference of the light waves scattered to the side, but would allow waves directed straight ahead to be transmitted.

The lattice theory of corneal transparency was totally accepted until the histology of the shark cornea was examined. As opposed to primate corneas, in the shark cornea the collagen fibers are randomly arranged. Happily, Einstein had helped develop mathematical techniques that permit the accurate characterization of particle distributions that range continuously from perfect randomness to a perfect order, like a lattice pattern. These techniques had been applied to problems of the superposition of the phases of light waves scattered from such quasi-random distribution. Thus, George Benedek of the Massachusetts Institute of Technol-

ogy was able to harness these techniques to explain the transparency of all ocular tissues.[2] The key to transparency is in the arrangement of the elements. Transparency can result from mixing two transparent elements of different refractive indices, if (1) the spacing between the elements is less than the distance of half a wavelength of light and (2) there is a recognizable pattern or predictable relationship between the fibers. For example, in Figure 3.1, right, the fluid pools between the lens fibers have a different refractive index and disrupt the proper arrangement and spacing. The result: increased light scattering and a cataract. A similar phenomena can be seen in Figure 3.2 (see Color Plate I)—the diver has been made invisible by a blanket of air bubbles in water.

When a transparent structure loses its clarity, the physicist describes it predominantly as a light scatterer rather than as a light transmitter. This concept is a bit foreign to the clinician, whose textbooks talk about opaque lenses and corneas. The word *opaqueness* conjures up the image of a cement wall, which stops light. Of all the experiments that demonstrate that most cataracts scatter light rather than stop light, the most graphic involves the relatively new science of holography. If it is true that a cataract splashes or scatters oncoming light so that a poor image is focused on a screen (the retina), then theoretically it should be possible to collect all the scattered light with a special optical element and recreate a sharp image. The essence of such an optical element, one that would take the scattered light of the cataract and rescatter it so that a proper image could be formed, would be a special inverse hologram of the cataract

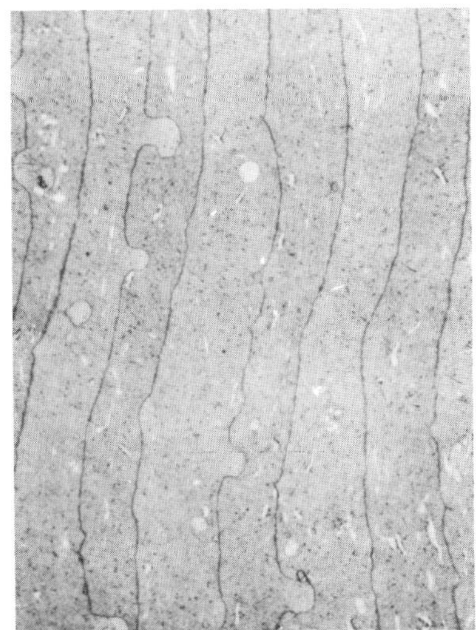

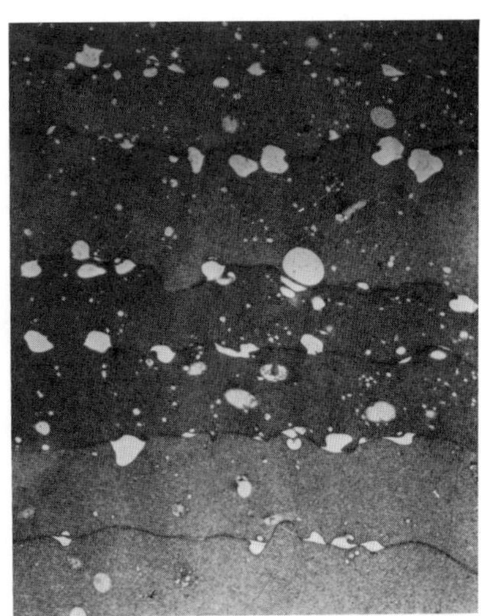

FIGURE 3.1. *Left*: Electron micrograph of the fiber pattern in a normal lens. *Right*: Fluid pools disrupting the fiber pattern in an early cataract. (From Miller and Benedek, p 64. Courtesy of Charles C Thomas, Publisher, Springfield, Illinois.)

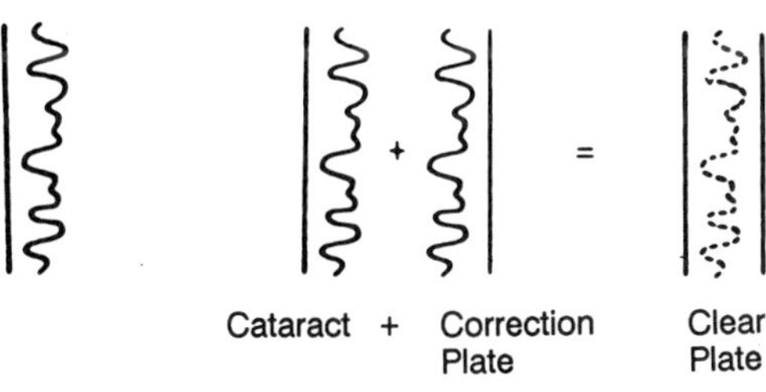

FIGURE 3.3. Method in which the inverse conjugate hologram of a cataract and the cataract itself could recreate a clear image. (From, Miller Zuckerman, and Reynolds, p 323.[3] Copyright 1973, American Medical Association.)

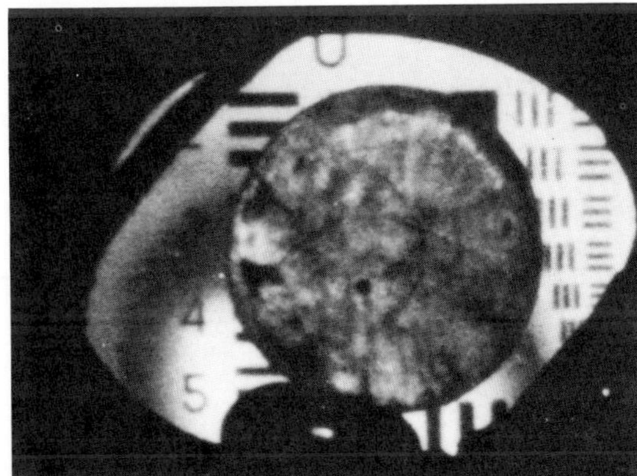

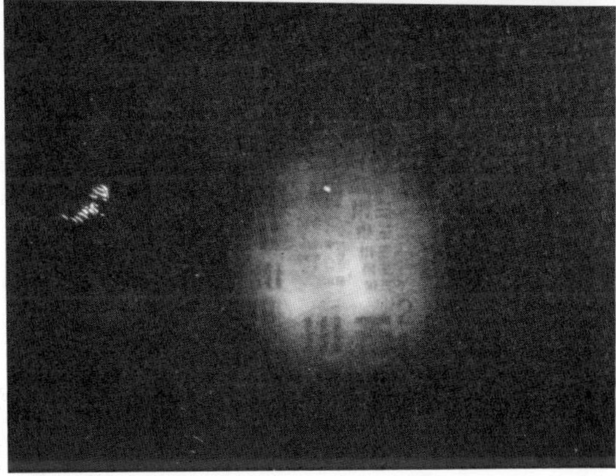

FIGURE 3.4. Photograph of an image degraded by an excised cataract (top) and the clearer image produced by the combination of cataract and holographic filter. (From Miller D, Zuckerman JL, Reynolds GO: Phase aberration balancing of cataracts using holography. *Exp Eye Res* **15**:157, 1973, Fig. 2)

itself. Figure 3.3 describes how such a filter would work. Figure 3.4 demonstrates how a cataract extracted from a patient who had worse than 20/200 visual acuity was made relatively transparent, on the optical bench, by registering a special inverse hologram of that specific cataract in front of the cataract.[3] A more thorough description of light-scattering optics can be found in Miller and Benedek.[4]

To follow the progress of conditions like cataracts or corneal edema, a measure of tissue transparency or tissue back-scattering is useful. Let us see how this can be done.

Glare and Contrast Sensitivity Testing

Although it is possible to quantitate the amount of light scattered by various ocular tissues by means of photoelectric devices, a subjective discrimina-

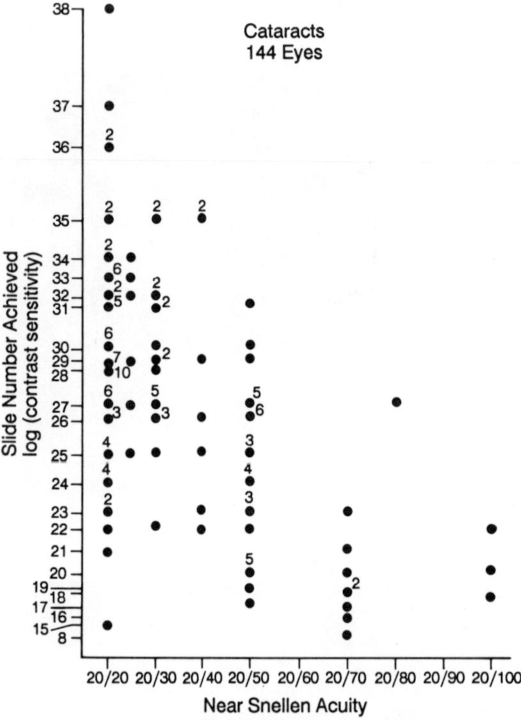

FIGURE 3.5. Study of 144 patients with cataracts in which visual acuity versus glare sensitivity was plotted. Many patients have good visual acuity. (From LeClaire et al, p 53.[11] Copyright 1982, American Medical Association.)

tion system would better relate such scattering to the patient's complaints. Snellen visual acuity has been the traditional index, but as more studies have been done, the sensitivity of this test has been found deficient. Figure 3.5 shows that many patients with cataracts have good visual acuity but poor contrast sensitivity in the face of a glare source. This should not come as a surprise, because the essence of vision is in discriminating the luminance (brightness) of one object as opposed to another, often with a natural glare source present. Thus a plane is seen against the sky because the retinal image of the plane does not stimulate the photoreceptor to the same degree that the image of the sky does. The glare from the sun might diminish the contrast further. Terms like *contrast, luminance,* and *intensity discrimination* are used to describe differences in brightness between an object and its background. How then could ocular light scattering, glare, and contrast sensitivity be linked to give the clinician a useful index?

The stage was set to solve this puzzle by an industrial scientist by the name of L. L. Holladay.[6] In 1926, he packaged the degrading effect of stray light on visibility for normal subjects into the concept of glare and glare testing. In the 1960s, Ernst Wolf, a visual physiologist working in Boston, realized that glare testing could be a useful way to describe the increase in light scattering seen in different clinical conditions.[7-9] How does increased light scattering produce a decrease in the contrast of the retinal image in the presence of a glare source? Figure 3.6 shows the way in which corneal edema splashes light from a far-off naked light bulb onto the foveal image, thus reducing the contrast of that image. Figure 3.7 (see Color Plate I) illustrates the way that a patient with a cataract or corneal edema sees a road sign in the presence of a glare source. Thus, several of us embodied the principles of a glare tester into a small device that could be used in a clinician's office.[10] Unhappily, the device was too compli-

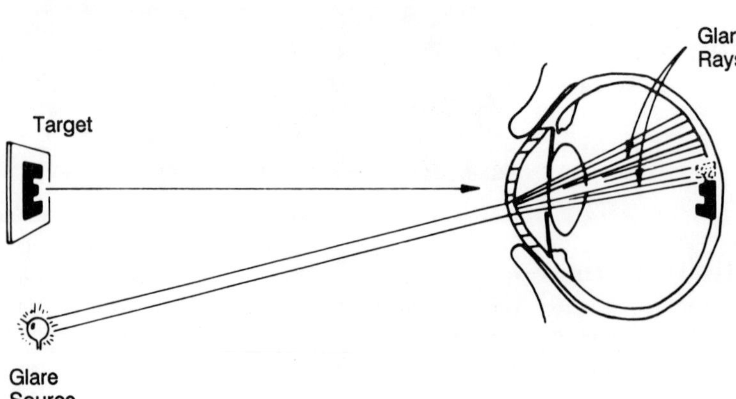

FIGURE 3.6. The eye with corneal edema scatters light from the peripheral light bulb onto the fovea, thus decreasing the contrast of the foveal image. This is known as glare degradation. (From Miller and Benedek, p 38.[4] Courtesy of Charles C Thomas, Publisher, Springfield, Illinois.)

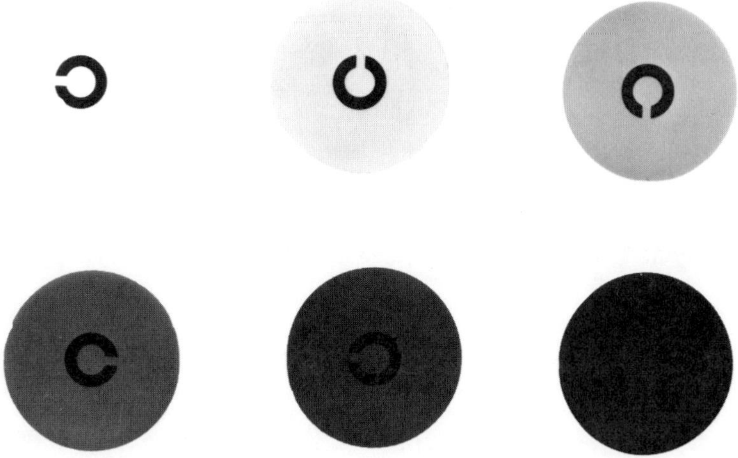

FIGURE 3.8. Example of variable contrast targets using the Landolt ring.

cated and expensive. When only three were sold, the idea simply sank out of view. In the mid 1970s, Princeton Nadler, an ophthalmologist practicing outside Pittsburgh, observed that many of his cataract patients complained of annoying glare. His observations and perseverance rekindled interest in glare testing, and a simpler, less expensive, clinical glare tester was designed (Miller-Nadler glare tester).[11]

Glare Testers

Since that time, many new glare testing devices have been offered to the clinician. Therefore, a discussion of the essential ingredients in any glare tester—the target and the glare source—might be helpful.

Present-day glare testers offer two types of targets—a standard Snellen visual acuity chart and a variable contrast sensitivity target. The variable contrast targets may be presented as (1) sinusoidal contrast gratings, (2) the Snellen chart printed in different contrasts, or (3) the Landolt ring presented in different contrasts (Fig. 3.8). To learn whether a variable contrast target or a standard visual acuity target would be more valuable in cataract testing, we designed an experiment using scattering filters of progressive severity (simulated cataracts). Normal subjects looked through these scatterers at both visual acuity charts and contrast sensitivity targets. In all testing situations a glare light was employed. Figure 3.9 shows that the contrast sensitivity function gradually decreases as the simulated cataract progresses, whereas visual acuity stays almost constant and then falls sharply when the filter has become 80% "cataractous."[10]

Thus, these laboratory experiments suggest that a variable contrast target in the face of a glare source follows cataract progression more smoothly than a conventional visual acuity target.

Now let us take a look at the glare source. Should it have a point configuration or surround the target? Our studies[10] showed that many subjects tend to look directly at the glare source if it is a point or a bulb. This alters the test results because the light both bleaches the macula and creates an afterimage. Therefore it seems more reasonable to surround the contrast target with a circular glare source.

How bright should the glare source be? We recall that even normal young eyes scatter 10% to 20% of the incident light.[4] One has only to consider a healthy young outfielder losing a flyball "in the sun" to appreciate that. Thus, the glare light should allow a normal subject to discriminate a target with a low contrast of 5% to 10%. Abrahmisson and Sjostrand[12] and others[11] found that a glare source of between 200 and 400 cd/m² would be an appropriate brightness for a glare source.

The final question is whether a contrast target is more useful in following cataract patients with or

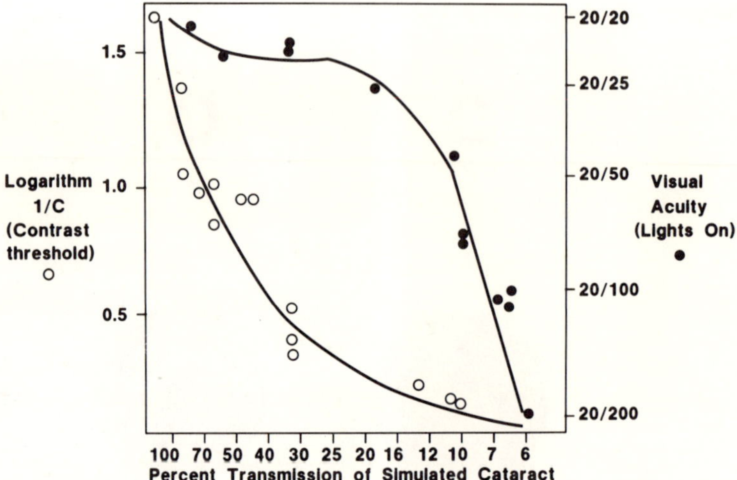

FIGURE 3.9. Results of normal subjects looking through progressive light-scattering filters (simulated cataracts) at a conventional visual acuity chart (solid circles) and a contrast sensitivity target (open circles). A glare source was employed in all cases. Contrast sensitivity gradually decreases as the simulated cataract progresses, whereas visual acuity stays almost constant and then falls steeply only when the filter has reached about 20% transmission (i.e., 80% simulated cataract). (From LeClaire et al, p 153.[11] Copyright 1982, American Medical Association, and Miller and Benedek, p 95.[4] Courtesy of Charles C Thomas, Publisher, Springfield, Illinois.)

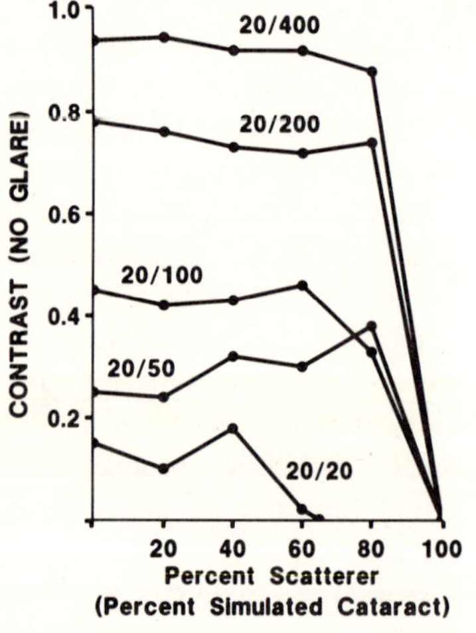

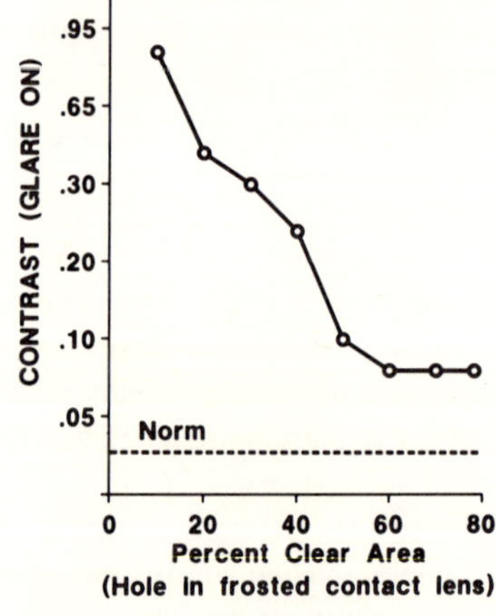

FIGURE 3.10. The curve on the left (filled circles) represents the progressive severity of a simulated cataract (percent of glass lens covered with vaselined finger blots) versus contrast sensitivity for different-sized letters. The experiment used *no* glare source. The curve on the right (open circles) presents the progressive severity of a simulated cataract (clear holes of different sizes drilled in frosted contact lens) versus contrast sensitivity, *with* glare source. To be noted is the gradual nature of the contrast sensitivity loss as "cataract" progresses, with glare light on. In the no-glare testing situation, contrast sensitivity remains stable until an "advanced simulated cataract" sets in. Then a sharp drop in contrast develops. (From Zuckerman JL, Miller D, Dyes W, et al: Degradation of vision through a simulated cataract. *Invest Ophthalmol* **12**:213, 1973, Fig. 13, used by permission)

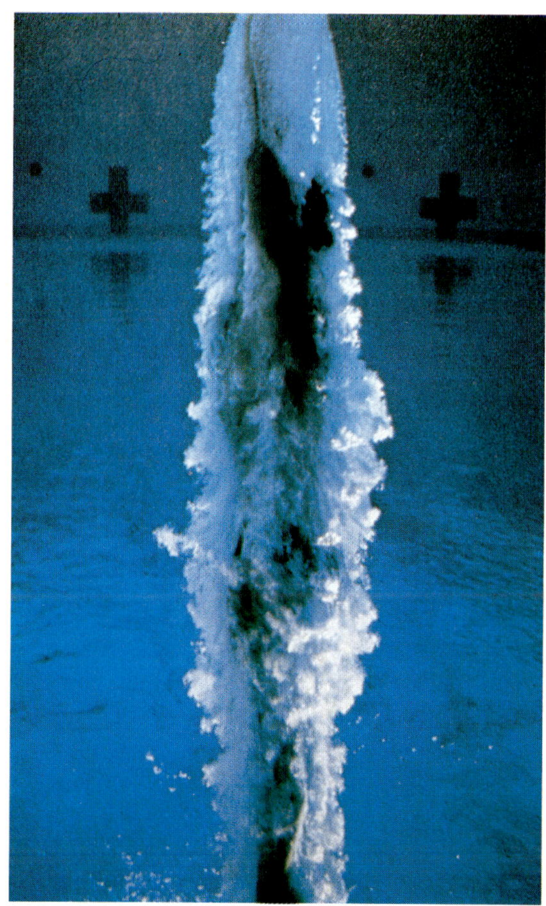

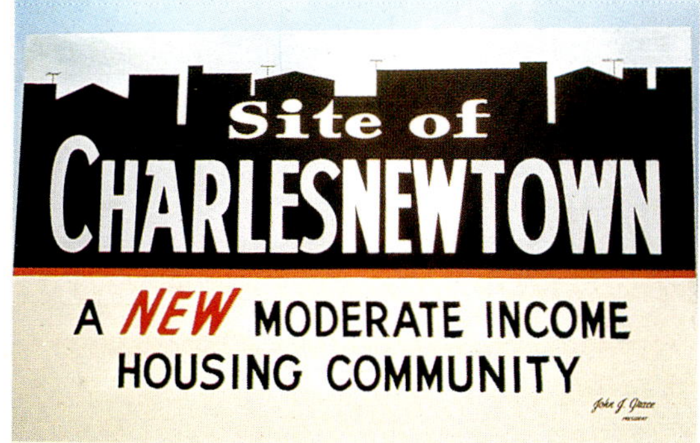

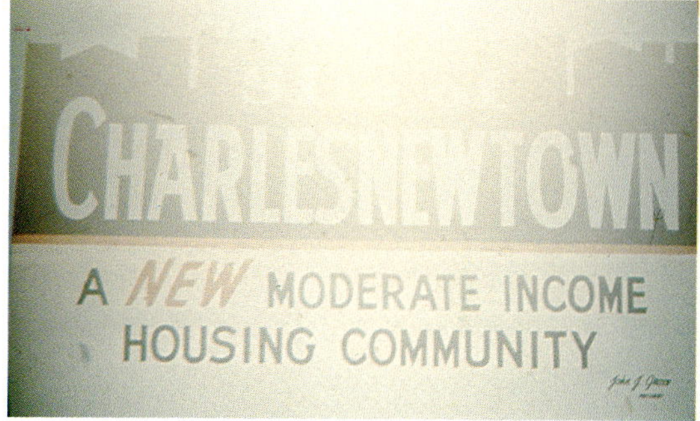

FIGURE 3.7. Photograph of the way a sign (A) would appear to a normal person (top) and (B) would appear to a patient with corneal edema in a glare situation (bottom).

FIGURE 3.2. The diver almost invisible, enshrouded in a blanket of air bubbles and water.

FIGURE 3.12. Artist's drawing of the ultimate glare test. The "jack-knifed" trailer-truck is rendered invisible to oncoming cars by the glare produced by the bright beams of the car in the adjacent lane. (Courtesy of L. Cook, Boston, MA)

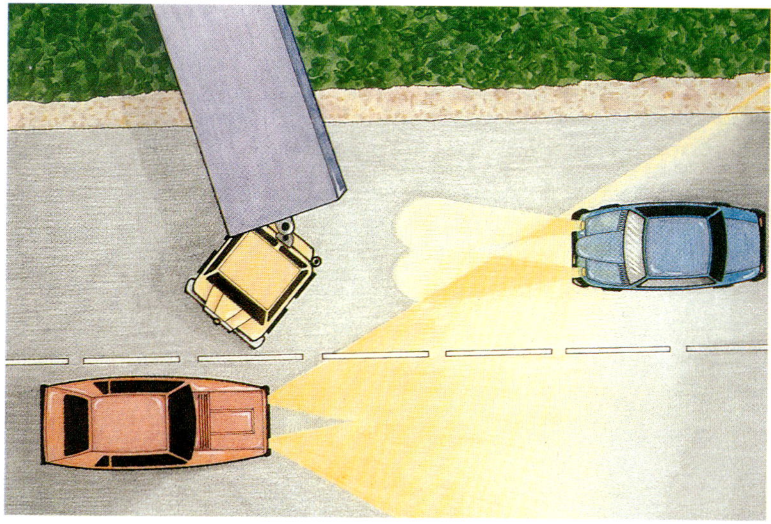

Color Plate II

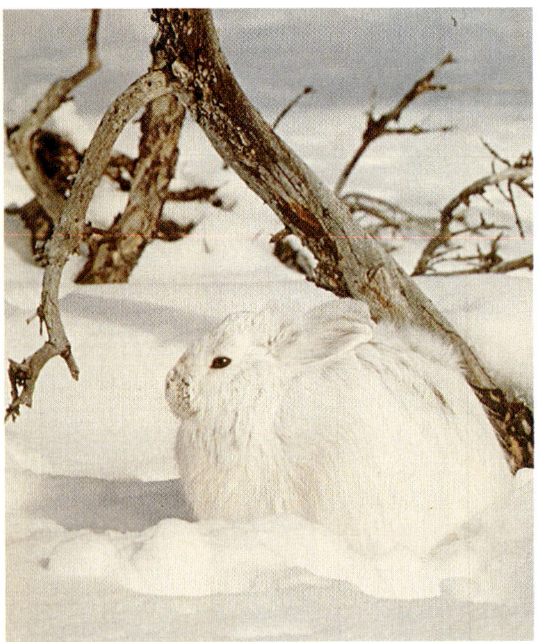

FIGURE 3.13. Arctic hare exploits glare and white background, becoming a low contrast object. (From Burton M, Burton J, Hughes D, World Encyclopedia of Animals, Octopus Books, Ltd., London, 1978, p. 17. Photograph courtesy of Bruce Coleman, Ltd., Uxbridge, England, and C. Ott.)

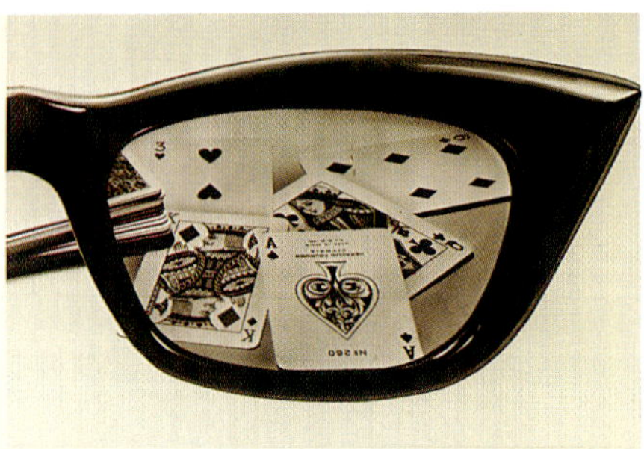

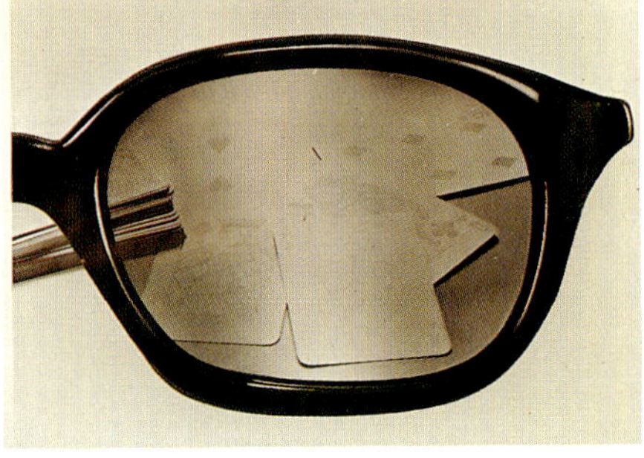

FIGURE 3.15. Illustration of the use of a polaroid filter to reduce glare from reflected lights and allow visualization of the details of playing cards. (Courtesy of Polaroid Corporation, Cambridge, Mass.)

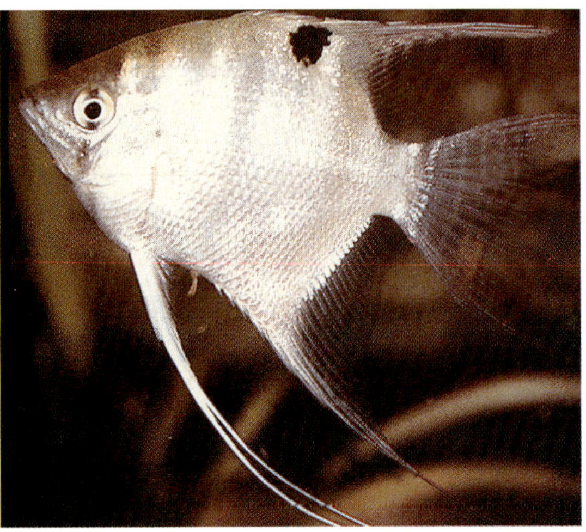

FIGURE 3.14. The silver shimmering body of this small tropical fish (P. dumeril) would be difficult to see against the noonday sun. (Courtesy of Dr. Herbert R. Axelrod, from Dr. Axelrod's Atlas of Freshwater Aquarium Fishes, 3rd ed. Neptune City, N.J., TFH Publications, 1989)

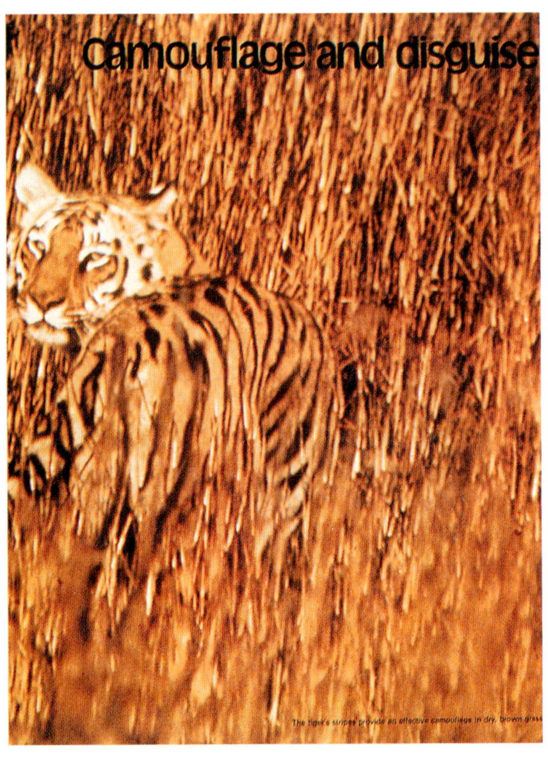

FIGURE 3.16. The striped tiger is rendered all but invisible by the surrounding vertical vegetation. (From Fogden M, Fogden I: Animals and Their Colors. New York, Crown Publishing, 1974, p. 30, used by permission of Life Picture Service, New York.)

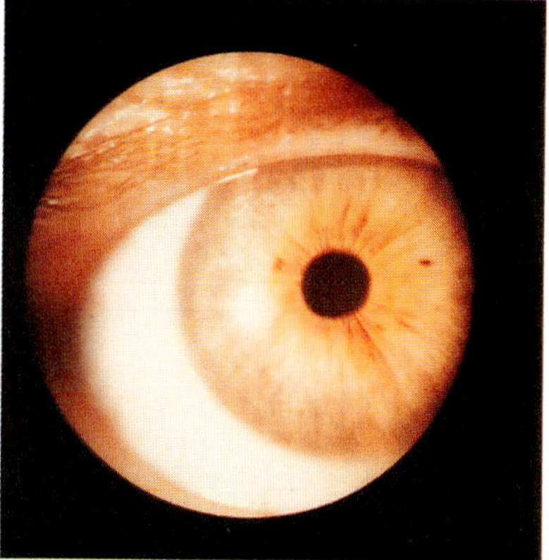 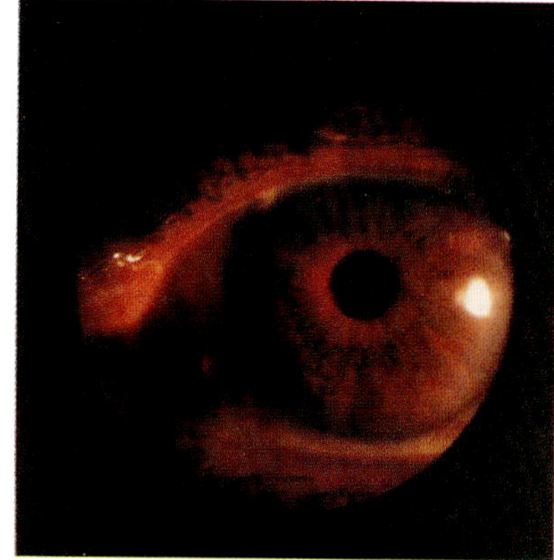

FIGURE 3.17. Difference in contrast between a dark pupil against a light iris (1) and against a dark iris (2). The test of contrast is made more difficult by dim illumination, and can be further obscured by light reflected from the patient's spectacles.

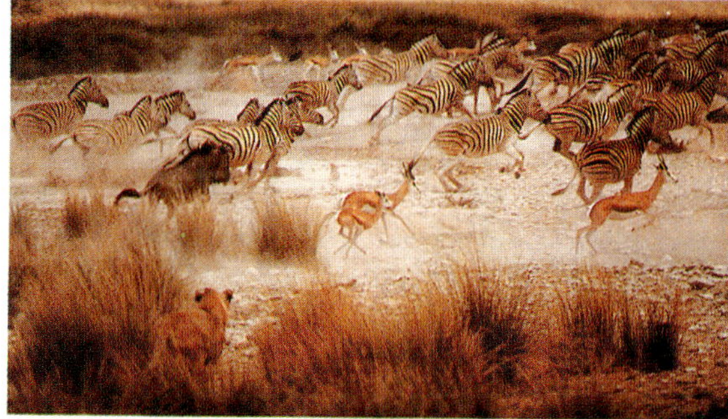

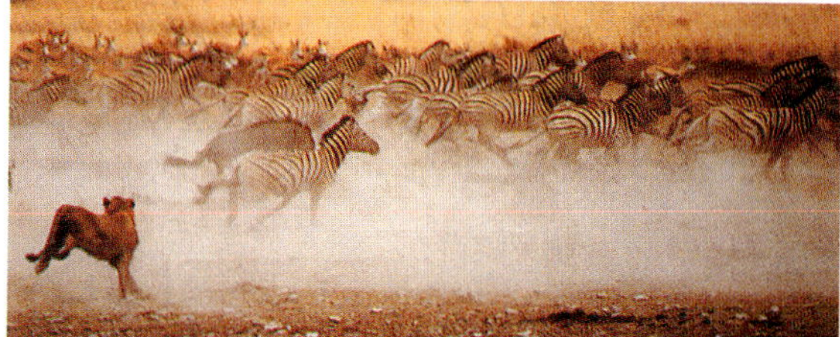

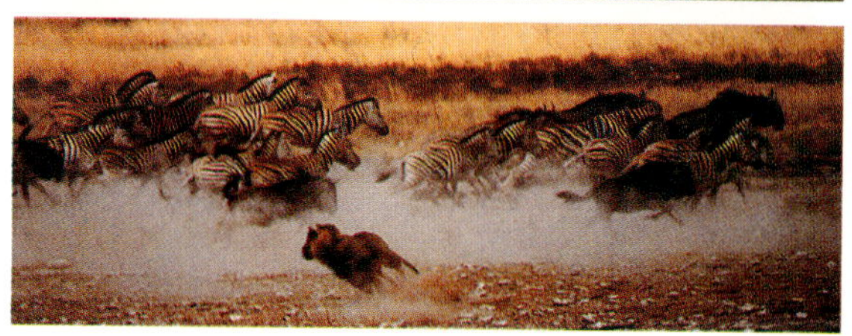

FIGURE 3.18. The background of a herd of moving zebras (1) makes it difficult for the lioness in the foreground (2) to determine the speed of an intended victim in the foreground (3). (From Reardon M: Etosha. Capetown, South Africa, 1981, p. 104, used by permission of Photo Researchers, Inc., New York.)

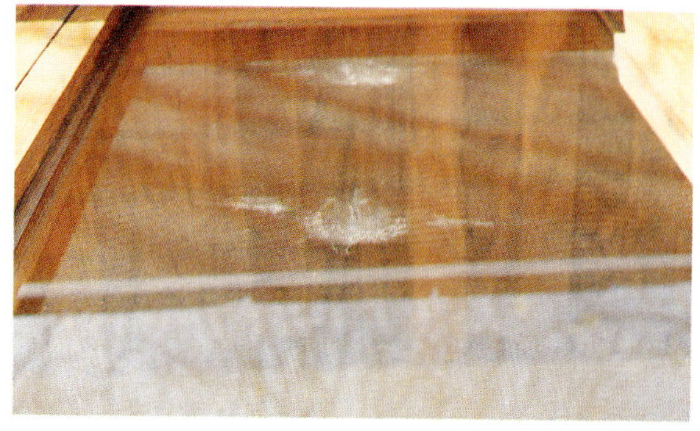

FIGURE 3.21. Photograph of the imprint of a bird that accidentally struck a freshly cleaned window. (Courtesy of R. Stegmann, Pretoria, South Africa)

Color Plate IV

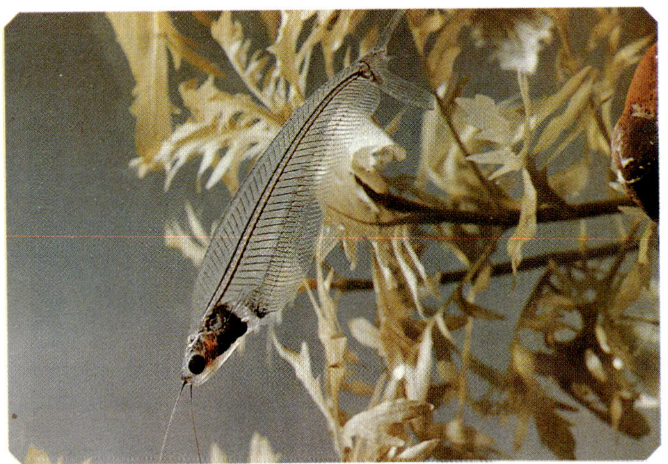

FIGURE 3.22. The glass catfish of the fresh waters of Southeast Asia. One can see leaves through its body. (From Burton M, Burton J, Hughes D: World Encyclopedia of Animals. London, Octopus Books Limited, 1978, p. 164. Courtesy of J. Burton and Bruce Coleman, Ltd., England.)

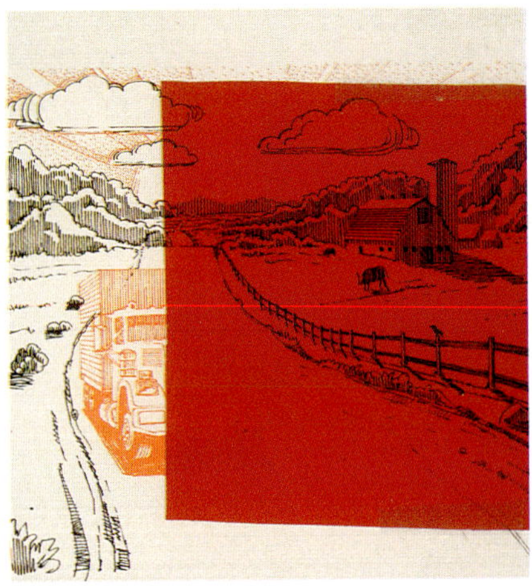

FIGURE 3.23. A scene drawn on white paper with red and black ink. When a red filter is placed over part of the picture, the objects drawn in red disappear.

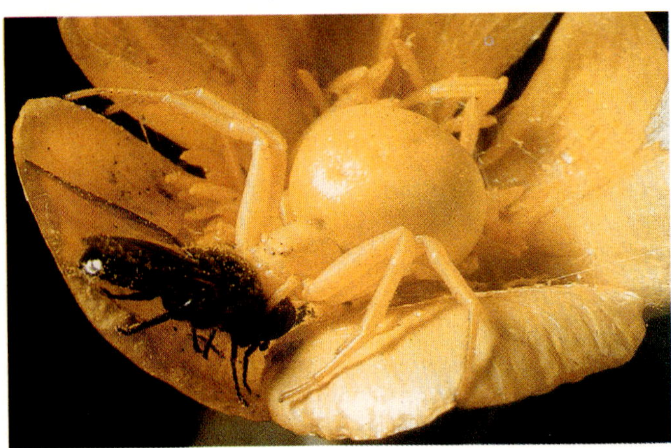

FIGURE 3.24. The yellow spider sitting on the yellow flower falls below the threshold of contrast for the unsuspecting bee. (From Hoyle F: The Intelligent Universe. New York: Holt Rhinehart and Winston, 1983, p. 119, used by permission of Natural History Photographic Agency, Sussex, England, and N.A. Callow.)

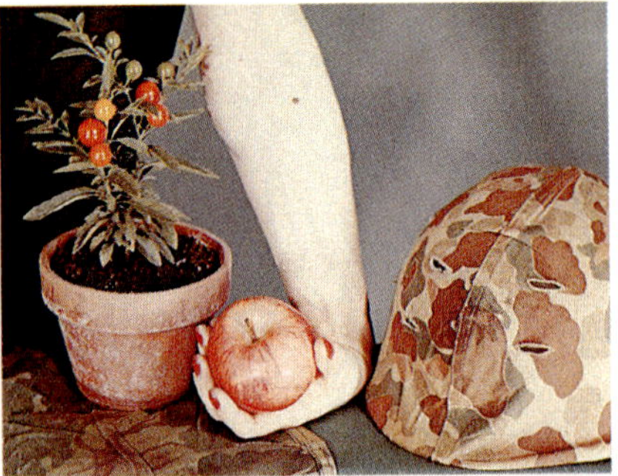

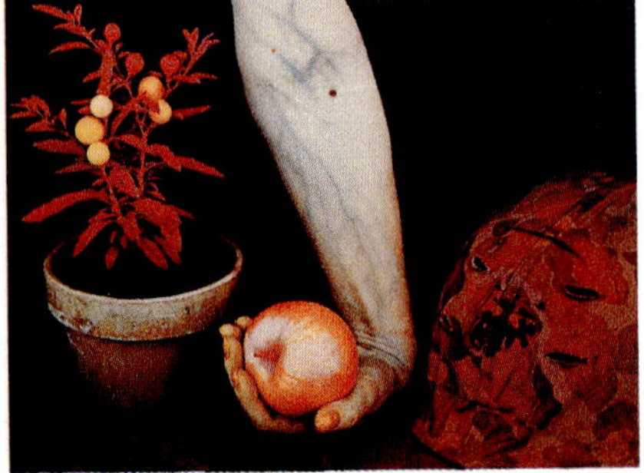

FIGURE 3.25. Photograph of scene taken with regular film (top) and with infrared-sensitive film (bottom). The blue veins emit a strong infrared radiation that is sensed much better by the IR-sensitive film. (From Kodak Publication No. M-28, Applied Infrared Photography, Eastman Kodak, 1972. Reprinted courtesy of Eastman Kodak Company.)

without a glare source. To answer this question, we again used normal subjects looking through a progressive series of light scatterers. Figure 3.10 shows that for five different spatial frequencies (equivalent to different Snellen lines), contrast sensitivity stayed constant until the filter was 80% "cataractous," when *no* glare light was used. On the other hand, the contrast sensitivity functions decreased gradually with filters of increased light scattering, when a glare light was used.

These experiments suggest that glare sources with contrast targets are more useful in following patients with cataracts than are contrast tests alone. This argument was partially supported, in another way, by a clinical study[13] of diabetic patients with retinopathy and cataracts. The investigators were unable to distinguish between contrast sensitivity losses in patients with cataracts and no retinopathy versus patients with clear lenses and retinopathy.

Contrast and Glare for Normal Eyes

For perspective, let us now discuss the limits of contrast and glare sensitivity in normally sighted creatures.

The term *glare* has been variously defined. Commonly it is used to describe an environmental situation such as a bright sunbathed beach or snowscape. In our mind's eye, we have no difficulty in picturing the scenes so described.

Among professionals, glare has also been defined as the contrast-lowering effect of stray light within the eye. This definition for many is faulted by the paucity of information it conveys to the clinician or student. It assumes a prior knowledge of contrast sensitivity and visual physiology. A more meaningful definition, which ties together environmental and optical factors with their impact on the visual mechanism, is presented in the 1984 reference volume of the Illuminating Engineering Society of North America:

Glare: the sensation produced by luminance within the visual field that is sufficiently greater than the luminance to which the eyes are adapted to cause annoyance, discomfort, or loss in visual performance and visibility.

Glare has been a visually troublesome problem to humans and their hominid ancestors for *2.8 million years*.* Surely the ancient hunter-gatherers cupped their hands above their squinting eyes as they scanned the surrounding sun-baked savanna. Their survival was dependent on the successful hunt for game and the avoidance or repelling of hostile intruders driven by similar survival instincts.

The first actual device to substantially reduce the disabling effects of glare was designed and made by the Eskimo as long as 2000 years ago.† Actual remnants were found and dated from early sites in Alaska and Siberia. Horizontally slotted ivory goggles (Fig. 3.11), held in place by a thong, quite effectively allowed peripheral vision while blocking out excessive light reflected by surrounding snow and ice during the long Arctic days. Survival for the hunter would have been impossible without such goggles to prevent snow blindness when hunting and traveling in the bright snowscapes of the Arctic parts of the Northern hemisphere. We may also presume that the first hominids to move into snowy winterlands, probably about 50,000 years ago,† would have had to use similar eye-shading devices.

Using Glare to Make Things Invisible

During the Second World War, one of the key strategic areas for the British was the Suez Canal. Yet the air superiority of the enemy made it all but inevitable that the canal would ultimately be destroyed by enemy bombs. If only the canal could be made invisible, mused British Intelligence. But the very size of the structure, as well as its high level of activity, made traditional camouflage cover impossible. Then someone had a good idea. If you want to make something disappear, turn to a professional magician. In this case, they turned to the famous performer Jasper Meskelyne, a fourth-generation magician.[14] By lining the canal with bright rotating searchlights he was able to create so

---

*Personal discussion (1988) with Steven J. C. Gauling, PhD, Associate Professor of Biologic Anthropology, Department of Anthropology, University of Pittsburgh, Pittsburgh, PA 15260.

†Personal discussion and correspondence (1988) with William W. Fitzburgh, PhD, Curator of Archeology, Department of Anthropology, Smithsonian Institute, Washington, D.C. 20560.

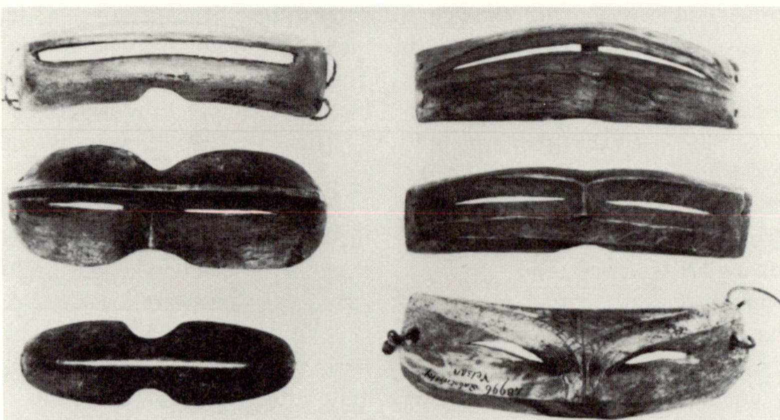

Figure 3.11. Snow goggles from Point Hope and northern Norton Sound "illustrate . . . forms common in northern Alaska and Canada." (From "inua," *spirit world of the bering sea eskimo*," Smithsonian Institution Press, Washington, DC, 20560, courtesy of William W. Fitzhugh and Susan A. Kaplan) (Catalogue No. 83-10674, Department of Anthropology, Smithsonian Institution)

much confusing glare that the canal was rendered invisible to the swarms of German bombers that appeared night after night. Was the Suez Canal made invisible by the searchlights? The normal cornea, lens, and vitreous scatter between 10% to 20% of light incident on the eye.[4] In fact, it is the back-scattered light that allows the clinician to see these structures in the slit lamp. Thus if a glare light is intense enough and close enough to the target, the contrast of the target becomes diminished or washed out and the target is rendered invisible to the bombardier. The same phenomenon is also the reason that a young tennis player may occasionally lose a high lob in the sun. Returning to the Suez Canal, it is only fair to admit that there may have been another mechanism that helped render it invisible. If the windshields of the bombers were pitted, scratched, or coated with rain or dust, they all became substantial light scatterers and further obscured the details of the canal when the bright lights were turned on.

During the day, fighter pilots used glare to tactical advantage by maneuvering to have the sun at their backs for strafing attack against enemy aircraft. And not too long ago, Archie Moore, former light heavyweight champion of the world (1952–1962), commenting on boxing tricks, was quoted as stating "outdoors I kept my opponents facing the sun."[15]

A real-life glare test is pictured in Figure 3.12 (see Color Plate I). As dusk approached on this particularly hot and steamy Louisiana highway, a large trailer-truck struck a bump and jackknifed while racing eastward. It came to a stop totally obstructing its lane. A "good Samaritan" traveling west noticed the crippled truck. With night setting in, he decided that the dark-colored truck would be difficult to see and thus pose a hazard to oncoming traffic. In an attempt to warn drivers in the truck's lane, he turned on his bright beams. At that moment a man driving a car with a scratched and pitted windshield approached the truck. The light from the bright beams was scattered across the driver's retina by the hazy windshield and he never knew of the presence of the truck as his car ripped into its side, killing him.

The world of nature is replete with examples of glare being used for the survival of one species against another. In the canopy of the rain forest in Central America lives an entire ecological society of plants, animals, and insects. In this environment, on the roof of the forest, so to speak, there is little escape from the bright sun. Thus, glare and low contrast are the way of life. Some creatures exploit the ambient glare to become invisible. For example, albino animals abound. Figure 3.13 (see Color Plate II) shows an Arctic hare, which becomes almost invisible at high noon. Clearly, the

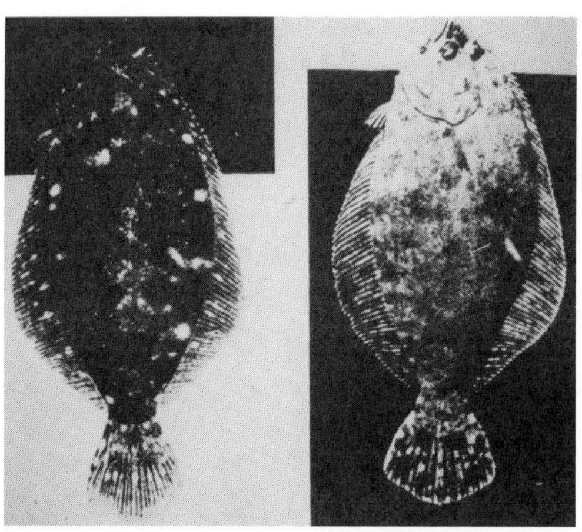

FIGURE 3.19. The paise is able to alter its body coloration to match the surroundings of its head. In this picture
the experimenter has also altered the background of the
body to show that the head controls the coloration of the
whole body. (From Hollwich F: *The Influence of Ocular
Light Perception on Metabolism in Man and Animals*.
New York, Springer-Verlag, 1979, p 5, used by permission)

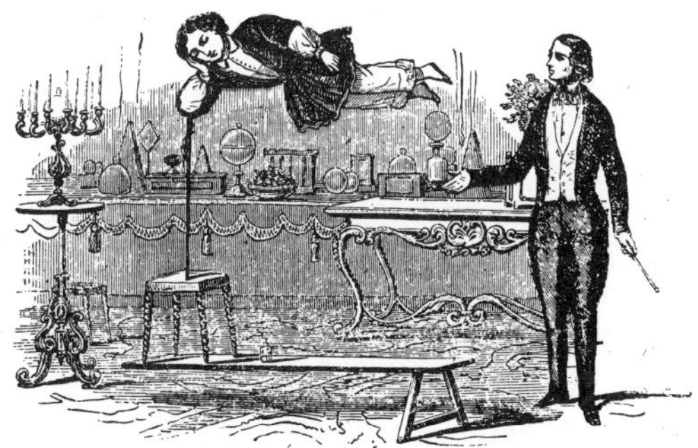

FIGURE 3.20. The magician used very thin "invisible"
wires to suspend the "levitating" subject. (From Char-
ney DH: *Magic*. New York, Strawberry Hill, 1975, p 67,
used by permission)

contrast of a white animal against the white background or bright sky can be close to or below
threshold visibility of most of its enemies. In the
same vein, one can also appreciate the difficulties
of seeing the glistening silver body of the fish from
below at high noon (Fig. 3.14, see Color Plate II).

The surface foam of the ocean is an excellent
hiding place for surface fish. Many small fish
escape their predators by swimming within or close
to the surface foam, which, of course, scatters light
much like a cataract and thus hides the fish during
the day.

Every fisherman reading this book knows how
difficult it is to see the bodies of fish below the
surface of clear nonfoamy water. The reason is that
the rippling water surface reflects back the light of
the sun and sky. These reflected glare sources
obscure a clear view of the fish below. One must
assume that this glare acts as protection for the
fish, who swim near the surface, against marauding
bears and other predators. As one pictures the bear
crudely poking its claws below the surface of the
water in the hope of snagging a fish, one is
reminded of the dive-bombing precision of peli-
cans, who seem to have an uncanny view of fish
below the surface. How does the pelican beat

glare? The best way to eliminate reflected glare is
to use polaroid filters. For example, in Figure 3.15
(see Color Plate II), polaroid glasses cancel out the
reflected glare of the shiny playing cards and allow
one to see the markings. Is it possible that these
birds have the equivalent of a polaroid filter some-
where in their eye?

The Natural Limits of Contrast Sensitivity

Many animals are clothed in a skin that places
them just below the contrast sensitivity threshold
of their enemies or unsuspecting victims. For
example, the striped tiger (Fig. 3.16; see Color
Plate II), hiding in the long vertical grass, is all but
invisible to its potential prey.

We, as clinicians, are often pressed to our own
contrast thresholds when we try to follow pupillary
movements in a dimly lit room. For example, the
black pupil is easily seen against the lightly colored
iris, but it is not readily seen against the dark iris
(Fig. 3.17; see Color Plate III).

Contrast is used not only to detect an object
against a background, but also to detect an object's
movement against a background. The phenomenon
is a sophisticated form of edge detection. Appreci-
ating this mechanism, one must sympathize with
the lioness in the foreground of Fig. 3.18 (see
Color Plate III) as she unconsciously attempts to
anticipate the speed of her zebra victim against a
background of other moving zebras.

Interestingly, contrast detection is not always
passively dependent on the circumstances of the

environment. Some natural creatures are able to actively lower their contrast level by altering themselves. For example, the paise in Figure 3.19 alters its coloration to match the surroundings of its head.

The leading magicians of the past century have often used the contrast sensitivity function of their audiences in creating their illusions. The trick of levitation, which has amazed so many audiences for years, was created by using a harness and two fine but strong supporting wires, as shown in Figure 3.20. The thinness of the wires and the compatible coloring of the stage flats or curtains pushed contrast sensitivity for objects of high spatial frequency beyond the threshold of the audience.

The Role of Transparency in Visibility

In terms of contrast sensitivity, a transparent object is invisible because it allows the background to show through. Thus, if there is no contrast between the object and the background, they become one and the same. For example, one can easily be injured by walking into a closed glass door. The reason we do not do that often is that light reflected off the surface of the glass door usually warns us of the door's presence. Children or animals that have not learned to use this clue are more apt to be injured by glass doors. In Figure 3.21 (see Color Plate III) one can see the imprint of a bird that has accidentally struck a freshly cleaned window.

Nature has also made use of transparency to protect some of its creatures from its enemies, for example, the glass catfish (Fig. 3.22; see Color Plate IV). Some of the background vegetation can be seen through the fish's body.

Wavelength Dependence Invisibility

In Figure 3.23 (see Color Plate IV), a scene has been drawn on a white background with both red and black ink. When half the picture is covered by a red filter, the red lines disappear. Giving the picture a red background pushes the reader's contrast threshold to the point where the red lines cannot be seen against the red background. In the same way, the yellow spider poised on the yellow leaf in Figure 3.24 (see Color Plate IV) falls below the contrast threshold of the eye of the unsuspecting bee, who probably is on its very last exploration for honey.

In Figure 3.25 (see Color Plate IV), the infrared-sensitive film "sees" the venous pattern of the subject's forearm much more vividly than the film that records only visible light. Thus, visibility involves not only contrast, but the ability to record the key wavelengths represented in the contrast pattern.* Therefore, the color-deficient patient will not see certain patterns obvious to the normal subject.

References

1. Maurice D: The structure and transparency of the cornea. *J Physiol* **136**:263, 1957.
2. Benedek GB: Theory of transparency of the eye. *Appl Opt* **10**:459, 1971.
3. Miller D, Zuckerman JL, Reynolds GO: Holographic filter to negate the effect of cataract. *Arch Ophthalmol* **90**:323, 1973.
4. Miller D, Benedek GB: Intraocular light scattering. Springfield, Ill., Charles C Thomas, 1973.
5. Hirsch RP, Nadler MP, Miller D: Glare measurement as a predictor of outdoor vision among cataract patients. *Ann Ophthalmol* **16**:965, 1984.
6. Holladay LL: The fundamentals of glare and visibility. *J Opt Soc Am* **12**:492, 1926.
7. Wolf E: Glare and age. *Arch Ophthalmol J* **64**:502, 1960.
8. Wolf E, Gardiner JS: Studies on the scatter of light in the dioptric median of the eye as a basis for visual glare. *Arch Ophthalmol* **37**:450, 1963.
9. Miller D, Wolfe E, Geer S, et al: Glare sensitivity related to the use of contact lenses. *Arch Ophthalmol* **78**:448, 1967.
10. Miller D, Wolf E, Jernigan ME, et al: Laboratory evaluation of a clinical glare tester. *Arch Ophthalmol* **87**:324, 1972.
11. LeClaire J, Nadler MP, Weiss S, et al: A new glare tester for clinical testing. *Arch Ophthalmol* **100**:153, 1982.
12. Abrahmisson M, Sjostrand J: Impairment of contrast function as a measure of disability glare. *Invest Ophthalmol Vis Sci* **27**:1131, 1986.
13. Howes SC, Caelli T, Mitchell P: Contrast sensitivity in diabetics with retinopathy and cataract. *Aust J Ophthalmol* **10**:573–578, 1982.
14. Fisher D: *War Magician*. New York, Coward-McCann, 1983.
15. Torres J: Champion's champion. Parade, *The Sunday Newspaper Magazine*, Pittsburgh Press, June 5, 1988.

---

*Some aphakic patients can see ultraviolet light.

4
Essential Factors in Testing for Glare

Thomas C. Prager

Introduction

High-contrast Snellen letters, which traditionally have been used to assess visual acuity, are usually presented in a darkened refracting lane. This testing situation provides incomplete information regarding the patient's ability to function in the multicontrast environment outside the examining room. Thus, this method of acuity measurement is a poor indicator of functional vision in the real world. How many cataract, corneal transplant, refractive surgery, and contact lens patients can see quite well in the dark confines of the examining room but later call to complain about poor vision as they try to function in the outside world? With the dramatic improvement in surgical technique, intraocular lens design, and successful outcomes, over 1.1 million cataract procedures are performed in the United States each year.[1] The need for precise determination of visual disability due to cataracts has provided the impetus for glare testing to move from the laboratory to the clinician's office.

Determining visual acuity in the presence of a glare field[2,3] is a quantitative method of objectively documenting the debilitating effect of light scatter due to media opacity. However, the patient should be the ultimate authority in assessing whether changing vision due to opacities, such as a cataract, impairs life-style. Since Miller and Nadler introduced the first commercial glare tester in 1983, a host of other instruments have appeared in the marketplace. Already these standardized instruments have become a valuable part of the visual assessment of many cataract patients. Although there is no question whether to remove a cataract causing 20/400 vision, the decision to operate on a patient with 20/50 acuity is not so clear. Numerical results from glare tests help substantiate the need for cataract extraction. Accurate documentation of functional visual loss is essential; studies that have sought to weigh the relative sensitivity of these various first-generation instruments have not been conclusive due to problems in experimental design. The field of glare testing is further complicated by lack of consensus on presentation target (optotype), contrast, and type and amount of glare.

This chapter introduces basic concepts of glare testing. It identifies several methodological factors to be considered before one designs a glare experiment or when one interprets other studies in the literature. These factors are potential sources of error in any glare study that compares indoor with outdoor acuity. They include the study population, visual stimuli (optotypes), and aspects of the outdoor testing situation. Statistical methods to accurately determine the overprediction and underprediction rates are also discussed. Findings from a recent study[4] will be used to illustrate major methodological points. This research compares the relative sensitivity of two commercial glare testers with two optotypes (sinusoidal grating at various contrasts versus high-contrast letters).

Terms and Concepts

Snellen Acuity

Routine Snellen acuity testing conducted under scotopic/mesoptic light conditions has been with us long enough to become an integral part of ophthalmology, even though its ability to predict outdoor vision is unreliable. The general ophthalmic community knows what 20/20 visual acuity means but may be unfamiliar with newer methods of visual assessment that include contrast sensitivity and glare testing.

Disadvantages of the Snellen Acuity Chart

Although entrenched as the standard in vision assessment, the conventional Snellen chart has the following disadvantages[5,6]:

1. The number of letters per line differ. Therefore, one mistake per line has a different meaning at different levels of visual acuity.
2. The size of the letters does not progress regularly. Therefore, a report of a loss of two lines of vision is misleading depending on which extreme of the chart the loss occurs.
3. The lines of the chart contain letters of differing perceptual difficulty. For example, an *A* or *L* is easier to perceive than an *E*. Each line should have letters of equal difficulty.

The National Eye Institute has developed a new high-contrast eye chart[5] based on the Bailey-Lovie chart that corrects these problems.* To translate results from the Bailey-Lovie chart to the Snellen chart, one determines the total number of letters correctly identified (X in the following equation[7]) and converts this score into a Snellen equivalent (Table 4.1).

Equivalent Snellen acuity

$$= 20 \text{ multiplied by } 10^{(55-X)/50}$$

Contrast Sensitivity

The problems inherent in the Snellen acuity chart have been addressed and perhaps overcome, but the ability to see outside in the multicontrast everyday world still must be taken into account. The capacity to discern the minimum difference in the luminance of two adjacent areas as a difference in brightness is termed *contrast threshold*. *Contrast sensitivity* is the reciprocal of contrast threshold.

---

*A set of three charts is available from Globe Screen Printing, 875 Hollins St., Baltimore, MD 21201, (301) 685-6750.

The perceptual extraction of figure from field is comparable to acoustical discernment of differences in loudness. An obvious high-contrast situation is a black dog in a snowbank. A subtle example of contrast is a drive-in movie at dusk. As the sunlight disappears, the picture on the movie screen becomes more vivid (higher contrast). This scenario can be recreated in the clinic. Measuring acuity with the lights on or off can directly affect the apparent contrast of the Snellen chart. In the following example the absence or presence of the overhead room lights in the refracting lane can reduce contrast from 94% to 31%. Contrast,[8] also known as *modulation contrast*, for periodic patterns is defined as a percentage:

$$\frac{\text{Luminance maximum} - \text{luminance minimum}}{\text{Luminance maximum} + \text{luminance minimum}}$$

The light reflected from the white background of the Snellen chart would represent the luminance maximum, whereas a dark letter would be measured to obtain luminance minimum. In a dark room the contrast of the Snellen chart is very high—94% (using arbitrary light units):

$$\frac{\text{White background} - \text{black letters}}{\text{White background} + \text{black letters}} = \frac{97 - 3}{97 + 3}$$

$$= 94\% \text{ contrast}$$

Perceptual contrast is reduced markedly with room lights on (an additional 100 light units are added to both white background and dark letters):

$$\frac{\text{White background} - \text{black letters}}{\text{White background} + \text{black letters}} = \frac{197 - 103}{197 + 103}$$

$$= 31\% \text{ contrast}$$

Even if the room lights are off, the contrast of the Snellen chart can change from room to room due to either smudges (fingerprints) or dust on the projector lens or on the slide itself.

Change in ambient light in everyday situations will similarly affect the apparent contrast of an object. Some of the variations in light levels[9] encountered include:

Operating table	2,500 foot candles (fc)
Office	200
Courtroom	70
Examining room	50
Nightclub	5

TABLE 4.1. Conversion table: Number correct ETDRS/Bailey-Lovie chart to Snellen equivalent

Number Correct ETDRS	Snellen Equivalent 20/	Number Correct ETDRS	Snellen Equivalent 20/
0	251.79	36	47.98
1	240.45	37	45.82
2	229.63	38	43.76
3	219.30	39	41.79
4	209.43	40	39.91
5	200.00	41	38.11
6	191.00	42	36.39
7	182.40	43	34.76
8	174.19	44	33.19
9	166.35	45	31.70
10	158.87	46	30.27
11	151.72	47	28.91
12	144.89	48	27.61
13	138.37	49	26.37
14	132.14	50	25.18
15	126.19	51	24.05
16	120.51	52	22.96
17	115.09	53	21.93
18	109.91	54	20.94
19	104.96	55	20.00
20	100.24	56	19.10
21	95.73	57	18.24
22	91.43	58	17.42
23	87.30	59	16.64
24	83.37	60	15.89
25	79.62	61	15.17
26	76.04	62	14.49
27	72.62	63	13.84
28	69.35	64	13.21
29	66.23	65	12.62
30	63.25	66	12.05
31	60.40	67	11.51
32	57.68	68	10.99
33	55.08	69	10.50
34	52.61	70	10.02
35	50.24		

The Relationship of Grating Acuity to Contrast

The resolution or acuity of an object is dependent on its contrast.[8,10-12] At contrast threshold, the human eye is most sensitive to medium-resolution targets (approximately 20/50 to 20/70). It is easier to see a grating composed of medium-width bars than one composed of broad or thin bars. For recognition of either a broad- or thin-bar grating, significantly more contrast is required than for detection of a medium-width grating. The psychophysical contrast sensitivity curve showing the preference for medium-width bar gratings is depicted in Figure 4.1. A patient who has visual acuity of 20/20 in the clinician's office but has impaired broad-bar contrast vision may be unable to see a truck in the fog. The patient with refractive error only would have contrast decrements to the thinner bars.

Bar gratings translate to visual acuity. A line pair of a black and a white bar makes up one cycle. The number of cycles per degree of arc subtended at the retina is roughly equivalent to a Snellen acuity. To convert from Snellen acuity to cycles per degree[13] one divides 600 by the Snellen line number. Thirty cycles (bar pairs) per degree approximates 20/20

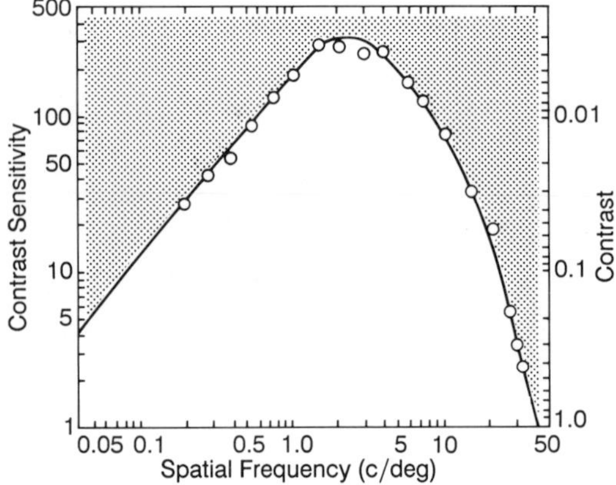

FIGURE 4.1. Contrast sensitivity (1/contrast) versus spatial frequency. This idealized plot for normal vision shows that less contrast is required to detect medium-resolution targets than to detect low- or high-resolution targets.

vision, whereas 3 cpd is approximately 20/200 acuity. This conversion cannot be exact, since varying amounts of contrast will change the perceptual recognition of a grating. With reduced contrast, 20/20 vision may be associated with as few as 18 cpd.[13]

The description and reduction of any optotype into its sinusoidal component parts is called Fourier analysis.[14] Bar gratings, that have a "fuzzy" appearance due to a gradual change in luminance profile, vary sinusoidally (Fig. 4.2A-C) and have the least complicated mathematical composition. More properly, there is only a fundamental frequency with no higher order harmonics (Fig. 4.3A). Since Snellen letters and square wave gratings (Figs. 4.2D and 4.3B) are composed of a fundamental and higher order harmonics, the correlation between letters and sinusoidal gratings

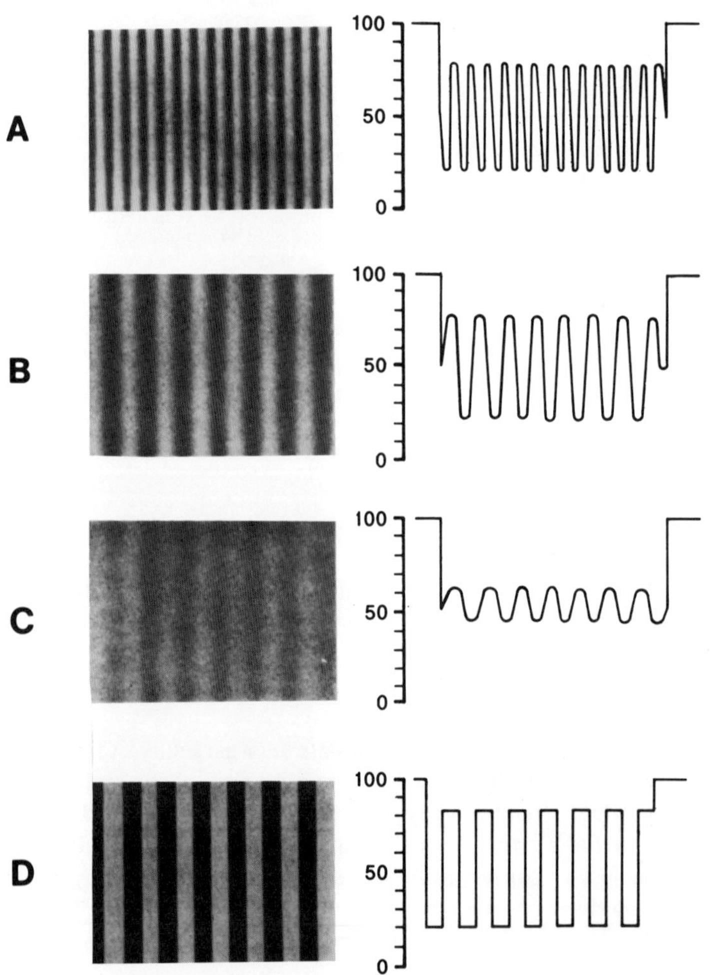

FIGURE 4.2. Examples of gratings. A, B, and C demonstrate sinusoidal variation in luminance, whereas D, a square wave, has an abrupt luminance onset and offset. A and B differ in spatial frequency; B and C differ in contrast ($L_{max} - L_{min}/L_{max} + L_{min}$).

can be only approximately equivalent. This difference in Fourier complexity, and hence perceptual difficulty, explains why patients may miss a few letters on a particular Snellen line and identify others on the same line or even on the next line that contains letters of reduced size.

In addition, the perception of a grating is related to the number of cycles, the field size, the bar length, and the patient's relative state of light adaptation.[15,16] The best sinusoidal gratings stimuli would have at least six repetitions, with each component bar being of equal length and the total grating area subtending greater than 6 degrees. When these criteria are met, the target may optimally stimulate receptive fields[17] located at the retina, the lateral geniculate body, and the occipital cortex. The difference in field size at different retinal locations means that various-sized targets are tuned to specific retinal areas. Generally, the peripheral retina responds quickly to flashing stimuli composed of large elements (low spatial frequencies), whereas the macula generates electrical impulses to finely detailed (high spatial frequencies), slow moving, sustained targets.[17] There appears to be a large array of specialized receptors sensitive to contrast, direction, and speed of movement.

Clinical Application of Contrast Sensitivity

In many cases, neurological or pathway problems[12,18-21] are more apt to be recognized by the clinician using a measure of contrast sensitivity than by using a standard high-contrast Snellen acuity chart. The same individual with optic neuritis who sees 20/20 high-contrast letters may be unable to see 20/80 with low-contrast letters. Contrast sensitivity may be altered in the following disorders, among others:

Amblyopia
Cystoid macula edema
Cortical lesions
Glaucoma
Multiple sclerosis/optic neuritis
Senile macular edema

The findings from contrast sensitivity tests overlap, and different neurological problems can generate the same contrast sensitivity curve.[12] A contrast loss to medium-width targets could indicate

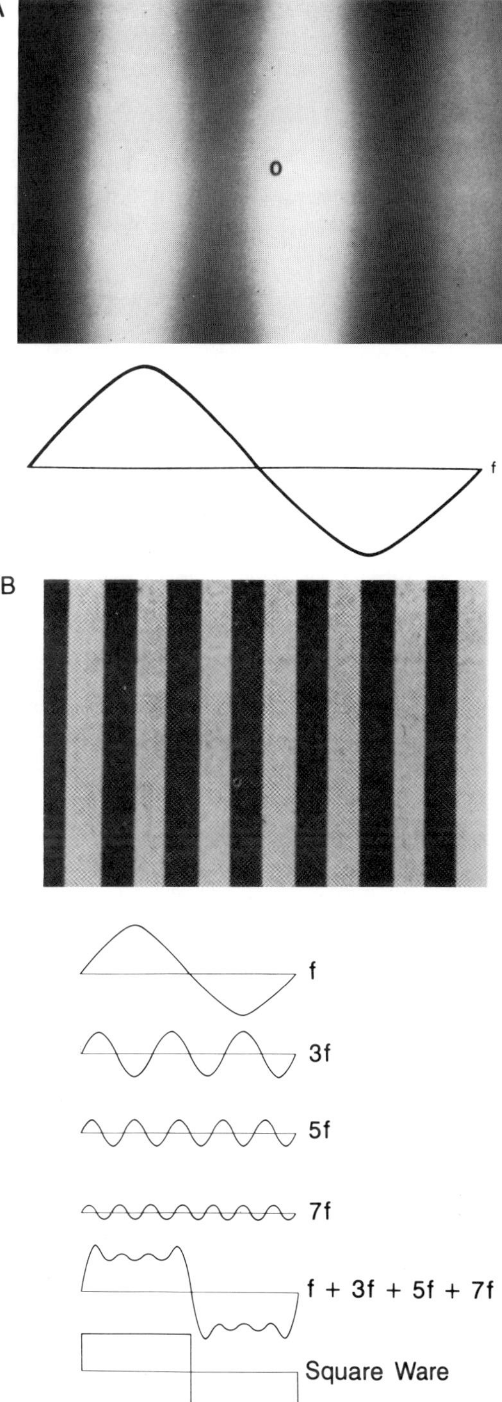

FIGURE 4.3. Fourier analysis of a sinusoidal grating (A) has a single component, the fundamental or first harmonic oscillation. Fourier composition of a square wave (B) contains an infinite number of harmonics but may be approximated by summing a finite number of sinusoids.

optic atrophy, glaucoma, cataract, or optic neuritis, whereas a high spatial frequency loss could be due to refractive error, corneal edema, cataract, macular degeneration, or amblyopia. The primary importance of this type of assessment is as a screening test, even though different diseases may yield similar contrast sensitivity functions. Impaired contrast sensitivity suggests further testing.

Instruments to Assess Contrast Sensitivity

The Arden plates[22] introduced more than 10 years ago were one of the first attempts to bring contrast sensitivity to the clinical level. Each plate had a different size bar grating that gradually became fainter (lower contrast) toward the top of the page. These plates were quite difficult to reproduce photographically. Reporting of contrast threshold was entirely subjective; thus a motivated individual could easily deceive the examiner because there was no check on accuracy.[23]

Nicolet introduced a sophisticated contrast sensitivity tester in 1981 that overcomes the problems encountered with the Arden plates. Bars are projected on a high-quality TV screen, and the beginning point for the test can be randomized. The results are automatically printed out. The system also can be used as a stimulator for visual evoked responses (VERs). Even though time-consuming tasks such as luminance calibration, data collection, and plotting are done automatically, the main drawback to this instrument is its cost.

An eye chart that combines both visual acuity and contrast sensitivity without the subjective limitations of the early Arden plates is manufactured by Vistech (Dayton, OH).[24] The chart is composed of vertical and oblique sinusoidal bar gratings that subtend approximately 1 degree of retinal area at 10 feet. Each of the five gratings is similar in visual angle to letters found in the standard Snellen acuity chart. Along each acuity line the bar gratings become lower in contrast by an average of 0.2 log units while maintaining the same spatial frequency. The bars are presented in three orientations as a means of reducing subjective responses. These visual targets or patches fall short of the theoretical "best" stimuli because the wide (low spatial frequency) stimuli do not have six repetitions and thus do not fill peripheral retinal receptive fields. With central fixation and a 1-degree target, it is debatable whether a peripher-

ally originating disease, such as glaucoma, could be detected early enough to be clinically relevant. The circular patches, by definition, have bars composed of unequal length, and the odds of *guessing* the correct bar orientation are high, 1 out of 3.

Glare

Glare is experienced every day. Examples include being dazzled by oncoming headlights, driving into the sun, following a baseball as it arches toward the sun, and reading a book with glossy pages. Veiling glare or disability glare is a specialized case of contrast degradation. Fry and Alpern in 1953[2] offered the stray-light hypothesis, which stated that the veiling luminance produced by stray light within the eye causes an actual and perceptual reduction in retinal image contrast. Opacities, like ground glass, act as point sources of light, causing light scattering and superimposing a veiling light on the retina. The more scattered light, the greater the reduction in real and apparent contrast. Ocular opacities include:

Cornea
    Microcystic epithelial edema
    Superficial punctate keratitis
    Anterior membrane dystrophies
    Stromal dystrophies
    Endothelial dystrophies
Cataracts or partially opacified capsules
Vitreous opacities (floaters)

Whereas standard contrast sensitivity tests are somewhat nonspecific in identifying the source of a disorder, an abnormal glare test strongly indicates an anterior segment problem. Experimentally induced corneal edema has been shown to have a small effect on contrast sensitivity but may increase glare sensitivity up to 300%.[25] The influence of retinal changes appears to have a minimal effect on glare disability. Diabetic patients with macular edema, a potential source of light scatter, have been shown to have glare sensitivity changes that correlate more closely to lens changes than to the degree of edema.[26]

Glare Types

The glare source may be a point source of light (Fig. 4.4A) that mimics the glare disability associated with an oncoming headlight. Patients

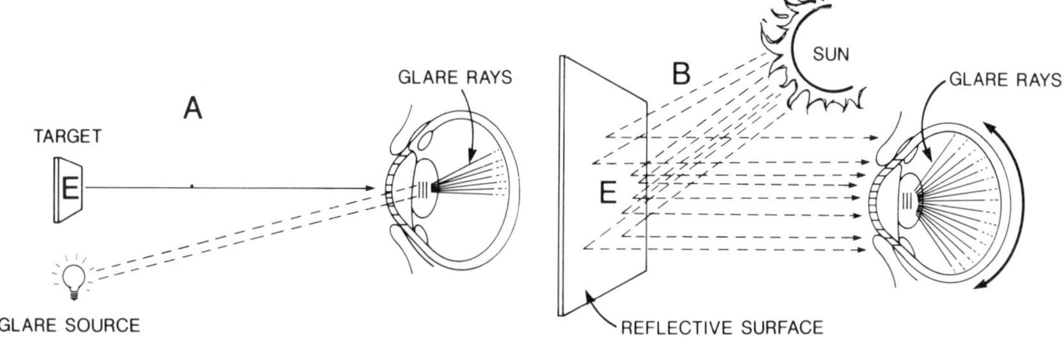

FIGURE 4.4. The effect of two types of glare, point source (A) and uniform field (B), on a lenticular opacity (small cataract). Veiling glare reduces contrast of the retinal image, but the edge detail may remain unblurred.

report, however, that it is difficult to maintain target fixation when the point source is off-axis because of the tendency to stare directly into the stimulating light. It is even harder for the experimenter to be sure that the patient is maintaining fixation. Results may be further confounded by the persistent afterimage, which may have an unpredictable debilitating effect. Bright hemispheres or light annuli that provide uniform light diffusion (Fig. 4.4B) overcome these drawbacks. Regardless of glare source, it is imperative that for each glare tester luminance remain consistent over time. Use of a decaying bulb that "grays out" or deposits tungsten on the inside of the bulb will confound the results of an experiment and introduce unspecified variability into them, since changing luminance results in a change in contrast. This problem is partially solved by use of a halogen bulb with binary response properties: either the bulb glows with 90% to 100% of its full capability or it ceases to function.

Glare Instruments

Although many commercial instruments are available, the following descriptions cover the major types of glare testers.

Miller-Nadler Glare Tester

This is a contrast test surrounded by a uniformly bright light source.[27-31] The instrument uses a 20/400 black Landolt C, with a background annulus that becomes progressively darker with subsequent slide presentations. The orientation of the C changes in one of four directions. A bright projec-

tor screen, which is equivalent to "new snow on a sunny day" (420 ft-lambert), serves as a constant glare source, surrounding both the target C and the annulus. The final glare disability score, expressed as a percentage, is converted to a Snellen equivalent from a table provided by the manufacturer.

Brightness Acuity Tester (BAT)

The BAT provides a uniform glare source by projecting light onto a 60-mm white diffusing hemisphere with a 12-mm viewing port.[32] The instrument resembles an ice-cream scoop with a hole in the center. Testing is conducted at three luminance settings. The BAT provides an average luminance of 400 ft-lambert at the highest luminance setting, an average luminance of 100 ft-lambert at the medium setting, and 12 ft-lambert at the lowest setting. These setting are roughly equivalent to brightness reflected from a white sand beach (high) or from the surrounding foliage (medium) on a clear day when the overhead illuminance is 10,000 FC. The lowest setting is equivalent to bright overhead fluorescent lighting (300 fc).

Vistech VCT8000

This instrument utilizes the previously described patches of sinusoidal gratings that are nominally equivalent to five Snellen acuities. The chart has been reduced in size and placed in a compact viewing system. Illuminance is held constant by a calibration circuit, and glare conditions may be readily changed by selecting from an array of high-intensity bulbs that surround the test card or by activating a central bulb that simulates an oncoming headlight.

EyeCon 5

Contrast and optotype on this IBM-PC-based instrument are software programmable, permitting custom protocols. Landolt *C*, sinusoidal gratings at four orientations, or Sloan letters are presented at a viewing distance of 12 ft on a high-quality monitor devoid of flicker and having uniform luminance. The optotypes are surrounded by a 130 cd/m² glare field, equivalent to a bright overcast day. The National Research Council's standards for assessment of distance acuity served as a guideline in the development of this instrument.

Experimental Design Considerations

Only a handful of experiments have attempted to analyze a glare tester's precision in predicting outdoor acuity/glare disability. Most glare test studies are conducted in cataract populations, since the greatest clinical application is substantiation of a patient's visual complaint prior to surgery. The results from these experiments are variable. The source of confusion is the greater variability surrounding the testing environment rather than the instruments themselves. Special consideration should be given to the study population, the optotype, and the outdoor testing situation, since each of these factors can significantly alter the experimental outcome. Our controlled study[4] sought to determine the relative sensitivity of two commercially available glare testers (Miller-Nadler and the BAT) in predicting outdoor acuity in patients with minimal cataracts. Although both instruments demonstrated a significant positive correlation between predicted and obtained outdoor acuity, they also showed a significant difference (with the Miller-Nadler instrument being less predictive than the BAT on the medium-luminance setting). This indicates that the instruments may predict better than random chance, but there is room for improvement.

Study Population

While our reported correlations are lower than others in the literature,[29,31,32] this may be due to our study population, which included only patients with minimal cataracts and moderately reduced visual acuity. Inclusion of patients with dense cataracts, who will not see well indoors or outdoors regardless of instrument, will result in an artificially high correlation coefficient and loss of instrument sensitivity. An appropriate study population is needed to validate functional complaints in patients with minimal pathological changes and abnormal glare results.

Carefully screened subjects were recruited from two populations: (1) patients who were found to have cataracts on routine screening and (2) patients without cataracts. All subjects had normal retinas, visual pathways, and visual cortical function. None of the subjects demonstrated corneal opacities or had had previous corneal surgery. The vitreous was examined for clarity by direct and indirect ophthalmoscopy; persons with vitreal changes were not included in the study. After optical correction for myopia, presbyopia, and hyperopia, the only ocular and functional difference between normal controls and study patients was the presence of an early cataract. For each patient, data from one eye only were used, and it was same eye in all testing conditions. This is an important consideration: including data from both eyes, which can be expected to correlate to each other, causes an unwarranted gain in statistical power.[33] Before they were enrolled in the study all patients received a detailed description of the study and their expected participatory role.

Optotypes

Scoring Data

In an evaluation of glare testers using letter stimuli, it is important to use a chart that corrects for the previously identified drawbacks of the traditional Snellen chart.[5] Accurate computation of line differences and visual acuity can only result from a chart that contains an equal number of letters per line and equal increments between the lines.

An outdoor vision score that is worse than predicted is considered to be a glare disability underprediction. Conversely, an outdoor vision score that is better than predicted is recorded as a glare disability overprediction. Figures 4.5 and 4.6 depict scattergrams with linear regression and labeling of areas of glare disability underprediction

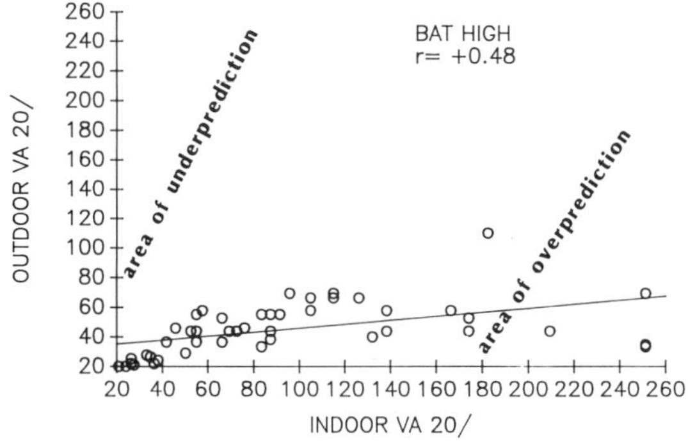

FIGURE 4.5. Scattergram of indoor visual acuity (VA) determined by the brightness acuity tester (BAT) on the high-luminance setting versus actual outdoor acuity for 47 subjects with minimal cataracts. A line of best fit is drawn through the data. The BAT was used in conjunction with high-contrast letter optotypes. Areas of glare disability underprediction and overprediction are indicated.

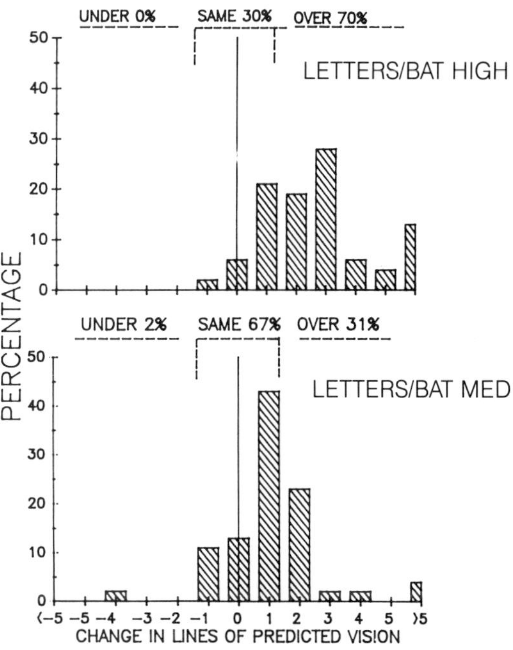

FIGURE 4.7. Percentage of the cataract population with outdoor vision better (glare disability overprediction), the same, or worse (glare disability underprediction) than predicted. Percent change is in lines of vision. A plus or minus one line of predicted vision equals no change. The top of the figure depicts data from letter optotypes and the brightness acuity tester (BAT) at the highest luminance setting. The bottom graphs data from letter optotypes and the BAT at medium intensity.

and overprediction at high glare luminance for 95% contrast letters (Fig. 4.5) and for varying contrast sinusoidal gratings (Fig. 4.6). Accurate instrument glare disability underprediction and overprediction rates, or line differences, are established for each individual by determining the total difference in the number of letters identified indoors and outdoors. This difference score is then divided by five, the number of letters per line on the Bailey-Lovie chart.

A graphic example of line differences is illustrated in Figures 4.7 and 4.8 for high-contrast letters and varying-contrast sinusoids at high- and medium-glare intensity. This histogram clearly summarizes glare disability underprediction and overprediction rates. The no change (or "same") category from predicted acuity to obtained outdoor vision includes plus or minus one line of vision.

The same type chart must be used in both indoor and outdoor testing conditions. Conclusions are confounded, for instance, if sinusoids are used indoors and Snellen letters outdoors.[34]

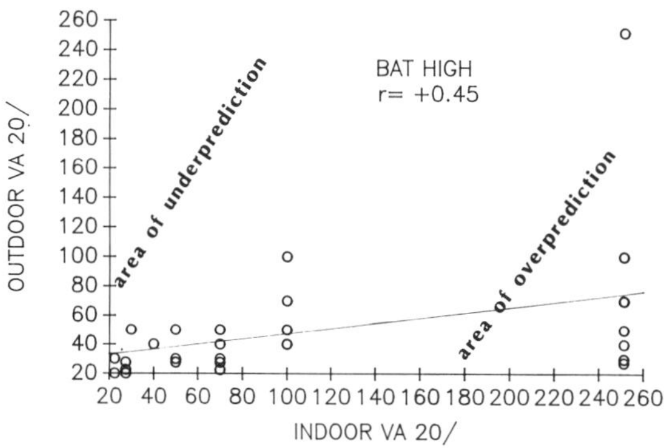

FIGURE 4.6. Scattergram of indoor visual acuity (VA) determined by the brightness acuity tester (BAT) on the high-luminance setting versus actual outdoor acuity for 47 subjects with minimal cataracts. A line of best fit is drawn through the data. The BAT was used in conjunction with varying-contrast sinusoidal gratings. Areas of glare disability underprediction and overprediction are indicated.

Effect of Glare on Contrast and Acuity

A recent article by Legge, Rubin, and Luebker[35] concludes that change in acuity or resolution is inversely proportional to the square root of contrast. Thus, glare should affect contrast more than

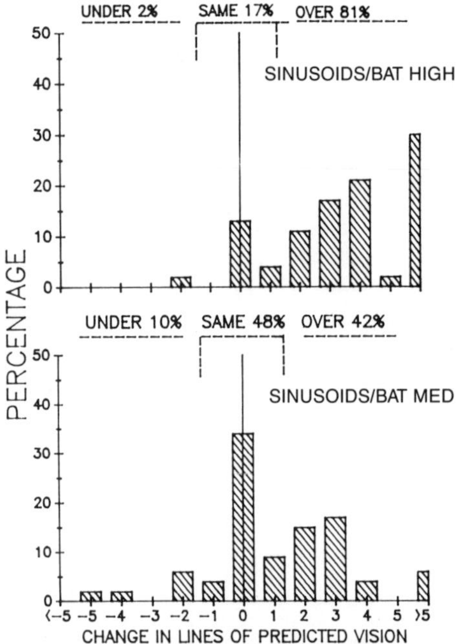

FIGURE 4.8. Percentage of the cataract population with outdoor vision better (glare disability overprediction), the same, or worse (glare disability underprediction) than predicted. Percent change is in lines of vision. A plus or minus one line of predicted vision equals no change. The top of the figure depicts data from sinusoidal grating optotypes and the brightness acuity tester (BAT) at the highest luminance setting. The bottom graphs data from sinusoids and the BAT at medium intensity.

letter perception. In our experiment we found that in the absence of a glare field, high-contrast letter stimuli demonstrated essentially the same visual acuity as found with multicontrast sinusoidal gratings (20/43 vs. 20/45). In the presence of the same medium-intensity glare source, the varying-contrast sinusoidal stimuli indeed did predict greater glare disability than the high-contrast letters (20/73 gratings, 20/59 letters). This same trend was noted outdoors, with patients demonstrating somewhat greater disability with the reduced-contrast bar gratings (20/56 gratings, 20/45 letters).

Gratings Versus Letters

Theoretical and clinical studies have proven the need for contrast sensitivity testing. However, the choice of the optimum target is open to speculation.

It is not clear that sinusoidal gratings are superior to letters. From a theoretical perspective, sinusoidal gratings are "simpler" than letters because sinusoidal grating stimuli contain only a fundamental frequency as opposed to letters composed of higher frequency harmonics. However, many cognitive skills used in educational and industrial situations center around the ability to read letters. In ophthalmology, Snellen letters have been used for over 125 years to measure visual acuity. The perception of letters, composed of many spatial frequencies, is less susceptible to the degrading effects of astigmatism than is perception of sinusoidal gratings presented at just three orientations. The sinusoidal grating chart has forced-choice alternatives, all within 45 degrees of one another, which could induce a bias against patients with astigmatism in the meridian being tested. The best chart for determining the effects of glare disability might use Bailey-Lovie letters, equated for equal line interval and letter difficulty, at varying contrasts.[12] Optimally these charts would be mounted on a projector slide with a calibrated light source for ease of presentation.

Outdoor Ambient Conditions

Light readings at the eye should be measured and equated among study patients. Just reporting the angle of the sun is not sufficient, since perceptual brightness changes with the angle of the sun, with cloud conditions, and with time of year. The influence of varying ambient light may be readily identified and minimized by stepwise regression analysis or analysis of covariance. Without a detailed description of the outdoor testing conditions it is impossible to equate glare test results collected in dissimilar environments, such as the parking lot of the Houston Astrodome, a blacktop parking lot bordered by pine trees, and a solid white concrete wall that diffuses light uniformly.

The essential aspects of the outdoor testing area are included in the following example:

Testing was conducted at the edge of a lightly pigmented concrete parking lot surrounded by a grass field extending 200 yds. The field abutted several two-story white apartments and four 30-ft trees. The background environment occupied an average of 15 degrees of visual field as determined by sextant measurement. We tested between 8:00 AM and 1:30 PM from August to October. The subjects all faced the eastern sun, which subtended an angle of 30 to 80 degrees above the horizon, producing light readings averaging 9277 fc overhead and 6376 fc at eye level. To minimize variability in ambient testing conditions, data were not collected if the direct eye level illuminance was less than 4000 fc. The light levels at the eye (along the patient's line of sight) ranged from 4200 to 8100 fc and did not differ significantly between cataract and normal populations: normal population 6296 fc (1039 SD), cataract patients 6316 fc (993 SD). To further assess the effect of variation in outdoor light levels among cataract patients, a stepwise regression was run with illuminance as the first stepwise predictor. The results of this analysis showed outdoor illuminance to be a poor predictor of outdoor acuity ($r = -.09, p = 0.73$), suggesting that the influence of outdoor light variability among cataract patients was minimal.

Research that clarifies and standardizes glare testing is important to allow accurate determination and documentation of a patient's visual complaint. However, to assess the validity/sensitivity of the various instruments, additional methodological considerations must be addressed and experiments designed and replicated to demonstrate that the theoretical issues found in the laboratory are clinically significant in the evaluation of cataract patients. The fact that these methodological considerations have by and large not been taken into account during the development of glare testing apparatuses should make us very cautious about accepting their results as valid documentation of functional disability.

The entire field of glare testing clearly is in a state of evolution. It is hoped that these first-generation instruments will lead to more sophisticated glare testers and/or calibration procedures that better correlate to real-world conditions. The varying results of these early experiments only underscore the fact that there are no standards for glare type, illuminance, or target configuration. The most important conclusion for the clinician is that impairment of a patient's life-style should remain the overriding consideration when discussing the possibility of cataract surgery. This is more important than just a score from an instrument.

References

1. Coopersmith LW, Carr MA: Forecasting intraocular lens implantation to 1990 using a model of population dynamics. *J Catar Refract Surg* **13**:302–308, 1987.

2. Fry GA, Alpern M: The effect of a peripheral glare source upon the apparent brightness of an object. *J Opt Soc Am* **43**:189–195, 1953.

3. Lie I: Visual detection and resolution as a function of adaptation and glare. *Vis Res* **21**:1793–1797, 1981.

4. Prager TC, Urso RG, Holladay JT, et al: Glare testing in cataract patients: Instrument evaluation and identification of sources of methodological error. *J Catar Refract Surg* **15**:149–157, 1989.

5. Ferris FL III, Kassoff A, Bresnick GH, et al: New visual acuity charts for clinical research. *Am J Ophthalmol* **94**:91–96, 1982.

6. ETDRS Coordinating Center: Early treatment diabetic retinopathy study, in *Manual of Operations*. Baltimore, Department of Epidemiology and Preventive Medicine, 1980; pp 1–15.

7. Personal communication, Jack T. Holladay, MD, University of Texas Medical School Houston, TX, October 1988.

8. Campbell FW, Green DG: Optical and retinal factors affecting visual resolution. *J Physiol* **181**:576–593, 1965.

9. Michaels D: *Visual Optics and Refraction: A Clinical Approach*. St. Louis, Mo.: CV Mosby, 1985, p 13.

10. Lie I: Visual detection and resolution as a function of adaptation and glare. *Vis Res* **21**:1793–1797, 1981.

11. Regan D, Raymond J, Ginsburg AP, et al: Contrast sensitivity, visual acuity, and the discrimination of Snellen letters in multiple sclerosis. *Brain* **104**:333–350, 1981.

12. Regan D, Neima D: Low-contrast letter charts as a test of visual function. *Ophthalmology* **90**:1192–1200, 1983.

13. Ginsburg AP: The evaluation of contact lenses and refractive surgery using contrast sensitivity, in *CLAO Guide to Basic Science and Clinical Practice*. Orlando, Fla., Grune and Stratton, 1987, p 56.17.

14. Campbell FW, Robson JG: Application of Fourier analysis to the visibility of gratings. *J Physiol* **197**:551, 1968.

15. Sjostrand J: Contrast sensitivity in macular disease using a small field and a large field T.V. system. *Acta Doc* **57**:832–846, 1979.

16. Corwin TR, Richman JE: Three clinical tests of the spatial contrast sensitivity function: A comparison. *Am J Optom Physiol Opt* **63**:413–418, 1986.

17. Hubel D, Weisel T: Brain mechanisms of vision. *Scientif Am* **241**:150–164, 1979.

18. Bodis-Wollner I: Visual acuity and contrast sensitivity in patients with cerebral lesions. *Science* **178**:769, 1972.

19. Regan D, Silver R, Murray TJ: Visual acuity and contrast sensitivity in multiple sclerosis—hidden visual loss: An auxiliary diagnostic test. *Brain* **100**:563–579, 1977.

20. Zimmern RL, Campbell FW, Wilkinson IMS: Subtle disturbances of vision after optic neuritis elicited by studying contrast sensitivity. *J Neurol Neurosurg Psychiat* **42**:407–412, 1979.

21. Arden GB, Jacobson JJ: A simple grating test for contrast sensitivity: Preliminary results indicate value for screening in glaucoma. *Invest Ophthalmol Vis Sci* **17**:23, 1978.

22. Sokol S, Domar A, Moskowitz A: Utility of the Arden grating test in glaucoma screening: High false-positive rate in normals over 50 years of age. *Invest Ophthalmol Vis Sci* **19**:1529–1533, 1980.

23. Ginsburg AP: A new contrast sensitivity vision test chart. *Am J Optom Physiol Opt* **61**:403, 1984.

24. Hess RF, Carney LG: Vision through an abnormal cornea: A pilot study of the relationship between visual loss from corneal distortion, corneal edema, keratoconus and some allied corneal pathology. *Invest Ophthalmol Vis Sci* **18**:476–483, 1979.

25. Rubin GS, Sunness JS: Assessing visual function in patients with macular edema, in *Noninvasive Assessment of the Visual System*, 1988 Technical Digest Series (Vol 3). Washington, D.C., Optical Society of America, 1988, pp 140–143.

26. Miller D, Nadler MP, LeClaire J, et al: A new clinical glare tester in assessment of corrected aphakia, in Emery JM, Jackson AC (eds), *Current Concepts in Cataract Surgery: Selected Proceedings of the Seventh Biennial Cataract Surgical Congress*. New York, Appleton-Century-Crofts, 1982, pp 257–262.

27. LeClaire J, Nadler MP, Weiss S, et al: A new glare tester for clinical testing. Results comparing normal subjects and variously corrected aphakic patients. *Arch Ophthalmol* **100**:153–158, 1982.

28. Hirsch RP, Nadler MP, Miller D: Glare measurement as a predictor of outdoor vision among cataract patients. *Ann Ophthalmol* **16**:965–968, 1984.

29. Nadler DJ, Jaffe NS, Clayman HM, et al: Glare disability in eyes with intraocular lenses. *Am J Ophthalmol* **97**:43–47, 1984.

30. Hirsch RP, Nadler MP, Miller D: Clinical performance of a disability glare tester. *Arch Ophthalmol* **102**:1633–1636, 1984.

31. Holladay JT, Prager TC, Truillo J, et al: Brightness acuity test and outdoor visual acuity in cataract patients. *J Catar Refract Surg* **13**:67–69, 1987.

32. Ederer F: Shall we count numbers of eyes or numbers of subjects? (Editorial) *Arch Ophthalmol* **89**:1–2, 1973.

33. Neumann AC, McCarty GR, Locke J, et al: Glare disability for cataractous eyes: A consumer's guide. *J Catar Refract Surg* **14**:212–216, 1988.

34. Legge GE, Rubin GS, Leubker A: Psychophysics of reading. V. The role of contrast in normal vision. *Vis Res* **27**:1165–1177, 1987.

5
Contrast Sensitivity and Glare Testing in Corneal Disease

David Miller and Suketu Sanghvi

Introduction

A variety of corneal lesions result in decreased sensitivity to contrast and increased sensitivity to glare. The purpose of this chapter is to show the clinician the physical basis for this finding, and to review the relationship between certain corneal lesions and their accompanying derangements of contrast sensitivity and glare disability.

The unifying thread of this chapter is the phenomenon of light scattering. Almost all corneal diseases convert the clear cornea to a light-scattering tissue. Because of this light scattering a diseased cornea appears cloudy to the observer. Why does a cornea that scatters light decrease contrast sensitivity and increase glare disability? In both cases, the cloudy cornea degrades the image received by the retina. The contrast of the retinal image is decreased because the cloudy cornea effectively disburses part of the light that would otherwise have produced a sharp image. Light from a peripheral or "glare" source intensifies the problem. Such light is normally focused onto the retinal periphery. A cloudy cornea, however, will splatter some of this light onto the foveal image, further decreasing the contrast (Fig. 5.1).

Basic Mechanisms

Light Scattering

Light scattering is a feature not only of the diseased cornea. In reality, a clear cornea is no more than about 90% transparent—it scatters about 10% of incident light.[1] If the cornea were 100% transparent, its gray-blue optical section would not be visible in the slit lamp.

Interestingly, Leonardo da Vinci noted the effect of light scattering and postulated a mechanism.[2] He observed that a far-off mountain peak looked blue. In advising his art students he wrote, "You must make the nearest building . . . its real color, but make the more distant ones less defined and bluer." It is fascinating to note how close to the truth Leonardo was in explaining the phenomenon:

The blueness we see in the atmosphere is not intrinsic color, but is caused by warm vapor evaporated in minute and sensible atoms on which the solar rays fall, rendering them luminous.

As "laboratory evidence" in support of his hypothesis, he recommended the following experiment:

If anyone wishes for a final proof, let him paint a board of various colors, . . . and over all let him lay a very thin and transparent coating of white. He will then see that this thin and transparent layer will show a . . . beautiful blue.

Leonardo's thin layer of white paint, a colloidal suspension of fine particles in a solvent, is, in a sense, much like a mildly edematous corneal stroma. Such a stroma is made of collagen fibrils (akin to Leonardo's paint particles) embedded in a mucopolysaccharide matrix (akin to the paint solvent). The scattering elements are spaced greater than half a wavelength of light apart, leading to visible light scattering (Fig. 5.2).[3]

We will now review three special features of light scattering with particular applicability to the cornea: wavelength dependence, polarization, and diffraction.

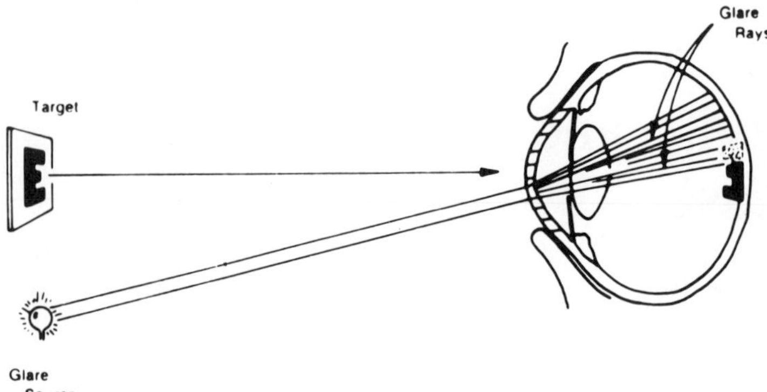

FIGURE 5.1. The eye with corneal edema scatters light from the glare source onto the fovea, thus decreasing the contrast of the foveal image. This is known as glare degradation. (From Miller and Benedek G, p 38.[8] Courtesy of Charles C Thomas, Publisher, Springfield, Illinois.)

Wavelength Dependence

If the components that produce light scattering are smaller than a wavelength of light, the scattered light is *wavelength dependent*. Known as Rayleigh scattering, this means that short wavelengths, such as blue light, are scattered more than longer (redder) ones. In fact, the scattering is inversely proportional to the fourth power of the wavelength. Thus, light in the ultraviolet range (wavelength 350 μ) is scattered 16 times more than light in the visible red range (wavelength 700 μ).

A portion of the light incident on the cornea is scattered in a wavelength-dependent fashion. The normal corneal stroma preferentially scatters short wavelengths, hence its bluish color in the slit lamp.[4] As the stroma becomes edematous, its color in the slit lamp becomes whiter. The observed white light implies that the incident slit beam must no longer be scattered in a wavelength-dependent fashion, and we infer that the scattering centers are now larger than the size of a wavelength of light. Clouds and ocean foam are other examples of this type of light scattering.

Polarization

In addition to being wavelength dependent, light scattered by particles smaller than its wavelength is polarized. The blue light of the sky, which is produced by the tiny particles of our atmosphere, is also polarized. Theory predicts that the direction of the plane of polarization depends on the angle of incidence of the light source. Thus, the direction of the plane of polarization of a patch of sky light can be used to deduce the position of the sun, and can be used as a navigation reference, even on a cloudy day. In fact, the eye of the honey bee registers the direction of the plane of polarization of a patch of sky and uses such a system of navigation to lead the other members of the hive to nectar-producing plants.[6]

Since the normal cornea scatters a small portion of incident light in a wavelength-dependent fashion, it also polarizes this portion of light. Unlike sky light, this light is primarily circularly polarized due to the arrangement of stromal fibers into an orthogonal array (different lamellae oriented in many different directions). Interestingly, the macular region of the retina also has polarizing elements (which produce the Haidinger brush phenomenon[7]). Perhaps this retinal polarizing system serves to cancel the polarized forward-scattered light produced by the normal cornea!

Diffraction

When the scattering elements are both small and ordered, they can produce a type of diffraction grating. For example, atmospheric ice crystals between the observer and the moon produce the colored halos around the moon that warn the sailor of an impending storm.

A similar effect occurs in corneal edema, in which edema fluid of one index of refraction becomes interspersed between corneal epithelial cells of a higher index of refraction, producing an ordered array of scattering elements. This takes place after a swim in a freshwater lake, and (as seen in Fig. 5.3), produces the colored halos that are also seen after prolonged wearing of a poorly fitting contact lens, in acute glaucoma, or in early bullous keratopathy.[8-10] It is interesting (in light of

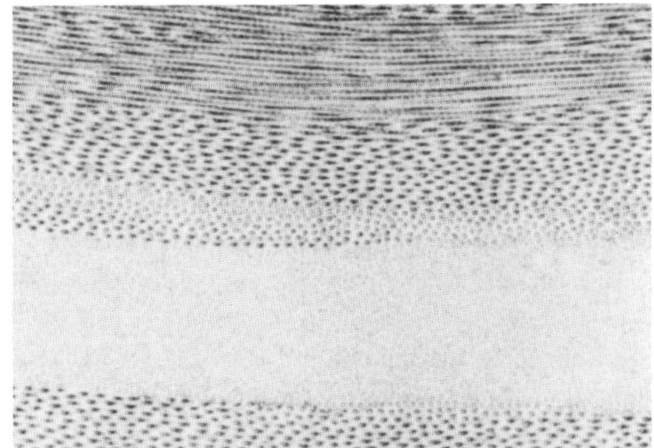

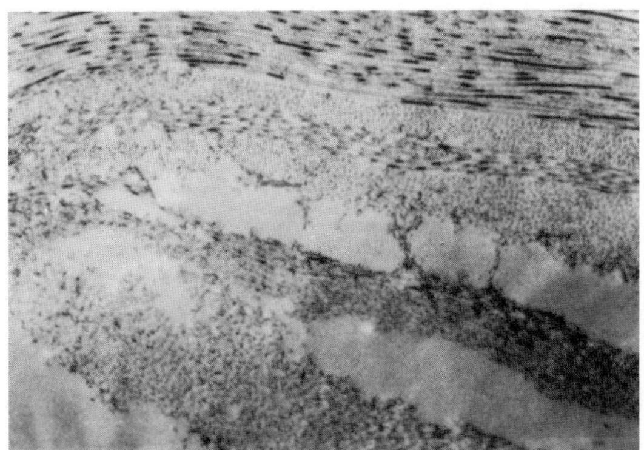

FIGURE 5.2. Electron micrographs. (a) Arrangement of collagen fibers in a normal corneal stroma. (b) A corneal stroma with edema. Note the irregular collection of fluid. (From Miller and Benedek, p 20.[8] Courtesy of Charles C Thomas, Publisher, Springfield, Illinois.)

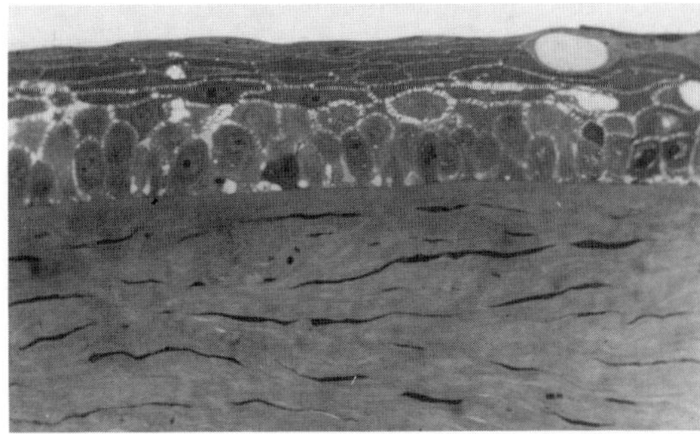

FIGURE 5.3. A light micrograph showing corneal epithelial edema. (From Miller and Benedek, p 54.[8] Courtesy of Charles C Thomas, Publisher, Springfield, Illinois.)

the foregoing discussion of wavelength dependence) that as cases like these progress and the fluid pools between the epithelial cells increase in size, the patient reports white halos rather than colored ones.

Extraneous Light and Contrast Degradation

We have asserted that corneal lesions that scatter light degrade contrast sensitivity by splashing extra, noninformation-containing light onto the retinal image. This can be demonstrated by a simple calculation, following Prager and colleagues.[11]

Suppose we wanted to measure the contrast of the standard projected Snellen chart in both a darkened examining room and a lighted one. Contrast is essentially the difference between the luminance of the target and its background, and can be expressed as a percentage, as follows:

$$\frac{\text{Background luminance} - \text{target luminance}}{\text{Background luminance} + \text{target luminance}} \times 100$$

To calculate the contrast of the projected Snellen chart in a darkened room, let us say the background illumination is 97 arbitrary light units and the target illumination (consisting of letters, and thus being darker) is 3 light units. This gives

$$\text{Contrast} = \frac{(97 - 3) \times 100}{(97 + 3)} = 94\%$$

Let us now turn the room lights on, thus placing an additional 50 light units onto both the background and letters of the projected Snellen chart. The new contrast is given by

$$\text{Contrast}' = \frac{(147 - 53) \times 100}{(147 + 53)} = 47\%$$

We see that this simple maneuver cuts the contrast in half. Just as the Snellen chart drops its contrast when extra light falls on it, so the retinal image loses contrast when a corneal lesion scatters extraneous light onto the retinal image.

Visual Function in Low-Contrast Situations

Fortunately, reduction in contrast is less debilitating than it might be, because the visual system is "tuned" to prioritize information in situations of low contrast. In a low-contrast situation, such as in rain or fog or through a mildly turbid cornea or lens, we see best objects 5 to 7 cycles per degree (cpd) in size. This is about the size of a 20/80 Snellen letter, an angular subtense of about 20 minutes, or the size of your thumb at arm's length. In fact, objects of this size are seen three times better than larger (20/200) or smaller (20/20) objects. It is interesting that this is roughly the scale of the movement of a person's eyes or lips at conversational distance.

The visual system not only prioritizes size (spatial frequency), but also colors. We recall that in many situations short-wavelength blue light is scattered more than visible light of greater wavelengths. Luckily, the eye is far less sensitive to blue than to yellow or green. Blue light is filtered out to some extent by the normal lens and xanthophyll macular pigment, and the retinal cones are less responsive to blue light than to other colors. As a result, we are less bothered by the scattered blue light produced by the air between ourselves and distant objects (although the observant da Vinci noticed the effect nonetheless). Patients with mild corneal edema, whose corneas scatter relatively more blue light, no doubt benefit from our reduced sensitivity to blue.

Clinical Applications

Corneal Edema

The term *corneal edema* includes a spectrum of corneal problems. We will focus first on the continuum of conditions that spring from endothelial decompensation, whether caused by the surgical trauma of cataract surgery, by a rejecting corneal graft, or by an inherited endothelial defect.

Current methods of following corneal edema include visual acuity testing (crude) and pachometry (more sensitive). Each of these techniques has significant limitations. Studies tracing the progression of corneal decompensation[12,13] have shown that the stroma increases in thickness (i.e., becomes waterlogged) before the epithelium does. In fact, the stroma increases in thickness by up to 30% before the epithelium becomes edematous. Interestingly, our studies[13,14] have shown that an increase in stromal thickness of up to 30% need not

influence Snellen acuity. Put another way, a patient may have edema with 30% stromal thickening and still maintain a visual acuity of 20/20, as long as the increased thickness does not involve the corneal epithelium! Unlike Snellen acuity, both contrast sensitivity and glare sensitivity are compromised as soon as the stroma thickens.

While pachometry may certainly be used to follow stromal thickening, it is of limited utility in epithelial edema, because epithelial edema does not add significantly to total corneal thickness until bullae form. Contrast sensitivity is reduced, however, and the change in contrast sensitivity seems to follow two different patterns.[15] Mild edema affects only the middle and high spatial frequencies, sparing the low frequencies. Incidentally, this effect can be mimicked by having a subject with a normal cornea look through a blurring $+1.25$ diopter (D) lens. With further edema, the sparing of low spatial frequencies disappears, and contrast sensitivity is decreased throughout the spatial frequency spectrum. The effect can no longer be simulated by dioptric defocus. Not surprisingly, the effect of an edematous epithelium gets larger and larger as the stroma thickens. Glare sensitivity measurements will also detect early epithelial edema: A mildly edematous epithelium is roughly equivalent to an increase of 10% in stromal thickness.

Contact Lens Usage

The wearing of contact lenses may reduce contrast sensitivity in many ways[16]:

1. Residual refractive error. For example, patients with significant corneal astigmatism wearing thin, soft contact lenses will experience a small blur, which will affect their performance on a contrast sensitivity test.
2. Spherical aberration. A spherical contact lens adds a small amount of spherical aberration to the ocular system by canceling the flattening of the peripheral cornea.[17] This effect is akin to a small amount of dioptric defocus.
3. Changes in the soft lens itself. Tonicity, pH, temperature, tear volume, or the plastic material itself can all affect soft lens hydration and thus ultimately change either lens thickness or curvature. These changes, in turn, might induce

a new refractive error and simulate dioptric defocus.

4. Lens deposits. It has been shown[18] that lens deposits function as light-scattering centers and therefore reduce contrast sensitivity. These degrading effects should be amplified in the presence of a glare light.

5. Corneal edema. It is known that oxygen deprivation of the cornea can produce edema. If all else is kept equal, the thicker the lens, the less oxygen is delivered to the cornea. In a recent study in which subjects were fitted with soft contact lenses of center thickness 0.03 mm, 0.07 mm, and 0.12 mm, loss of contrast sensitivity was proportional to lens thickness and was detectable after just one hour.[16] Studies on patients wearing hard contact lenses also showed increased glare disability when corneal epithelial edema was present.[19]

Keratoconus

Keratoconus is a prototypical example of the limitations of routine visual acuity measurement in corneal disease. As patients with keratoconus develop irregular myopic astigmatism, they note a decrease in the quality of their vision even before the change can be documented by a decrease in Snellen visual acuity.[20,21]

Patients with keratoconus demonstrate attenuation of contrast sensitivity with relative sparing of low spatial frequencies despite normal Snellen acuity.[16] However, once scarring develops in the keratoconic cornea, high spatial frequencies are also attenuated.[20,22] One would also expect an acute increase in glare sensitivity as soon as scarring developed. Thus, contrast sensitivity testing at a number of spatial frequencies may be an excellent way of following the progression of keratoconus.

Nephrotic Cystinosis

Cystinosis is a rare autosomal recessive metabolic disorder in which cystine accumulates in most bodily tissues due to a defect in lysosomal cystine transport. The ocular changes in cystinosis include distinctive refractile crystals in the cornea and a pigmentary retinopathy.

In a study of patients with infantile-onset cystinosis, contrast sensitivities were reduced at all

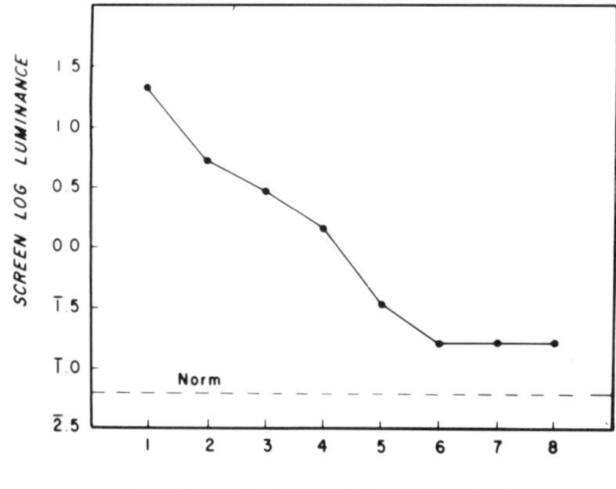

FIGURE 5.4. A subject wore a frosted scleral contact lens with different-sized holes, thus simulating different sizes of clear grafts surrounded by a hazy cornea. The subject's pupil measured 7.5 mm. The graph shows the relationship between graft size and glare (screen log luminance). (From Miller D, Dohlman CH: Optical properties of buried corneal silicon prostheses. *Am J Ophthalmol* **66**: 638, 1968. Published with permission from *The American Journal of Ophthalmology*. Copyright by The Ophthalmic Publishing Company and from Miller D and Miller R.[27] Copyright 1981, American Medical Association.)

frequencies, although the loss at high frequencies was greatest.[23] Ten of twelve subjects showed glare disability compared with a control population. Since these patients have stromal crystals as well as increased stromal thickness (edema?),[24] one speculates that both of these changes produced increased light scattering and thus a glare disability.

Penetrating Keratoplasty

As a sensitive measure of visual performance, glare testing has been used to tackle the question of optimal graft size. The experimental model[25] simulated different-sized clear grafts with either a frosted plastic disk or a frosted scleral contact lens with different-sized holes in the center. Visual acuity and glare measurements were recorded for each size hole, with the subjects' pupils dilated to different sizes.

Although visual acuity remained 20/20 for all hole sizes greater than 1 mm, glare sensitivity varied, as shown in Figure 5.4. The glare performance was determined by the percentage of clear cornea versus the percentage of hazy cornea (for a particular pupillary size). For example, a clear

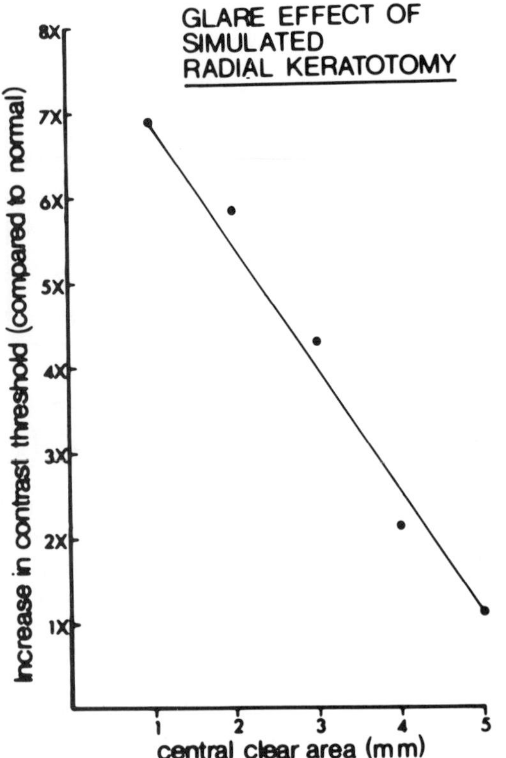

FIGURE 5.5. Results of a study using etched acetate sheets with different radial keratotomy patterns to simulate keratotomized corneas. The curve shows that glare disability increases as the central optical zone decreases. (From Miller and Miller.[27] Copyright 1981, American Medical Association.)

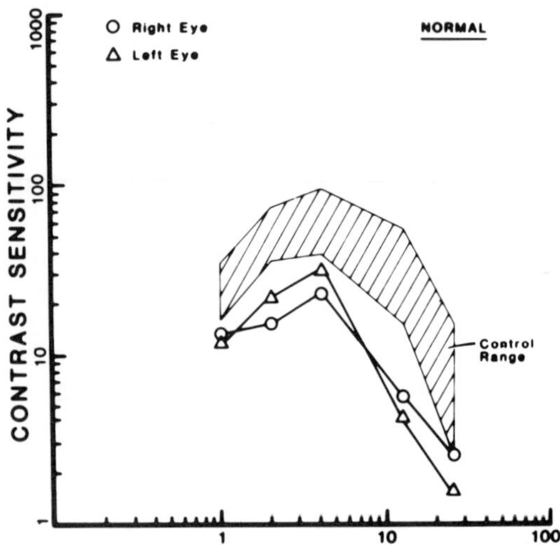

FIGURE 5.6. Contrast sensitivity results from a 25-year-old patient who underwent bilateral myopic epikeratoplasties for a −8.25-D myopic error. Two years postoperatively, uncorrected visual acuity in the OD, is 20/50 and in the OS is 20/20-3. The contrast sensitivity function for each eye is below the central zone, which represents the 95-percentile range for normal subjects. (From Kelley and Carney,[33] used by permission)

5-mm graft (area 19.6 mm²) surrounded by hazy cornea over a 7.5-mm pupil (area 44.0 mm²) occupies less than 50% of pupillary area. In this case, the glare sensitivity did not become normal until the simulated graft was about 7 mm in diameter (area 38.5 mm²), or almost 100% of the pupillary area. These results help explain the reduced visual performance of graft recipients under low light conditions.

Contrast sensitivity or glare testing may also be useful in detecting the earliest signs of graft rejection. In such cases, the earliest corneal change is stromal edema. Although visual acuity may remain normal, contrast and glare performance will start to slip. As the edema progresses to involve the epithelium, the degradation of these functions is accentuated. Similarly, reversal of graft rejection may be followed by an improvement in the contrast sensitivity function.[26]

Radial Keratotomy

In theory, the healing scars following radial keratotomy should produce light scattering. The thicker the scars and the closer they are to the corneal center, the worse should be contrast sensitivity and glare disability. This prediction was confirmed in a study using simulated keratotomized corneas made of clear acetate sheets with patterns of radial keratotomies etched on the surface.[27] The patterns had both narrow and wide simulated "scars" (0.1–0.3 mm) and central optical zones ranging from 1 mm to 5 mm in diameter. Experimental subjects held these patterns 5 mm from their corneas while their glare sensitivity was tested. The relationship between the thick simulated scars and the size of the optical zone is shown in Figure 5.5. The closer the "scars" are to the clear central zone, the worse the glare disability.

Most early studies of patients who had undergone radial keratotomy simply asked if they were bothered by glare. At the 3-month postoperative mark, 30% complained of annoying glare. At 6 months, 45% to 74% complained of glare.[29,30] At 1 year, 14% complained of glare, mostly "mild."[31]

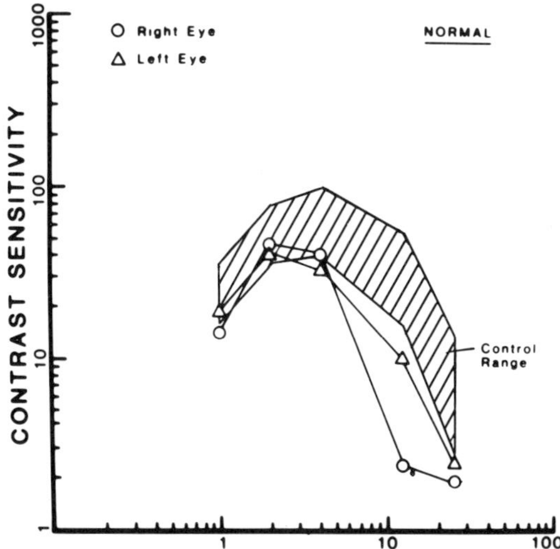

FIGURE 5.7. Contrast sensitivity results from a 29-year-old patient who underwent a 16-incision RK with two astigmatic incisions in the OS and an 8-incision RK in the OD. Her uncorrected visual acuity is 20/25 in each eye. The contrast sensitivity tests were performed 3 years after surgery.

At 1 year postoperation in the PERK study,[32] less than 1% of patients reported glare at night, and no cases of disability glare were found using the Miller-Nadler glare tester. Thus, it seems that the incisions scatter light and produce glare symptoms in the early postoperative period. As healing progresses and the scars shrink in size, however, they produce less light scattering. Should an incision be ragged or become infected, the healed scar may remain wide enough to produce glare symptoms.

To get a clearer idea of how refractive surgery that has had a chance to heal affects contrast sensitivity, we turn to a preliminary study by Kelley and Carney of Ohio State University.[33] They showed that for patients who had undergone myopic epikeratophakia, diminished visual performance was evident despite close-to-normal visual acuity and an otherwise successful outcome (Figs. 5.6, 5.7). Similar (but smaller) losses were also evident in the representative patient following radial keratotomy. In both instances the visual performance was similar to that known to exist for the contact lens-corrected keratoconic patient. The visual losses could be a result of disturbances in the shape, surface regularity, or transparency of the cornea following refractive surgery.

While losses were present in the glare-sensitized case, in general they were no more dramatic than in the baseline contrast sensitivity measurements. The primary mechanism of the visual losses is, therefore, not from increased intraocular scattering. Rather, the fidelity of information transmission through these surgically modified corneas is altered and leads to image aberration. [See *Modulation transfer function*. Ed.]

References

1. Feuk T, McQueen D: The angular dependence of light scattering by rabbit cornea. *Invest Ophthalmol* **10**:294, 1971.
2. Hey JD: From Leonardo to Graser: Light scattering in historical perspective. Part 1. *S Afr J Sci* **79**:11, 1983.
3. Benedek GB: The theory of transparency of the eye. *Appl Opt* **10**:459, 1971.
4. Farrell R, McCally RL, Tatham PER: Wavelength dependences of light scattering in normal and cold swollen rabbit corneas and their structural implications. *J Physiol (Lond)* **233**:589, 1973.
5. Stratton JA: *Electromagnetic Theory*. New York, McGraw Hill, 1941, p 563.
6. Frisch K von: The dance language and orientation of bees. Cambridge, Mass., Harvard University Press, 1967.
7. Hallden U: An explanation of Haidinger brushes. *Arch Ophthalmol* **57**:393, 1957.
8. Miller D, Benedek G: *Intraocular Light Scattering: Theory and Clinical Implications*. Springfield Ill., Charles C Thomas, 1973, pp 82–87.
9. Finkelstein IS: The biophysics of corneal scattering and diffraction of light induced by contact lenses. *Arch Am Acad Optom* **92**:231, 1952.
10. Lambert SR, Klyce SD: The origins of Sattler's veil. *Am J Ophthalmol* **91**:51, 1981.
11. Prager TC, Holladay JT, Ruiz RS: The other side of visual acuity testing: Contrast sensitivity. *CLAO J* **12**:230, 1986.
12. Dohlman CH: Physiology of the cornea: Corneal edema, in Smolin G, Thoft RA (eds), *The Cornea*. Boston, Little, Brown, 1983, pp 3–17.
13. Miller D, Dohlman CH: The effect of cataract surgery on the cornea. *Trans Am Acad Ophthalmol Otol* **74**:369, 1970.
14. Lancon M, Miller D: Corneal hydration, visual acuity and glare sensitivity. *Arch Ophthalmol* **90**:227, 1973.
15. Hess RF, Garner LF: The effect of corneal edema on visual function. *Invest Ophthalmol Vis Sci* **16**:35, 1977.

16. Grey CP: Changes in contrast sensitivity during the first hour of soft lens wear. *Am J Optom Physiol Opt* **63**:702, 1986.

17. Woo GCS, Sivak JG: The effect of hard and soft contact lenses (soft lens) on the spherical aberration of the human eye. *Am J Optom Physiol Opt* **53**:456, 1976.

18. McClure DA, Ohota S, Eriksen SP, et al: The effect on measured visual acuity of protein deposition and removal in soft contact lenses. *Contacto* **21**:8, 1977.

19. Miller D, Wolf E, Greer J, et al: Glare sensitivity related to the use of contact lenses. *Arch Ophthalmol* **65**:448, 1967.

20. Carney LG: Visual loss in keratoconus. *Arch Ophthalmol* **100**:1282, 1982.

21. Zadnik K, Mannis MJ, Johnson CA, et al: Rapid contrast sensitivity assessment in keratoconus. *Am J Optom Physiol Opt* **64**:693, 1987.

22. Hess RF., Cerney LG: Vision Through an abnormal cornea: A pilot study of the relationship between visual loss from corneal distortion, corneal edema, keratoconus and some allied corneal pathology. *Invest Ophthalmol Vis Sci* **18**:476, 1979.

23. Katz B, Melles RB, Schneider JA: Contrast sensitivity in nephrotic cystinosis. *Arch Ophthalmol* **105**:1667, 1987.

24. Katz B, Melles RB, Schneider JA: Glare disability in nephrotic cystinosis. *Arch Ophthalmol* **105**:1670, 1987.

25. Miller D, Wolf E: A model for comparing the optical properties of different sized corneal grafts. *Am J Ophthalmol* **67**:724, 1969.

26. Zadnik K, Mannis MJ, Johnson CA: Contrast sensitivity after penetrating keratoplasty. *Arch Ophthalmol* **105**:1220, 1987.

27. Miller D, Miller R: Glare sensitivity in simulated radial keratotomy. *Arch Ophthalmol* **99**:1961, 1981.

28. Hoffer KJ, Darin JJ, Pettit TH, et al: The UCLA clinical trial of radial keratotomy: Preliminary report. *Ophthalmology* **88**:729, 1981.

29. Deitz MR, Sanders DR, Marks RG: Radial keratotomy, an overview of the Kansas City Study. *Ophthalmology* **91**:467, 1984.

30. Rowsey JJ, Balyeat HD: Preliminary results and complications of radial keratotomy. *Am J Ophthalmol* **93**(4):437, 1982.

31. Arrowsmith PN, Marks RG: Visual, refractive and keratometric results after radial keratotomy. *Arch Ophthalmol* **102**:1612, 1984.

32. Waring GO, et al: Results of the PERK study one year after surgery. *Ophthalmology* **92**:177, 1985.

33. Kelley CG, Carney LG: Visual performance after refractive surgery: Effect of disturbed corneal optics. *Invest. Ophth Vis Sci* **29**:281, 1988.

6
Glare and Contrast Sensitivity in Cataracts and Pseudophakia

Daniel J. Nadler

Helen Thurber and I have just returned from dinner at the Elm Tree Inn in Farmington (New York) about 25 miles from our little cottage. It was such a trip as few have survived. I lost eight pounds. You see, I can't see at night and this upset all the motorists in the state tonight, for I am blinded by headlights in addition to not being able to see anyhow. It took us two hours to come back, weaving and stopping now and then, stopping for every car that approached, stopping other times just to rest and bow my head on my arms and ask God to witness that this should not be. A further peril of the night road is that flecks of dust and shreds of bug blood on the windshield look to me often like old admirals in uniform or crippled apple women, or the front end of barges, and I whirl out of their way thus going into ditches and fields and up on front lawns.... In every other way I am fine. I am very happy when I am not driving at night.... Even when I grope along, honking and weaving, stopping and being honked at by long lines of cars behind me, my wife is patient and gentle and kind. Of course, she knows that in the daytime I am a fearless, skillful driver who can hold his own with anyone. It is only after nightfall that this change comes upon me.[1]

Introduction

As clinicians we not infrequently encounter cataract patients who have given up driving at night. Few verbalize their complaints as amusingly as James Thurber has in the above paragraph, but the gist of what they observe is the same.

Why are measurements of glare disability and contrast sensitivity important in cataract patients? The answer lies in the very nature of these parameters. Although detailed descriptions of glare disability and contrast sensitivity appear elsewhere in this text, a brief review follows.

When we measure visual acuity we measure a person's ability to resolve fine spatial detail. Measurement is usually done using high-contrast targets (black figures on a white background) such as Snellen letters, numbers, or Landolt C rings. The contrast level of these targets approaches 100%. In the real world we rarely encounter such high contrast, and frequently we see patients who score well on standard acuity measurements but complain of blurred vision in everyday situations (see Fig. 6.1). It is for these patients that our standard measurements fall short. One cannot extrapolate how a patient might see in situations of reduced contrast simply by knowing the patient's acuity at nearly 100% contrast.

For over 200 years, grating patterns have been used to measure visual function and acuity (called *grating acuity*). These patterns consist of vertical alternating light and dark bars. A sinusoidal grating is one where the transition from light to dark bar is gradual, as opposed to the sharp margins on the bars of a square wave grating. The *spatial frequency* of the pattern refers to the number of cycles (pairs of alternating bars) subtended by 1 degree of visual angle at the observer's eye. Contrast (modulation) is defined as the luminance difference between two adjacent bars divided by the sum of the luminance of two adjacent bars (Chap. 9, Fig. 9.2). The minimum contrast at which the grating pattern is detectable is the *contrast threshold*, and the inverse of this is the *contrast sensitivity*. Figure 6.2 shows the plot of a typical contrast sensitivity curve. One can see that there is an optimal spatial frequency for contrast detection. For humans this is around 5 cycles per degree. Gratings *larger* and *smaller* than this require more contrast to be

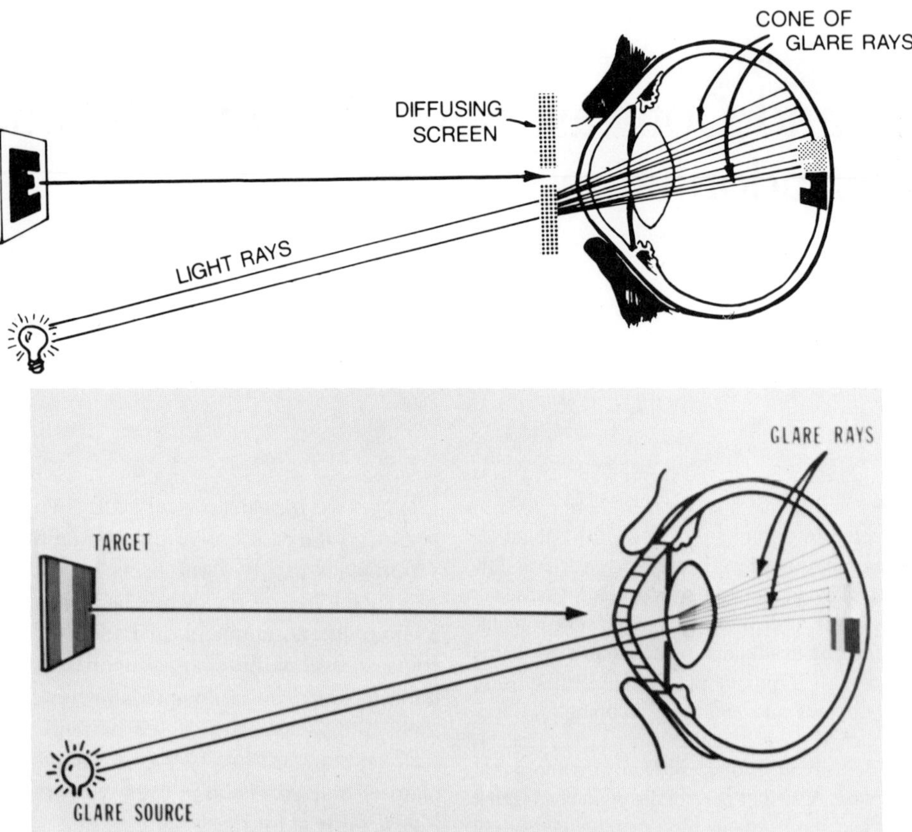

FIGURE 6.1. Schematic representation of the effects of glare in reducing the contrast of the focused retinal image. Both high (top) and average (bottom) contrast targets are proportionally affected, the latter suggesting more serious visual disability in real-life situations.

detected. It is important to recognize that a contrast sensitivity function (profile of the contrast sensitivity curve) cannot be established unless the mean luminance remains constant throughout the test. The last point on the spatial contrast sensitivity curve represents the finest pattern that an observer could detect at a theoretical 100% contrast, the so-called *cutoff frequency*. This is roughly equivalent to the Snellen acuity. One can therefore appreciate that a measurement of Snellen acuity represents only one point on the contrast sensitivity curve. Our visual performance, however, requires acceptable functioning for the *entire* contrast sensitivity curve.

The effect of glare is to reduce contrast. Contrast detection is the basic task from which all other visual behaviors are derived. The visual system is highly specialized to inform about luminous discontinuities and gradients in the visual field. It gives virtually no useful information when the retina is uniformly illuminated. When patients complain of glare, we cannot quantitate their visual disability unless we in some way measure contrast. It is well established that cataracts and other opacities of the media can profoundly reduce contrast and increase glare disability. For this reason it is important for us as clinicians to have a basic understanding of these phenomena in evaluating our patients with cataracts as well as those who have undergone cataract surgery.

Historical Background

Even the earliest discussions of glare alluded to the fact that cataractous changes might be a major cause of this condition. L. L. Holladay, whose observations were reported in 1926,[2] observed that

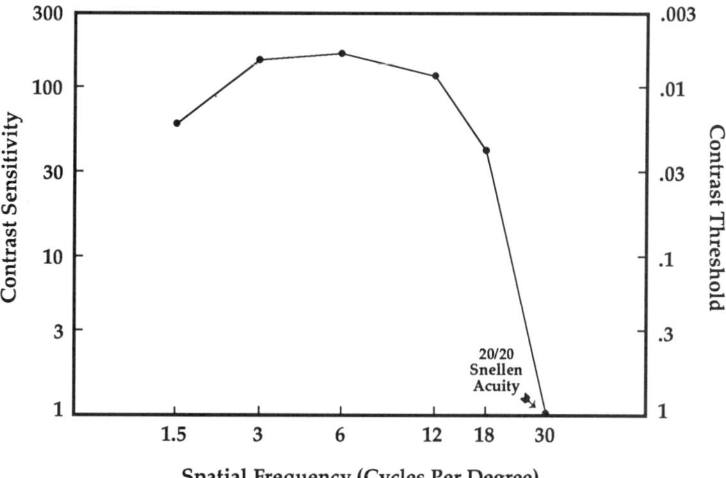

FIGURE 6.2. Typical contrast sensitivity curve showing a maximum contrast sensitivity at about 6 cycles per degree. The Snellen acuity roughly represents the theoretical cutoff frequency. (From ref. 19, with permission.)

the effects of glare were more pronounced in older individuals with "muddy" eyes. He further observed that the effects of glare caused by a point source of light were apparent even when this light source was *focused on the optic nerve*, thus eliminating the retinal photoreceptors as the only cause of glare. A detailed discussion of the historical background of the events leading to the development of the first clinical glare tester has been previously published.[3] The report of the first clinical glare tester[4] did not receive wide acceptance clinically due to a general lack of understanding of the importance of glare and to a failure to appreciate that standard vision tests do not measure visual image degradation due to glare.

A series of experiments designed to determine exactly how cataracts affect vision were reported in 1973.[5] These demonstrated the relationship between image contrast and resolution for different degrees of cataract by covering the lens of a model eye to varying degrees with an image degrader (vaseline). Zuckerman and colleagues showed that a cataract occupying up to 80% of the lens will allow visualization of larger test objects before contrast is lost. For smaller test objects, however, contrast is lost with as small as a 40% cataract. These investigators concluded that cataract disability comes from aberrations caused by adjacent areas of the lens having different refractive indices. These areas scatter rather than focus light within the eye and reduce overall contrast by washing out the retinal image. The investigators further suggested that eye charts with variable contrast targets

would better describe the quality of vision in cataract patients. Such charts are presently available commercially.

A similar investigation of human cataracts was reported by Hess and Woo in 1978.[6] Sensitivity functions were compared with Snellen acuity for ten patients with uniocular senile cataract. Contrast loss occurred in some patients for all measured frequencies and in other patients for only high frequencies. The amount of contrast loss was not related to the type of cataract. High-frequency contrast loss was shown to be similar to simple defocusing of the optical image, whereas low-frequency loss was shown to be far more visually disabling and not correlated with the degree of high-frequency loss. Measurements of acuity give no information regarding the type or the band of frequencies involved in the visual loss.

Glare testing and contrast sensitivity testing can be done in many ways. One innovative approach for evaluating low-contrast vision was reported by researchers who presented subjects with a series of slides picturing human faces.[7] The subjects controlled the amount of contrast for the slides and were measured for their ability to first detect the appearance of a face, then to discriminate between two faces to determine if they were the same or different. (Clinicians will appreciate this unique approach—some patients present to the doctor with complaints of inability to perceive or identify friends under various conditions.) Contrast sensitivity loss in the elderly cannot be explained completely by media opacities. Retinal luminance and

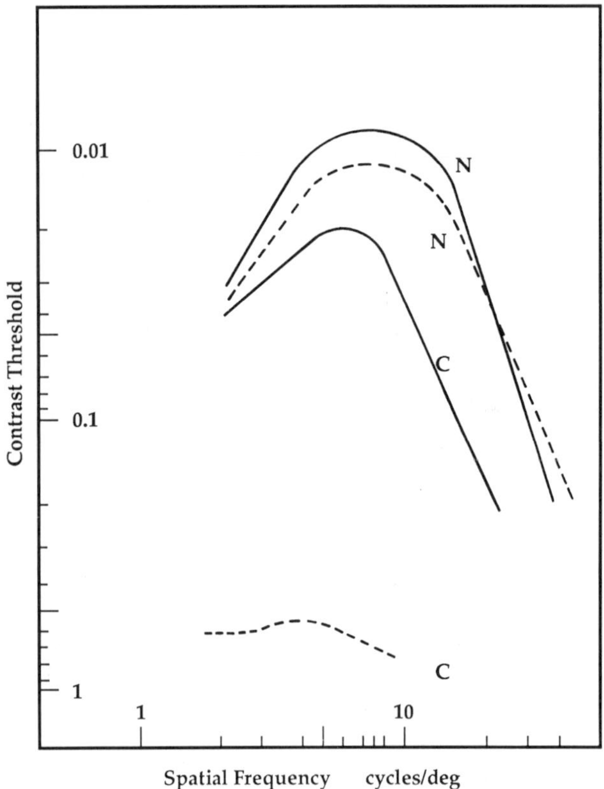

FIGURE 6.3. A typical contrast sensitivity function plotted for a normal subject (N) and a cataract subject (C). The contrast sensitivity function was plotted in the usual fashion and then with a superimposed glare source (dotted line). Contrast sensitivity for the cataract patient is markedly reduced when a glare source is included, e.g., the Brightness Acuity Tester (BAT). (From ref. 10, with permission.)

unidentified neural changes in the senescent visual system almost certainly play a role[7,8] (see Chap. 9).

Contrast Sensitivity Testing and Glare Testing for Cataracts

It is well established that cataracts affect the contrast sensitivity function even in the absence of glare.[6] The Arden grating test, when applied to evaluation of early posterior subcapsular cataracts, sometimes demonstrates profound loss of contrast sensitivity in patients who maintain relatively good high-contrast Snellen acuity.[9] Measurements of contrast sensitivity are often better correlated with patients' complaints than are Snellen acuity measurements.

Including a glare source in contrast sensitivity measurements can result in dramatic effects (see Fig. 6.3). Paulsson and Sjostrand[10] were among the earliest investigators to demonstrate the devastating effect that a glare source can have on the con-

trast sensitivity curve when an early cataract is present. Their initial findings were confirmed in subsequent experiments on larger numbers of cataract patients.[11] Widespread understanding and acceptance of the importance of these findings by the clinical community has been slow in coming because of a general lack of familiarity with the principals of contrast sensitivity testing. Few clinicians routinely test contrast sensitivity.

In an effort to familiarize the clinical community with the importance of this subject, Miller and Nadler collaborated to develop a simple and easily applied glare tester for clinical settings. Their tester is in many ways similar to that described in 1972.[4] It consists of a tabletop slide projector used to display a series of specially prepared 35-mm slides (see Fig. 6.4). Each slide contains a central black Landolt *C* ring surrounded by a gray background that is surrounded by a glare source. On each successive slide the background of the ring is progressively darkened until the orientation of the ring opening can no longer be identified. This represents the contrast threshold.

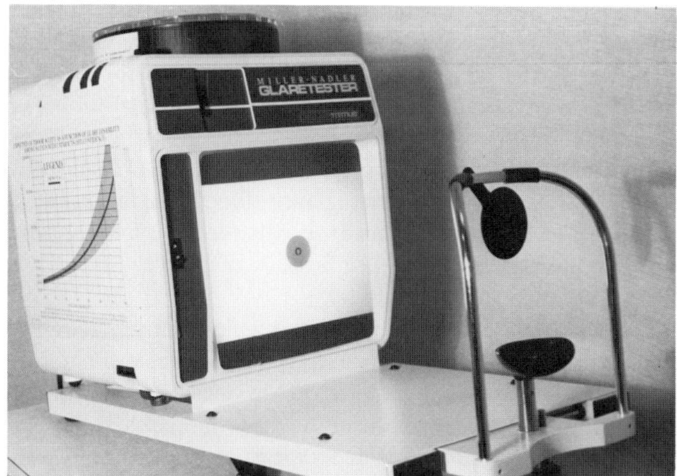
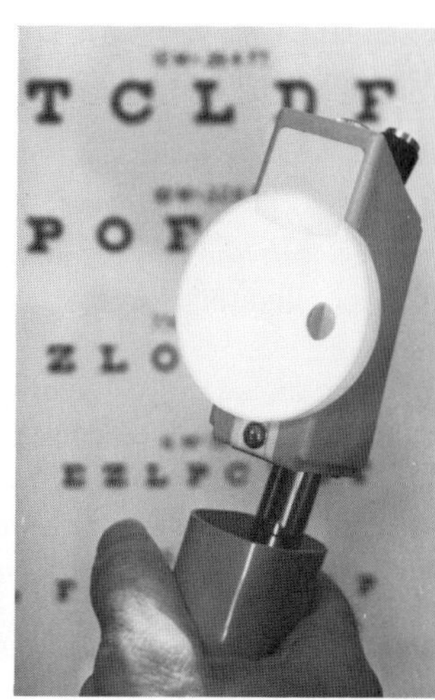

FIGURE 6.4. The Miller-Nadler glare tester (left) quantitates glare disability by measuring contrast sensitivity. The Brightness Acuity Tester (BAT) (right) quantitates glare disability by measuring its effect on Snellen acuity (left, courtesy of Titmus Optical, Inc., Petersburg, VA; right, courtesy of Mentor O&O, Inc., Norwell, MA).

The initial experience with this glare tester was with normal subjects, cataract patients, and patients with aphakia corrected in various ways.[12] The patients with aphakia, regardless of the mode of correction, were more sensitive to glare than were normal subjects. Among the latter, glare increased with age; among cataract patients there was no correlation between near visual acuity and glare sensitivity. LeClaire and co-workers also observed that centrally located subcapsular cataracts were among the most disabling from the standpoint of glare. Cortical spokes encroaching on the visual axis can also produce glare. Pure nuclear sclerosis, however, was not as likely to increase glare sensitivity as were the other forms of opacity.

Subsequent reports on the performance of this glare tester[13,14] established several important findings. Glare scores were significantly better predictors (nearly twice as predictive) of outdoor visual acuity among cataract patients facing the sun than was Snellen acuity. When patients faced away from the sun, however, glare testing was no better at predicting vision outdoors than was measurement of acuity in the refracting lane. Furthermore, results of glare testing with this device were as reproducible as results with acuity testing using standard methods, but were not so adversely affected by uncorrected refractive errors. Undercorrecting presbyopia by as *much as 2 diopters* resulted in

an increase in glare disability score averaging only 4.5% (roughly one slide on the test series).

During the testing process, when the subject finally could not identify any lower contrast targets, an opaque mask with a central target-size hole was placed over the screen to block out the surrounding glare source. The subject was then able to identify multiple additional targets of diminishing contrast (sometimes as low as 5–10% contrast). Thus glare was shown to be the cause of the diminished contrast sensitivity. This finding was so consistent that if a patient showed no multiple target improvement, other causes of impaired contrast sensitivity such as retinal disease (e.g., cystoid macular edema, macular degeneration) and neurologic disease (e.g., glaucoma, multiple sclerosis) were highly suspect.

Other glare testers have subsequently become available that document the need (or lack of need) for surgical intervention when cataracts are present. Presentation of a low-contrast optotype to patients with and without an accompanying glare source has been proposed as a faster and easier to use method for glare determination than measurement of contrast sensitivity function.[15]

The Brightness Acuity Tester (BAT)[16] further simplifies interpretation of glare testing for clinicians and patients by allowing subjects to view the standard eye chart, a familiar target, in the refracting lane (see Fig. 6.4). The glare source on the BAT has an illuminated hemisphere bowl 60 mm in diameter with a 12-mm aperture through which the patient views the eye chart. The bowl is illuminated by a shielded bulb. Three luminance settings are provided to simulate conditions of bright indoor lighting, overcast skies, and bright sunlight.

A problem encountered in comparing results of the various methods of measuring glare is the lack of standardization among these devices (see Chaps. 4 and 10). Sensitivity of the tests will vary depending on the type of target and the brightness and design of the glare source. A similar problem exists with automated perimetry. There is limited value in producing machines that are internally consistent (reproducible) if their results cannot be meaningfully compared with those of other devices intended to measure the same thing. A published comparison of the Miller-Nadler glare tester and the Brightness Acuity Tester[17] illustrates this problem. The two devices showed similar decreases in Snellen acuity when eyes with cataracts were compared; however, the BAT showed greater glare disability than the Miller-Nadler test when eyes with posterior capsule opacities were compared. Personal experience with the BAT suggests that on the "high" luminance setting, patients will usually demonstrate excessive disability when they will score relatively well on the Miller-Nadler test.

Only for the Miller-Nadler glare test and the BAT have data been published associating glare scores with outdoor acuity[13,16] (see Fig. 6.5). Both devices showed good statistical correlation. A more recent investigation[18] using the Miller-Nadler test to correlate glare score and outdoor acuity for different types of cataract found predictability differences for the different types of opacity. Patients with pure nuclear sclerosis often did not have reduced glare scores but did have poor acuity when measured with the Snellen chart outdoors. Although glare scores are sometimes an imprecise predictor of outdoor acuity in cataract patients, they remain *considerably more predictive* than outdoor Snellen acuity. More work needs to be done in developing devices that are accurate predictors of outdoor acuity for all types of cataract and media opacities.

Several recently developed glare testing devices use a *single bright light* just off the visual axis as a glare source.[19] The justification for this is that it most closely simulates certain real-life situations (e.g., oncoming headlights). Past research experience, however, has shown that if subjects even momentarily glance directly at this point source they may inadvertently receive a "photo stress test" that is more a measure of macular function than of glare disability.

Probably one of the most utilized glare tests for evaluating cataracts involves the examiner shining a penlight, held off the visual axis, at the observers eye while he or she reads the eye chart.[20] While this test undoubtedly measures glare disability, it lacks precision and reproducibility. Factors such as the intensity of the penlight, the angle and distance at which it is held, and the ambient room light are all important yet are impossible to standardize and control with this test.

The renewed interest in modern glare testing that has developed over the past ten years has been partially motivated by political and economic factors. Ophthalmology has found itself the object of increased scrutiny from the government and other third-party insurance payors of cataract surgery. The financial incentive for certain surgeons to perform large numbers of cataract procedures has been questioned by a U.S. Senate subcommittee report entitled *Cataract Surgery Fraud, Waste and Abuse*. This procedure has become one of the most common operations performed on elderly individuals today, with well over 1 million operations performed yearly. The large number of operations is due to a variety of factors. Surgical techniques and improved instrumentation have made cataract surgery a highly successful operation. People are living longer, and increasing numbers are demanding good vision to maintain active life-styles.

Nonsurgical Treatment of Cataracts

The high degree of light transmission of the human lens results from the spatial ordering of the lens fibers. As cataracts develop, soluble lens proteins become insoluble. Aggregates of these insoluble proteins destroy the spatial orderliness and are manifested as opacities. These opacities serve to

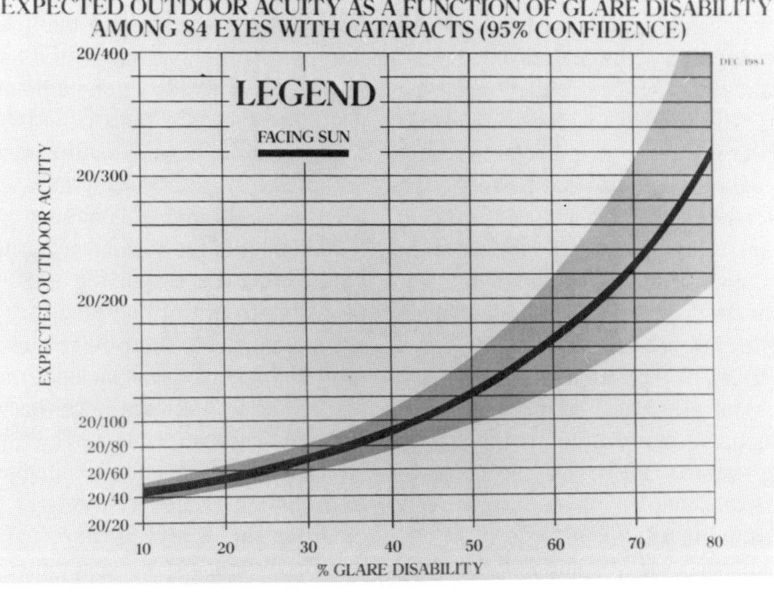

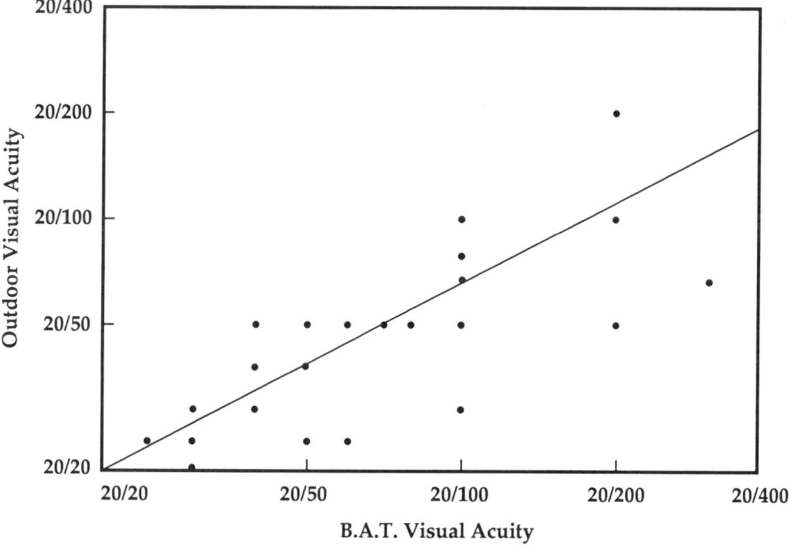

FIGURE 6.5. Only for the Miller-Nadler glare tester (left) and the brightness acuity tester (BAT) (right) have data been published attempting to correlate glare disability with outdoor visual acuity (Snellen) for cataract patients. Both devices are statistically better predictors of outdoor acuity than are measurements of indoor acuity. (Top, from Holladay et al.,[16] used with permission; bottom, courtesy of Titmus Optical, Inc., Petersburg, VA.)

scatter light, reduce contrast, and thus impair vision. Even the noncataractous human lens absorbs light in the blue spectrum and has a distinct yellow color. Absorption increases with age and results in less light being available for retinal imagery.[21] Patients will often observe that their ability to discriminate blues, greens, and purples is reduced or even lost as their lenses brunesce. Elderly women who select a hair color that appears bluish to other observers do so not out of a desire to have blue hair, but because their own color discrimination has been tainted by their brunescent lenses. They think their hair is silver gray. To a certain degree, the image degradation produced by cataracts can be modified with spectacle lenses that change (filter) the light rays before they reach the cataractous lens. This can be done in several ways.

Ultraviolet filters can be helpful for cataract patients.[22] Whereas the normal person can see the electromagnetic spectrum from only 410 to 720 nanometers (nm), ultraviolet light ranging from 310 nm to 410 nm will *induce* a certain fluorescence with a spectral peak of 530 nm on striking the lens. This fluorescence acts as a glowing green light source that bathes the retina with stray light and tends to degrade other focused retinal images. This phenomenon can increase up to three times with advancing age and can be very bothersome when the ultraviolet content of light is strong (e.g., at high altitudes and in snowfields).

Sunglasses can also have a beneficial effect for cataract patients, but the effect is best appreciated in bright environments.[3] When the retinal luminance level is high, the "retinal noise" level is also high, and discrimination of some subtle objects against a background can be difficult. A reduction in overall illumination also reduces retinal noise, and the visual mechanism functions at greater efficiency. Sunglasses also improve the ability to adapt to darkness. Individuals who spend long hours in the sun without sunglasses will have reduced dark adaptation that can last hours and even days.

The color (tint) of sunglasses is of no particular importance except for individuals who have a color deficiency. These persons should be advised to wear gray lenses[23] so that their color deficiency does not worsen.

The overall darkness of sunglasses should ideally depend on the brightness of the environment in which they are used. A transmission level of 10% to 25% is generally recommended for phakic patients in a bright setting; however, in dim illumination the transmission of light ideally should be more. Photochromic sunglasses offer a good solution to this problem. The silver halide crystals embedded in these lenses will change to pure silver and darken when exposed to light. When the light stimulus is removed, the crystals revert to silver halide and the lenses lighten.

Last, a polarizing filter can help reduce glare for both cataract patients and normal individuals. Certain reflecting surfaces such as bodies of water, pavement, automobile hoods, and beaches act as glare sources by reflecting the light in a polarized fashion. This light tends to wash out retinal images. A vertically oriented polarizing filter can neutralize the reflections from these surfaces and reduce stray light, thus improving contrast. Other antireflective coatings on lenses have similarly been shown to improve contrast sensitivity.[24]

A number of the above features have been incorporated in a lens employing a 550-nm cutoff filter (available from Corning Medical Optics[25]). These lenses effectively filter all frequencies below 550 nm (see Fig. 6.6). This includes the UV frequency and its induced fluorescence that can result from UV stimulation of the lens. The Corning lenses are also photochromic and provide optimum levels of transmission related to the light intensity of the environment. The yellow-orange color of these lenses perceptually darkens blues and greens yet allows yellows, oranges, and reds to appear naturally (unfiltered), thus augmenting the contrast of a natural visual scene before it is degraded by the cataract. The effectiveness of the lenses has been quantitated in a laboratory setting[26]: Improvements in acuity of selected patients with cortical cataracts was as great as 300%. Case reports in the literature further support the effectiveness of these lenses.[27]

Contrast Sensitivity Testing and Glare Testing in Pseudophakia

The increasing prevalence of extracapsular cataract surgery and lens implantation has taught us that these procedures and devices are imperfect. Capsular opacification, problems with intraocular lens design, and malpositioned lens implants can all sometimes result in conditions that are no better than the cataracts they replace. Glare and contrast sensitivity testing is often the best means of evaluating patients with complaints related to pseudophakia or aphakia.

In 1977 Miller and Lazenby[28] reported results of glare testing in patients with corrected aphakia using a device similar to the present Miller-Nadler tester. Patients wearing contact lenses, aphakic spectacles, and lens implants were compared with a group of phakic controls. All groups showed

Color Plate V

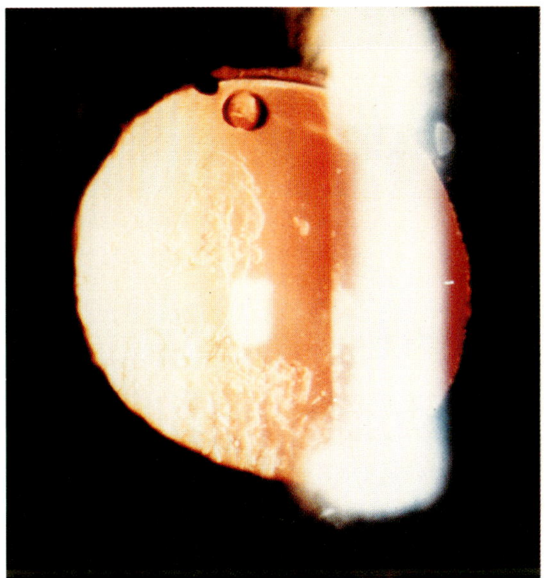 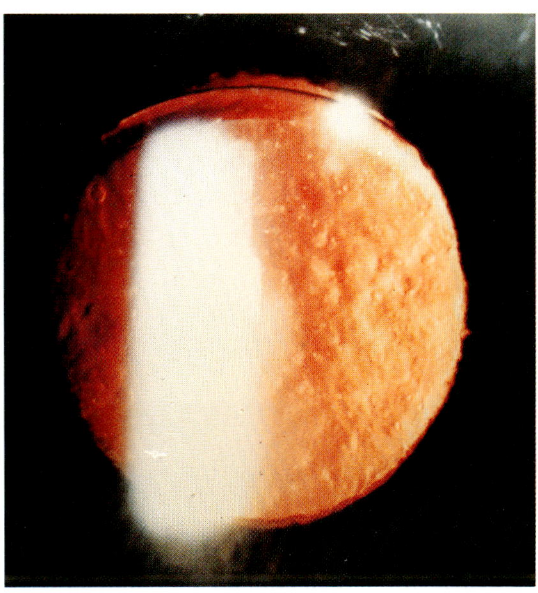

FIGURE 6.7. Elschnig pear information in this patient (left) was outside the visual axis and not visible when the pupil was undilated (acuity 20/20). Progression of pearl formation (right) resulted in a drop in acuity to 20/100. (From SA Obstbaum: The posterior capsule. *Implants in Ophthalmology* **2**(1):111, 1988.)

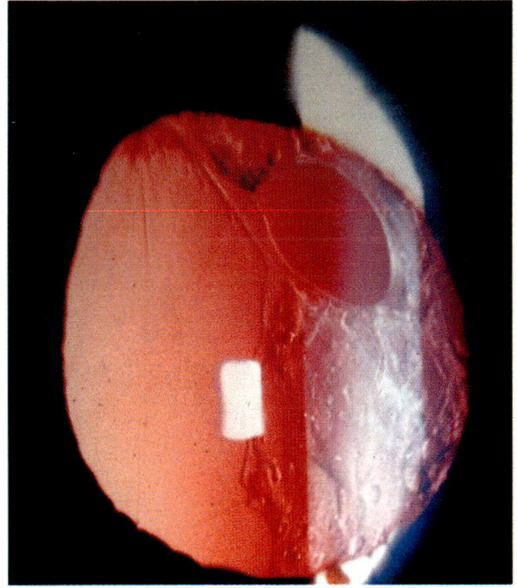 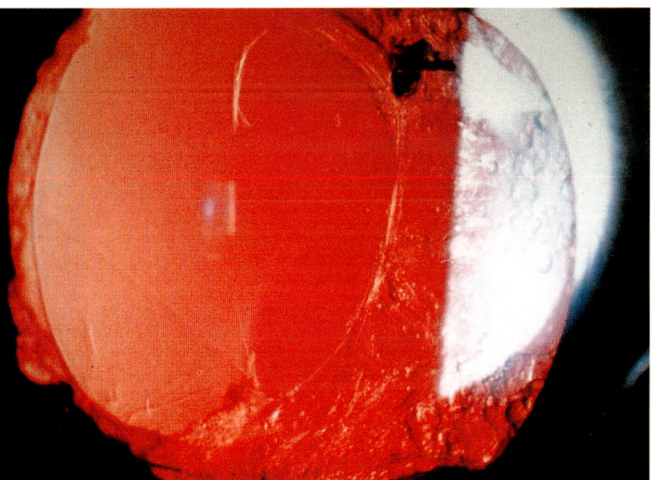

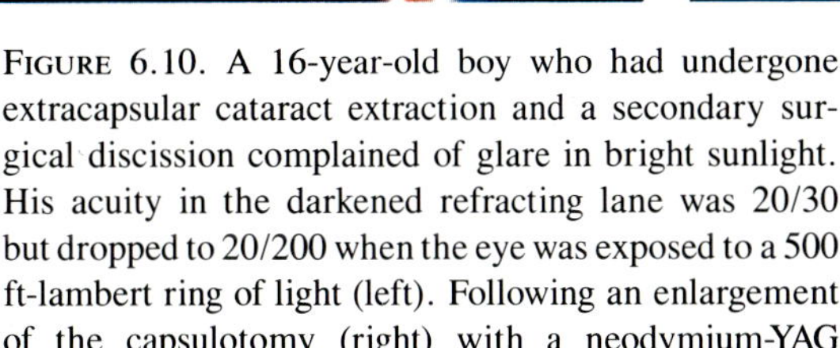

FIGURE 6.10. A 16-year-old boy who had undergone extracapsular cataract extraction and a secondary surgical discission complained of glare in bright sunlight. His acuity in the darkened refracting lane was 20/30 but dropped to 20/200 when the eye was exposed to a 500 ft-lambert ring of light (left). Following an enlargement of the capsulotomy (right) with a neodymium-YAG laser, his acuity improved to 20/25 and dropped to only 20/40 when exposed to a glare light. (From Koch D: The role of glare testing in managing the cataract patient. In *Focal Points 1988: Clinical Modules for Ophthalmologists*, American Academy of Ophthalmology, vol. 6, mod 4. San Francisco, American Academy of Ophthalmology, 1988.)

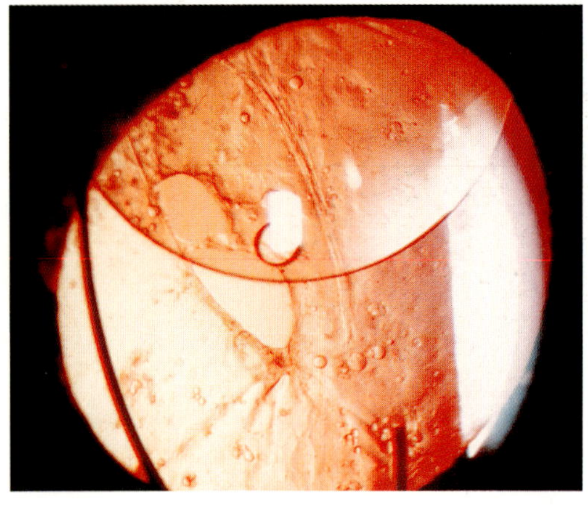

FIGURE 6.11. A 45-year-old man complained of glare and multiple images at night. His decentered implant exposed a positioning hole and optic edge in the visual axis. Although treatment with miotics partially improved his symptoms, the associated dimming of vision was unacceptable to him and ultimately the lens was repositioned surgically and a posterior capsulotomy was done. (From Koch D: The role of glare testing in managing the cataract patient. In *Focal Points 1988: Clinical Modules for Ophthalmologists*, American Academy of Ophthalmology, vol. 6, mod 4. San Francisco, American Academy of Ophthalmology, 1988.)

FIGURE 6.12. (*below*) Discrete striations in the posterior capsule seen by directed illumination (left) and retroillumination (right) can result in glare and unwanted images. If the capsule becomes thickened in the troughs of these striations, the patient will have symptoms suggesting an intraocular "Maddox rod." (From Obstbaum SA: The posterior capsule. *Implants in Ophthalmology* 2(1):111, 1988.)

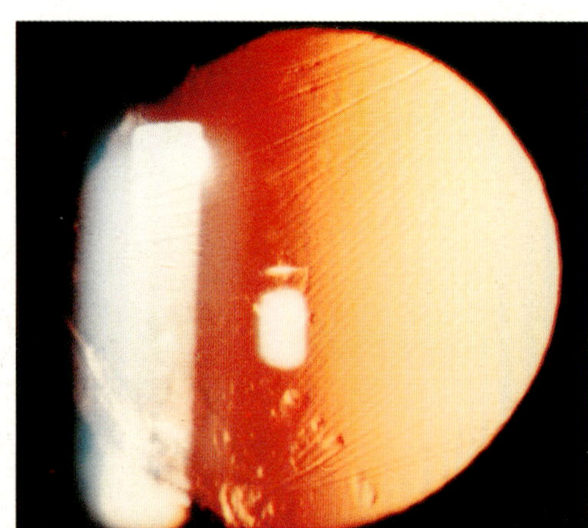

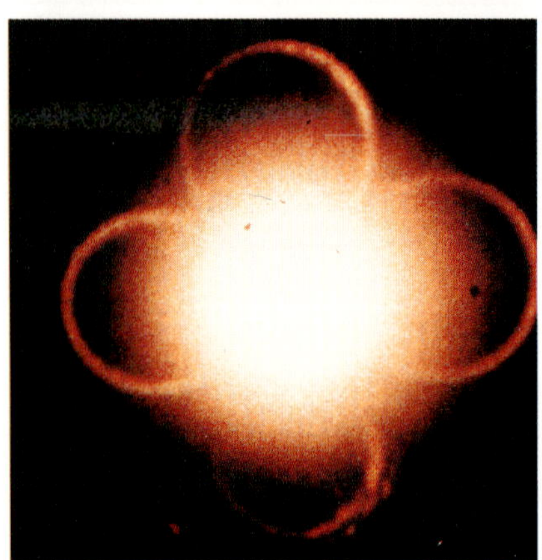

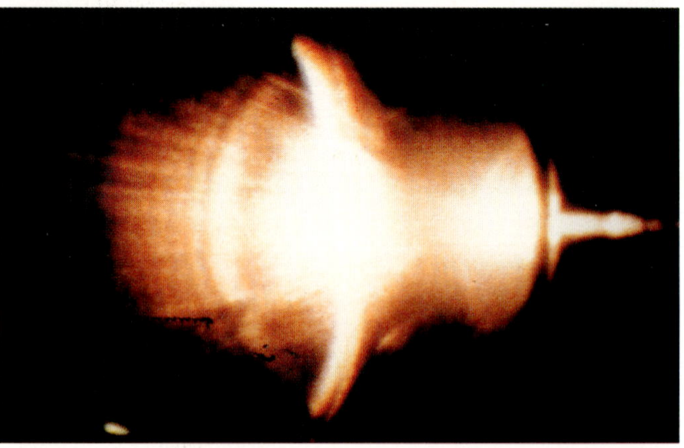

FIGURE 6.13. Photographic illustration of an experimental model designed to illustrate the unwanted images that can result from exposed positioning holes (left) and decentered lens implants with edges in the visual axis (right). These patients may score well on conventional glare tests but may be extremely bothered by these images. (Courtesy of Iolab Corporation)

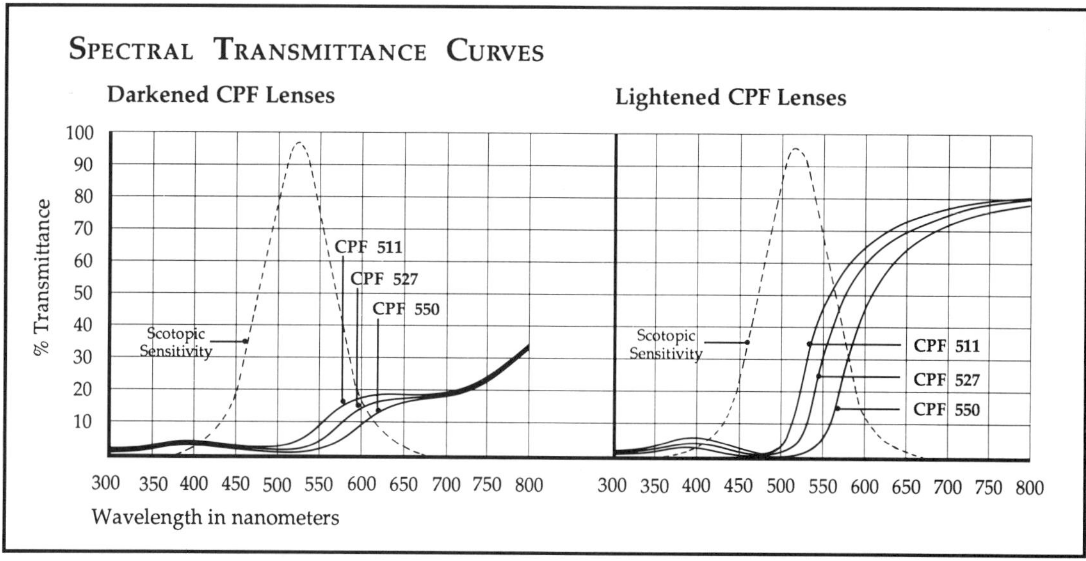

FIGURE 6.6. Spectral transmission curves for the Corning CPF lenses. The lenses are photochromic and can be obtained in three different cutoff frequencies (511 nm, 527 nm, 550 nm). Cutoff frequency selection is based on symptoms, diagnosis, and results with trial lenses. (Courtesy of Corning Medical Optics, Technical Products Division, Corning Glassworks, Corning, New York.)

comparable glare sensitivity, but six patients who had had extracapsular extractions resulting in capsular opacification were statistically more glare sensitive. This subgroup would not have been detected by Snellen acuity measurements alone, because their average acuity was 20/40.

Results comparing aphakic spectacle patients, patients with Copeland-style plastic lens implants, those with Lynell glass lens implants, and normal phakic subjects[12] using the Miller-Nadler tester showed that the patients with corrected aphakia were all more glare sensitive than the phakic controls. The patients had undergone intracapsular cataract extraction, so capsular opacification would not explain the differences. However, both styles of lens implant were of the iris-supported variety, which can sometimes demonstrate optical edges in the pupillary area and produce intraocular light scattering.

In another study, four pseudophakic eyes with a clear visual axis showed 2.3 times more light scattering than normal phakic eyes.[24] Differences in refractive index of the lens implants (1.492) versus the mean value of the human lens (1.386) have been offered as a possible explanation for this observation. Another possibility lies in the structure of the human lens. Its refractive index increases gradually toward the core, an optical feature minimizing reflections.

Contrast sensitivity measurements of pseudophakic eyes have nicely illustrated the inadequacies of Snellen acuity measurements. Hess, Woo, and White[30] evaluated nine patients with iris clip lens implants. Seven patients showed large and highly significant losses of contrast sensitivity. The spatial frequencies affected were variable and were not predictable from conventional acuity testing.

With visual loss due to optical anomalies, any threshold loss can have consequences for suprathreshold contrast targets. If the contrast threshold is raised by a factor of 10, suprathreshold contrast will be similarly reduced (a 100% contrast target will be perceptually reduced to 10%) (see Fig. 6.1).

Contrast loss in pseudophakic eyes is probably not related to lens style. Weatherill and Yap[31] found no differences among 73 patients receiving anterior-chamber iris-supported or posterior-chamber intraocular lenses. This is not to suggest that different styles of intraocular lenses are comparable under all conditions. A photographic comparison demonstrated that the scattered light from a four-loop Binkhorst anterior-chamber lens

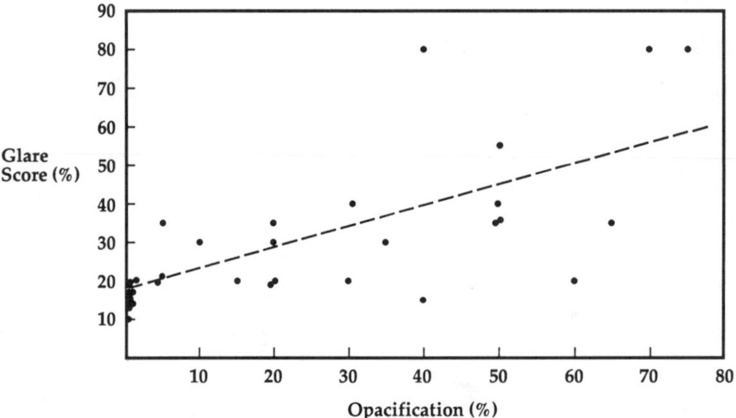

FIGURE 6.8. Glare score (percent contrast needed) plotted as a function of posterior capsule opacification in 32 pseudophakic subjects. Glare disability using the Miller-Nadler glare tester was highly correlated with degree of posterior capsule opacification: $r = .72$, $p < .00001$. (From ref. 34. Published with permission from *The American Journal of Ophthalmology*. Copyright by The Ophthalmic Publishing Company.)

exceeded that produced by a Kratz elliptical posterior-chamber lens.[32] The ends of the loops of the Binkhorst lens are situated in the pupillary axis and can act as tiny light pipes under certain angles of illumination (this can be easily demonstrated at the slit lamp).

The contrast sensitivity of patients receiving ultraviolet-absorbing lens implants has not been demonstrated to differ from that of patients receiving non-UV-absorbing lenses,[33] at least in the short term. UV-absorbing lenses do show different transmission patterns from clear crystalline lenses, and these transmission differences are accentuated when compared with crystalline lenses with nuclear sclerosis. These findings should not be interpreted as suggesting that there are no benefits to UV absorption, as the effects on the macula remain unanswered. However, one might reasonably speculate that the ideal intraocular lens should mimic the crystalline lens in spectral transmission characteristics.

Presently, from a clinician's viewpoint the most common cause of glare disability or impaired contrast sensitivity in pseudophakic patients is due to capsular opacification (see Fig. 6.7; see Color Plate V). The first effort to correlate the amount of capsular opacification with glare disability was published by Nadler and associates.[34] A group of patients receiving extracapsular cataract extraction and posterior chamber lens implants with intact capsules were examined 7 to 41 months postopera-

tively. They showed a highly statistically significant association between glare score and degree of opacification (see Fig. 6.8). The nature of the opacification was found to be important. Mild to moderate nonuniform clouding and Elschnig pearl formation on the capsule produce more intraocular light scattering than do dense fibrous plaques, which serve mainly to attenuate the light. Plaques are the greatest problem when they are within the pupillary aperture. Drill holes and edges from decentered lens implants were also shown to produce glare disability.

An investigation of patients examined 6 to 12 weeks after surgery and studied with both the Miller-Nadler glare tester and the Baylor visual function tester[35] produced statistically similar glare scores but results were generally less affected by glare due to the short postoperative period (most capsular clouding is not present immediately after surgery). Koch and colleagues further demonstrated no measurable differences between spheric and aspheric intraocular lenses (IOLs) and no measurable advantage of UV filtration using the above glare testers.

The widespread availability of the neodymium-YAG laser has greatly simplified the management of capsular opacification. Investigators from the Bascom Palmer Eye Institute[36] documented the substantial improvements in both glare score (using the Miller-Nadler test) and Snellen acuity following YAG capsulotomies. The authors could

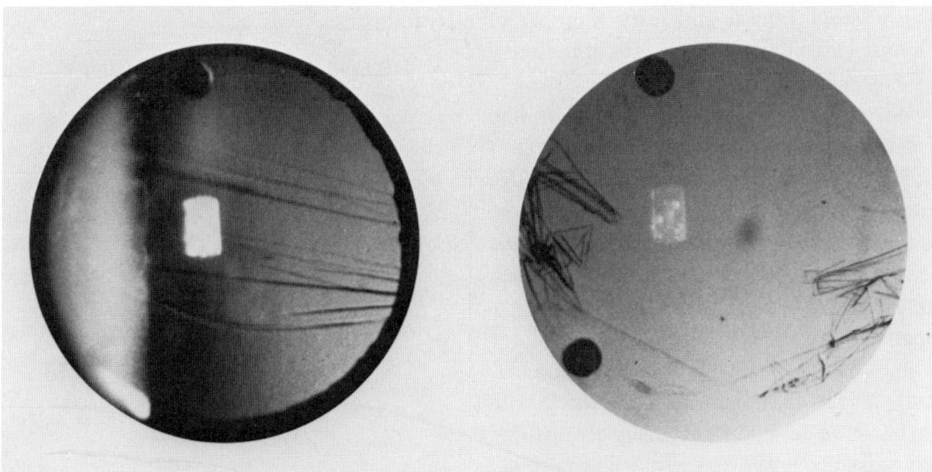

FIGURE 6.9. Intact posterior capsule with wrinkles (left) caused a patient to experience streaks around bright lights. This patient scored well with the Miller-Nadler glare tester. His bothersome symptoms were relieved by a laser capsulotomy (right). (From RK Parrish: Glare measurements before and after neodymium-YAG laser posterior capsulotomy. *Amer J Ophthalmol* **100**:712, 1985. Published with permission from The American Journal of Opththalmology. Copyright by The Ophthalmic Publishing Company.)

not recommend minimum glare thresholds to serve as an indication for capsulotomy, as some patients were more disturbed by capsular imperfections than others (see Fig. 6.9).

The optimal size of a posterior capsulotomy has been addressed by Holladay, Bishop, and Lewis.[37] Strict guidelines are not practical because of individual variations in pupil size under photopic and scotopic conditions. Theoretically, larger capsulotomies are advantageous because they will not limit acuity by diffraction and will allow the pupil to regulate image intensity (see Fig. 6.10; see Color Plate V). In general the posterior capsulotomy should equal or exceed the diameter of the pupil in scotopic conditions and remain within the border of the IOL. A capsulotomy extending beyond the edge of the implant may result in vitreous prolapse around the lens and potential complications more serious than glare.

Treatment of opacified capsules with the YAG laser is not totally without risk. When an intraocular lens is present, damage to the implant reportedly has an incidence of approximately 30%.[38] Frequently the small defects or "pits" caused by the laser are not bothersome, but case reports of two patients requiring IOL exchange to alleviate symptoms of extensive lens damage have been published.[39] One of these patients received a total of 216 bursts ranging from 0.5 to 5 millijoules (mJ) in two treatment sessions. YAG procedures should include minimizing the laser energy, maximizing the focus (with a contact lens), and shifting the point of optical breakdown posteriorly to avoid IOL damage. While injection-molded implants have been shown to be more prone to YAG laser damage, the defects in lathe-cut lenses have a greater potential for light polarization[40] and possible glare-related problems (although this has not been established as clinically important).

The problem of glare related to lens decentration is more difficult to manage than capsular opacification (see Fig. 6.11; see Color Plate VI). While lasers are good for opening capsules they are rarely helpful in repositioning IOLs. Lens decentration is not an uncommon problem. One autopsy review of 75 eyes with posterior chamber intraocular lenses observed that in 71% of cases a lens edge or element of the optic, such as a positioning hole, was situated either within the pupillary aperture or within 0.5 mm of the pupillary margin.[41] In 92% of the decentered lenses, one haptic was placed in the ciliary sulcus and the other in the capsular bag. The recent widespread availability and use of viscoelastic substances has probably served to reduce the incidence of asymmetric haptic placement. Furthermore, consideration of certain factors in the design of intraocular lenses will help reduce the problems of lens decentration when it occurs. Large lens diameters, fewer or no positioning holes, and possibly a matte finish for the edge of the lens implant are all potential means of reducing problems associated with decentered lenses.

Even well-centered lenses can create glare and other visual symptoms if, during periods of maximum pupillary dilation, portions of the lens edge or positioning holes are exposed. A 58-year-old pilot required lens exchange because his scotopic pupil measured 6 mm, exposing three drill holes. The resultant visual symptoms forced him to leave his occupation until the lens was exchanged.[42]

The symptoms of exposed lens elements and certain capsular defects are not always measurable with conventional glare or contrast sensitivity testing. Clinicians must be careful not to dismiss patients' complaints simply because they score well on a glare tester. The observation of light streaks similar to those seen with a Maddox rod or a Bagolini lens can result from spindle-shaped deposits of epithelial cells on the posterior capsule or with wrinkling of the capsule and thickening of the capsule in the troughs of these wrinkles (which creates an intraocular Maddox rod)[43] (see Fig. 6.12; see Color Plate VI). Other causes of light streaks include scratched intraocular lenses, scratched spectacles, eyelashes in the visual axis, and an enlarged tear meniscus.

A laboratory study entitled "Unwanted Optical Images Created by Posterior Chamber Intraocular Lenses" conducted by Iolab Corporation[43] photographically illustrates how exposed lens elements (such as positioning holes, annular ridges, and posterior optic bosses) may create visual symptoms (see Fig. 6.13; see Color Plate VI). Glare and contrast sensitivity testing may be helpful in detecting and quantitating these symptoms, but such testing is no more important than a careful history and detailed ocular examination.

Most clinicians realize that the value of glare testing and contrast sensitivity testing in cataract and pseudophakic patients lies in the ability of these tests to document and quantitate legitimate disability when standard vision testing does not. These devices were never intended to "create" disability for asymptomatic patients. The impact of patients' visual complaints on their desired lifestyle remains the bottom line in the decision to perform cataract surgery or laser capsulotomy.

Acknowledgment. I wish to thank Patty Miller for her help in preparing this manuscript and Saul Weiss for preparing the illustrations.

References

1. Bernstein G: *Thurber: A Biography.* New York, Dodd Mead & Co, 1975, pp 275–276.
2. Holladay LL: The fundamentals of glare and visibility. *J Opt Soc Am* **12**:271–319, 1926.
3. Miller D, Nadler D: Glare disability: Its measurement and correction. *Ophthalmol Ann* **3**:101, 1987.
4. Miller D, Jernigan M, Molnar S, et al: Laboratory evaluation of a clinical glare tester. *Arch Ophthalmol* **87**:324–332, 1972.
5. Zuckerman JL, Miller D, Dyer W, et al: Degradation of vision through a simulated cataract. *Invest Ophthalmol* **12**:213–224, 1973.
6. Hess R, Woo G: Vision through cataracts. *Invest Ophthalmol* **17**:428–435, 1978.
7. Owsley C, Sekuler R, Boldt D: Aging and low-contrast vision: Face perception. *Invest Ophthalmol* **21**:362–365, 1981.
8. Owsley C, Gardner T, Sekuler R: Role of the crystalline lens in the spatial vision loss of the elderly. *Invest Ophthalmol* **26**:1165–1170, 1985.
9. Skalka H: Arden grating test in evaluating "early" posterior subcapsular cataracts. *South Med J* **74**:1368–1370, 1981.
10. Paulsson L, Sjostrand J: Contrast sensitivity in the presence of a glare light. *Invest Ophthalmol* **19**:401–406, 1980.
11. Abrahamson M, Sjostrand J: Impairment of contrast sensitivity function as a measure of disability glare. *Invest Ophthalmol* **27**:1131–1136, 1986.
12. LeClaire J, Nadler MP, Weiss S, et al: A new glare tester for clinical testing: Results comparing normal subjects and variously corrected aphakic patients. *Arch Ophthalmol* **100**:153–158, 1982.
13. Hirsch R, Nadler MP, Miller D: Glare measurement as a prediction of outdoor vision among cataract patients. *Ann Ophthalmol* **16**:965–968, 1984.
14. Hirsch R, Nadler MP, Miller D: Clinical performance of a disability glare tester. *Arch Ophthalmol* **102**:1633–1636, 1984.
15. Sjostrand J, Abrahamson M, Hard A-L: Glare disability as a cause of deterioration of vision in cataract patients. *Acta Ophthalmol* **65**:103–106, 1987.
16. Holladay JT, Prager TC, Irajillo J, et al: Brightness acuity tester and outdoor visual acuity in cataract patients. *J Catar Refract Surg* **13**:67–69, 1987.
17. Smith P, Pratzer K, Webster N, et al: A clinical comparison of two methods of glare testing. *Ophthal Surg* **18**:680–682, 1987.
18. Neumann A, McCarty G, Steedle T, et al: The relationship between cataract type and glare disability as measured by the Miller-Nadler glare tester. *J Catar Refract Surg* **14**:40–45, 1988.
19. Koch D: The role of glare testing in managing the cataract patient. In *Focal Points 1988: Clinical*

Modules for Ophthalmologists, American Academy of Ophthalmology, vol 6, mod 4. San Francisco, American Academy of Ophthalmology, 1988.

20. Maltzman B, Horan C, Rengel A: Penlight test for glare disability of cataracts. *J Ophthal Nurs Technol* 7:137–139, 1988.

21. Trokel S: The physical basis for transparency of the crystalline lens. *Invest Ophthalmol* 1:493–501, 1962.

22. Miller D: The effect of sunglasses on the visual mechanism. *Surv Ophthalmol* 19:38–44, 1974.

23. Clark BAJ: Color in sunglasses. *Am J Optom* **46**: 825–840, 1969.

24. Coupland S, Kirkham T: Improved contrast sensitivity with antireflective coated lenses in the presence of glare. *Can J Ophthalmol* 16:136–140, 1981.

25. Corning's CPM$_{TM}$ 550 spectacles: Corning Glassworks, Technical Products Division. Corning, NY: OPM-40-20M-MP 386.

26. Tupper B, Miller D, Miller R: The effect of a 550 nm cutoff filter on the vision of cataract patients. *Ann Ophthalmol* 17:67–72, 1985.

27. Rutkowsky W: Light filtering lenses as an alternative to cataract surgery. *J Am Optom Assoc* 58:640–641, 1987.

28. Miller D, Lazenby G: Glare sensitivity in corrected aphakes. *Ophthal Surg* 8:54–57, 1977.

29. Heijde G, Weber J, Boukes R: Effects of stray light on visual acuity in pseudophakia. *Docu Ophthalmol* 59:81–84, 1985.

30. Hess R, Woo G, White P: Contrast attenuation characteristics of iris clipped intraocular lens implants in situ. *Br J Ophthalmol* 69:129–135, 1985.

31. Weatherill J, Yap M: Contrast sensitivity in pseudophakia and aphakia. *Ophthalmol Physiol Optics* 6: 297–301, 1986.

32. Aust W: Streulicht bei implantierten Kunststofflinsen im Modellversuch. *Klin Mbl Augenheilk* **188**: 69–71, 1986.

33. Hammer H, Yap M, Weatherill J: Visual performance in pseudophakia with standard and ultraviolet-absorbing intraocular lenses: A preliminary report. *Trans Ophthalmol Soc UK* **105**:441–446, 1986.

34. Nadler D, Jaffe N, Clayman H, et al: Glare disability in eyes with intraocular lenses. *Am J Ophthalmol* **97**: 43–47, 1984.

35. Koch D, Emery J, Jardeleza T, et al: Glare following posterior chamber lens implantation. *J Catar Refract Surg* **12**:480–484, 1986.

36. Knighton R, Slomovic A, Parrish RK: Glare measurements before and after neodymium-YAG laser posterior capsulotomy. *Am J Ophthalmol* **100**:708–713, 1985.

37. Holladay J, Bishop J, Lewis J: The optimal size of a posterior capsulotomy. *Am Intra-Oc Implant Soc J* **11**:18–20, 1985.

38. Stark WJ, Worthen D, Holladay JT, et al: Neodymium-YAG lasers; an FDA report. *Ophthalmology* **92**:209–212, 1985.

39. Bath PE, Hoffer K, Aron-Rosa D, et al: Glare disability secondary to YAG laser intraocular lens damage. *J Catar Refract Surg* **13**:309–313, 1987.

40. Path PE, Dang Y, Martin W: Comparison of glare in YAG-damaged intraocular lenses: Injection molded versus lathe-cut. *J Catar Refract Surg* **12**:662–664, 1986.

41. Brems R, Apple D, Pfeffer B, et al: Posterior chamber intraocular lenses in a series of 75 autopsy eyes. 3. Correlation of positioning holes and optic edges with the pupillary aperture and visual axis. *J Catar Refract Surg* **12**:367–371, 1986.

42. Apple D, Lichtenstein S, Heerlein K, et al: Visual aberrations caused by optic components of posterior chamber intraocular lenses. *J Catar Refract Surg* **13**:431–435, 1987.

43. Holladay JT, Bishop J, Lewis J: Diagnosis and treatment of mysterious light streaks seen by patients following extracapsular cataract extraction. *Am Intra-Oc Implant Soc J* **11**:21–23, 1985.

44. Unwanted optical images created by posterior chamber intraocular lenses. *Iolab*, 2153-3/86-992, 1986.

7
Diabetes Mellitus and Visual Function

Jerry D. Cavallerano and Lloyd M. Aiello

Introduction

The National Diabetes Advisory Board reports that nearly 6 million Americans have been diagnosed with diabetes mellitus. An additional 5 million Americans are estimated to have undiagnosed diabetes.[1] The majority of the latter has non-insulin-dependent diabetes mellitus (NIDDM), with a strong likelihood of having some degree of diabetic retinal disease at the time of diagnosis.

Diabetes, with its attendant diabetic retinopathy, remains the leading cause of new legal blindness in the United States for individuals between the ages of 20 and 74 years.[1] Blindness results from either proliferative diabetic retinopathy and its complications or from diabetic macular edema. There are presently an estimated 200,000 Americans with diabetic macular edema (DME) who are at risk of moderate visual loss (best corrected vision at the 20/200 level). Another 200,000 have proliferative diabetic retinopathy (PDR) without macular edema and are at risk for severe visual loss (best corrected vision at the 5/200 level). An estimated 200,000 individuals have both PDR and DME and are at risk for both moderate and severe visual loss.[2,3] This risk can be reduced by approximately 50% if timely panretinal laser photocoagulation or focal laser treatment is initiated, according to the established guidelines of the Diabetic Retinopathy Study and the Early Treatment Diabetic Retinopathy Study.[3]

While the relationship between diabetes mellitus and blindness is well established, many health practitioners do not recognize that diabetes sometimes poses more subtle disturbances in a person's vision.

These effects frequently remain unmentioned by the patient and unrecognized and untreated by the doctor. Specifically, diabetic eye disease or the treatment for diabetic retinopathy may result in alterations in visual function that are difficult to measure or monitor objectively. Clinically, we can categorize some of these alterations as glare disability, decreased visual function, reduction of contrast sensitivity, and decreased color sensitivity.

Difficulties in visual function may make it impossible for a person with 20/20 vision to drive at night, correctly interpret color shades, or read fine print. Such an individual may experience difficulty in dark or light adaptation or gross loss of visual field or fine disturbance in image size or shape while performing near-vision tasks. The person may be unable to perform tasks of daily living or maintain gainful employment, even while consistently showing a Snellen visual acuity of 20/20 or better.

This chapter discusses visual function problems resulting from diabetes and from the treatment of diabetic retinopathy. The importance of considering these visual disturbances in the decision to treat or withhold treatment in the presence of diabetic macular edema will be discussed. Possible ocular sources of these visual disturbances, as well as potential remedies for them, also will be presented.

What Is Visual Function?

Several terms and concepts need to be defined before we discuss diabetic effects on visual function. Visual function refers to a person's ability to use his or her eyes to perform particular tasks. Eleanore Ebert and her study group[4] measure functional vision as a person's ability to identify correctly currency denomination and color, to read a clock accurately, and to read large print comfortably.[4] Visual function, however, goes beyond the level of visual acuity alone. It takes into consideration the task a person is performing, the effects of ambient light, the level of a person's color vision, the extent of the visual field, and even the posture a person must assume to perform a given task.

Unfortunately, visual function is not a parameter that can be measured easily in a laboratory or examination room. The components contributing to visual function are numerous, varied, and interrelated. Visual acuity is certainly one component. Hue discrimination is another. Clearly, the effects of glare and light sensitivity need to be factored into the equation of visual function.

Two major components dealing with visual function include *glare* and *contrast sensitivity*. Webster's dictionary defines glare as a "strong usually unpleasant light, as from sunlight reflected from a shiny surface." Anyone who has tried to read with a bright light reflected from a glossy page knows how debilitating glare can become. There are several factors related to the ocular effects of diabetes and the treatment for diabetic retinopathy that contribute to glare, as will be discussed here.

The effects of glare impact on contrast sensitivity. It is reasonable to expect that if we establish an accurate and easily obtainable measurement of contrast sensitivity, we may obtain a useful index of visual function. If we add to this contrast sensitivity measurement an evaluation of color vision and performance on an Amsler grid testing chart, we will have a more complete understanding of visual function, although we are still unable to fully measure visual function itself.

One method to attempt to measure the effects of glare is to measure *contrast sensitivity*. Although the measurement of contrast sensitivity is by no means new,[5] Vistech Inc. has recently introduced an inexpensive, easy-to-administer pasteboard chart for doing so[6] (Fig. 7.1). Test charts are available for both near and distance measurements. The charts consist of five rows of circles containing sinusoidal gratings of different spatial frequencies. Nine columns make up each row, with gradually decreasing contrast of the targets going from left to right on the chart. The orientation of the gratings varies from straight vertical to slightly left or slightly right. Under controlled illumination and with best correction, a patient is asked to identify the orientation of the gratings. The targets become smaller as the patient works down the charts, and the contrast is diminished as the patient works to the right on the chart.

A range of normal and a conversion chart to indicate a patient's function expressed in comparable Snellen acuity levels are provided by the manufacturer. By measuring contrast sensitivity, therefore, we are measuring more than the ability to recognize sharp boundaries or high-contrast targets; in essence, by measuring contrast sensitivity we are measuring the ability to detect slight changes of luminance in targets without high border contrast.

Another test to measure contrast sensitivity is the Pelli-Robson letter-sensitivity chart.[7] The Pelli-Robson chart uses letters that all subtend an angle of 0.5 degree at 3 m. The letters are arranged in groups of three, and each subsequent group has a lower contrast. The observer's threshold log contrast is measured by determining the group in which he or she is last able to identify two of the three letters in the group. A key is then used to calculate the observer's log contrast sensitivity threshold.

Visual Function and Diabetic Retinopathy

At present no cure is known for diabetic retinopathy or diabetic macular edema. The Diabetic Retinopathy Study (DRS), however, demonstrated that panretinal photocoagulation can reduce the risk of severe visual acuity loss by at least 50%.[8] The Early Treatment Diabetic Retinopathy Study (ETDRS) demonstrated that properly applied focal laser photocoagulation reduces the risk of moderate visual acuity loss by 50% compared with indefinite withholding of laser treatment.[9]

Focal laser treatment for macular edema and panretinal laser photocoagulation, however, do have side effects that may change visual acuity and visual function.[10] The survey of Russell, Sekuler, and Fetkenhour illustrates that patients who had panretinal laser photocoagulation recognized a

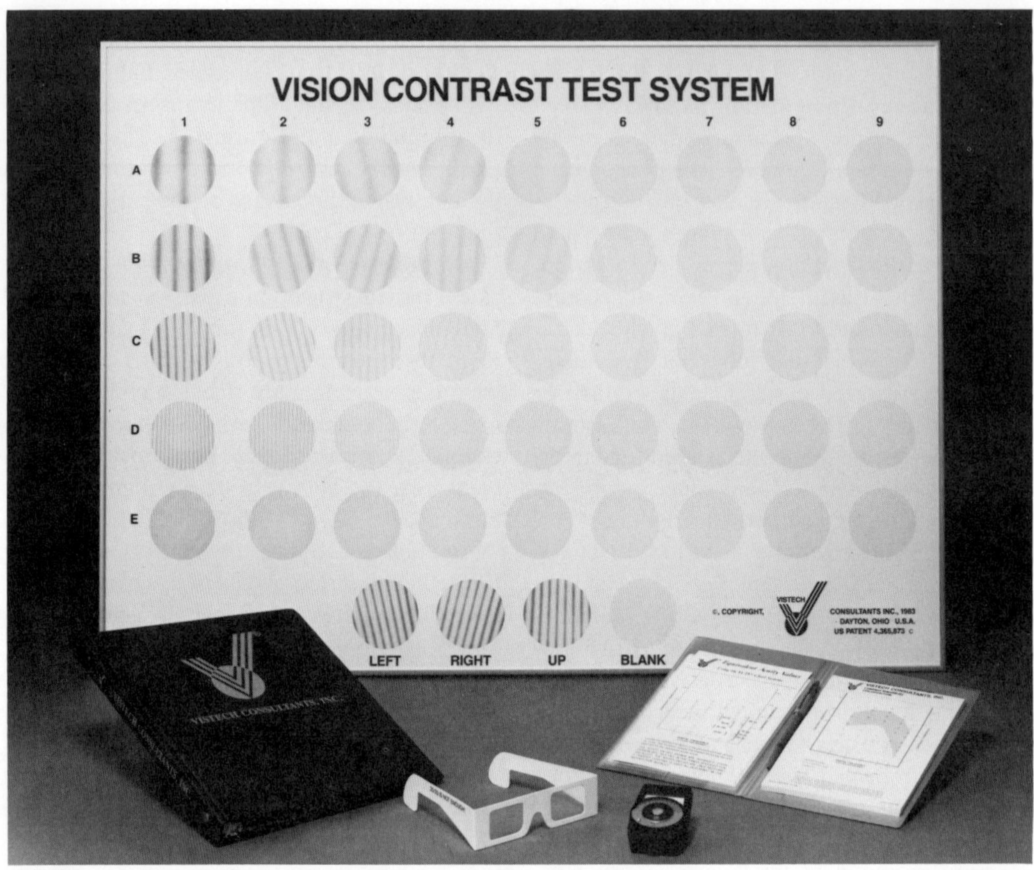

FIGURE 7.1. Vistech's distance contrast sensitivity chart and testing system. (Reproduced with permission of Vistech Consultants, Inc., Dayton, Ohio.)

distinct subjective change in visual function, evidenced by difficulty in adjusting to both bright and dim lights, in judging distances, and in accurately identifying colors (Table 7.1). Such changes were not always correlated with decreased acuity as measured on Snellen acuity charts.

Results of the DRS show that panretinal photocoagulation as applied according to study guidelines could result in a minor loss of visual acuity and constriction of peripheral visual field. Eyes treated with xenon-arc photocoagulation showed a more substantial loss of visual field.[8] The ETDRS demonstrated small but statistically insignificant differences in central visual field scores resulting from focal laser treatment. No treatment differences in color vision as measured by the Farnsworth-Munsell 100-hue test were found between the treated group and the untreated group.[9]

An understanding of visual function in relation to diabetic retinopathy can be valuable on a number of levels. Perhaps through the measurement of contrast sensitivity and/or color vision, in conjunction with conventional visual acuity readings, we might come to better understand the natural history of diabetic eye disease. This understanding could enhance our ability to predict diabetic retinal changes through the measurements of some visual function parameters. Furthermore, the measurement of visual function elements may be instrumental in determining the most appropriate time to intervene in treating diabetic macular edema according to the guidelines of the ETDRS.[11-13] The measurement of contrast sensitivity and color vision, in conjunction with visual acuity measurements and Amsler grid testing, provides a comprehensive means of monitoring a patient's progress,

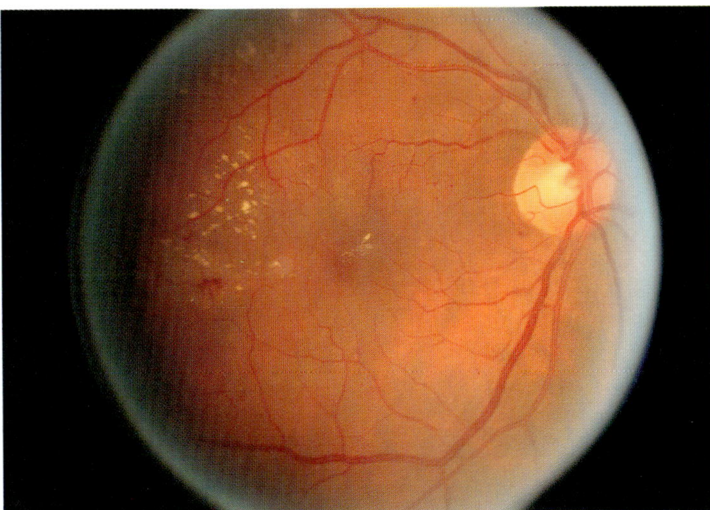

FIGURE 7.2. Eyes of a 54-year-old patient with insulin-dependent diabetes for 18 years. (A) Right eye with retinal thickening more than 500 μ from center of the macula with hard exudates less than 500 μ from center of the macula. Visual acuity is 20/15.

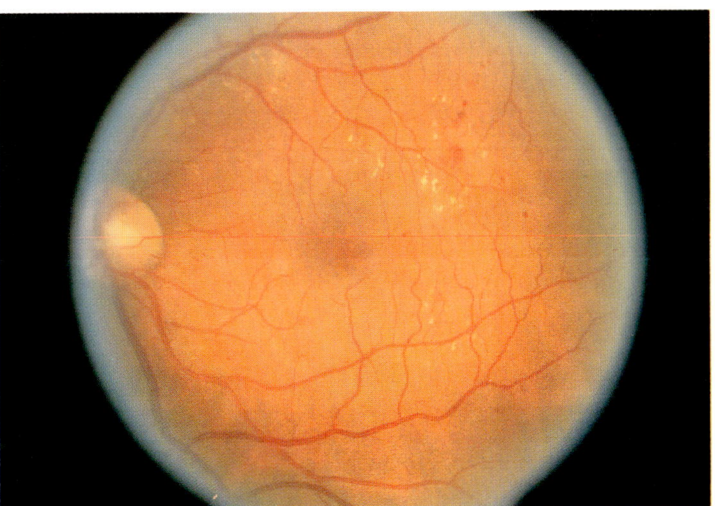

FIGURE 7.2 (B). Left eye with retinal thickening more than 500 μ and less than 1 disk diameter from center of the macula with hard exudates more than 500 μ from center of the macula. Visual acuity is 20/13.

Color Plate VIII

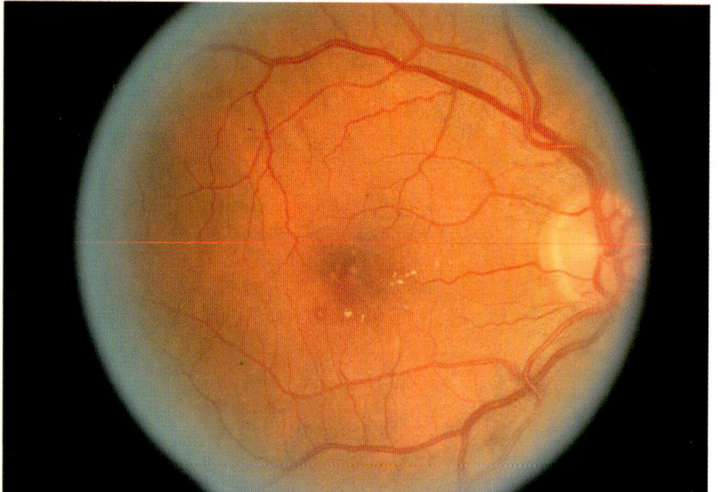

FIGURE 7.3. Eyes of a 58-year-old patient with insulin-dependent diabetes for 18 years. (A) Right eye showing drusen in the macular area with minimal retinal thickening less than 500 μ from the center of the macula. Waxy exudates are present less than 500·μ from center of the macula. Visual acuity is 20/15.

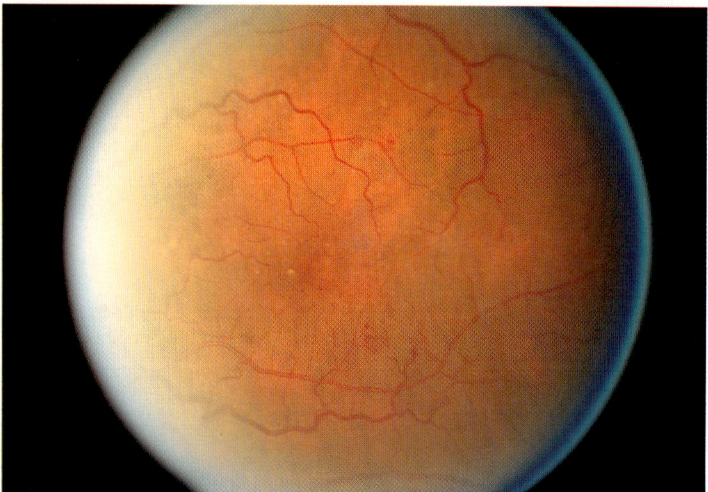

FIGURE 7.3 (B) Left eye with macular thickening less than 500 μ from center of the macula with cystoid changes. Pinpoint waxy exudates are also present less than 500 μ from center of the macula. Visual acuity is 20/20+.

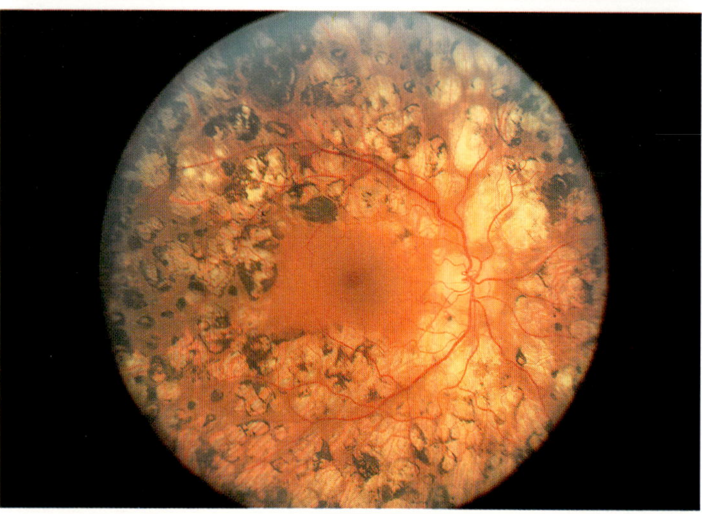

FIGURE 7.4. Left eye of patient with visual acuity of 20/20. Extensive scarring from panretinal laser coagulation is apparent. There is residual neovascularization on the disk. The macular area shows no thickening or hard exudates, but there is mild pigment mottling centrally.

TABLE 7.1. Self-reported visual function before and after binocular or monocular panretinal photocoagulation.

Have you noticed difficulty in:	Combined (%)		Binocular treatment		Monocular treatment	
	Before	Now	Correlation[a]	p	Correlation[a]	p
1 Adjusting to bright sunshine or bright indoor lighting?	14.3	68.6	0.53	0.025	0.41	0.073
2 Adjusting to dark indoor lighting?	25.7	85.7	0.34	0.119	0.46	0.047
3 Driving in the daytime?	17.1	31.4	0.78	0.001	0.52	0.043
4 Driving at night?	31.4	68.6	0.46	0.059	0.36	0.123
5 Recognizing scenes on TV?	11.4	34.3	0.48	0.043	0.34	0.117
6 Other problems with TV viewing?	20.0	37.1	0.40	0.076	0.41	0.071
7 Going down steps?	17.1	65.7	0.56	0.019	0.61	0.010
8 Losing your place while reading?	14.3	34.3	0.08	0.393	0.84	0.001
9 Sorting dark colors (as with black and navy blue socks)?	31.4	68.6	0.44	0.059	0.36	0.104
10 Athletic endeavors?	11.4	51.4	0.08	0.396	0.60	0.015
11 Recognizing friends' faces at a distance?	34.3	60.0	0.58	0.014	0.31	0.139
12 Recognizing friends' faces close up?	17.1	20.0	−0.18	0.274	0.42	0.065
13 Recognizing scenes at a distance in the daytime?	25.7	57.1	0.61	0.010	0.59	0.013
14 Recognizing scenes at a distance at night?	31.4	65.7	0.54	0.024	0.51	0.037
15 Telling how far from you an object is?	11.4	62.9	0.15	0.303	0.31	0.143
16 Dark spots that move when you move your eyes?	54.3	62.9	−0.02	0.472	−0.31	0.142
17 Blurry vision in distance (with glasses)?	40.0	62.9	0.54	0.023	0.26	0.181
18 Blurry vision in reading?	20.0	54.3	0.07	0.418	0.47	0.053
19 Lines you know are straight appear curved or distorted?	11.4	17.1	−0.11	0.36	−0.10	0.373
20 Car headlights are often blinding or annoying?	31.4	80.0	−0.05	0.431	0.56	0.024
21 Flickering spots before your eyes?	20.0	57.1	0.1	0.369	0.08	0.388
22 Parts of visual scene missing?	14.3	45.7	0.01	0.482	0.89	0.001
23 Running into doors, posts, walls?	8.6	60.0	−0.04	0.447	0.39	0.092
24 Bumping your head often?	5.7	37.1	−0.15	0.3	−0.20	0.251
25 Accidentally running into or hitting people in crowded places?	14.3	54.3	−0.21	0.243	0.31	0.138
26 Things appearing different using one eye compared with the other?	28.6	57.1	0.35	0.12	0.82	0.001
27 A tendency to close one eye to do things that would normally be done with both eyes open?	11.4	28.6	−0.15	0.309	0.46	0.056

Source: Russell, Sekuler, and Fetkenhour.[10] Reproduced with permission of the American Diabetes Association, Inc.
[a]Coefficient of correlation between each complaint's severity and visual acuity.

either before or after laser treatment. Furthermore, by testing these parameters we avail ourselves of the opportunity to advise a patient and demonstrate any weak points in visual function of which he or she is not yet aware.

At the William P. Beetham Eye Research and Treatment Unit of the Joslin Diabetes Center we routinely utilize traditional visual acuity testing with best correction for both distance and near vision to monitor visual status. We frequently augment these measurements, however, with the measurement of color vision with a D-15 color vision panel, Amsler grid testing, and contrast sensitivity testing using the Vistech acuity chart. The following case reports will demonstrate the role that these kinds of measurements can play in the management of patients with diabetic retinopathy and macular edema.

Case Reports

Case Number 1

Patient NP is a 54-year-old Caucasian man who has had insulin-dependent diabetes mellitus for 18 years. On examination on August 19, 1988, he had no subjective complaints. Best visual acuity with refraction of $+0.25\ -0.25 \times 90$ in the right eye (OD) and $+0.50\ -0.25 \times 90$ in the left eye (OS) was $20/15-1$ and $20/13-2$, respectively, on standard Snellen acuity charts. Anterior segment evaluation was unremarkable, with only mild lens changes consistent with the patient's age and duration of diabetes. Amsler grid testing showed no distortions or scotomata in either eye.

Color vision testing with an unsaturated D-15 color vision panel with appropriate near correction and using Macbeth easel lamp with daylight blue filter of standard illuminant C showed errors and reversals greater in the left eye than in the right, suggesting early tritan (blue-yellow) defects in each eye but without definite pattern. Contrast sensitivity testing on Vistech contrast sensitivity chart at 10 ft using full distance correction and appropriate chart illumination measured acuity at the 20/25 level in the right eye and at the 20/20 level in the left eye (Vistech conversion tables).

Retinal examination showed transitional background diabetic retinopathy in each eye (OU) (Fig. 7.2; see Color Plate VII). In the right eye there was thickening of the retina *greater* than 500 µ but less than 1 disk diameter from the center of the macula and less than 1 disk area in extent. Hard exudates were present less than 500 µ from the center of the macula. No neovascularizations were present. In the left eye there was retinal thickening greater than 500 µ from the center of the macula and less than 1 disk area in extent. Hard exudates were more than 500 µ but less than 1 disk diameter from the center of the macula. There were scattered retinal microaneurysms throughout the posterior pole but no neovascularizations. Although clinically significant diabetic macula edema was present in the right eye as defined by the ETDRS, it was decided to observe the maculopathy at regular intervals while withholding treatment.

Three months later patient NP was reexamined. He felt that he needed a stronger prescription for reading. Acuity with refraction of plano -0.25×90 OD and $+0.50\ -0.25 \times 90$ OS was 20/15 and 20/13, respectively. A reading add of $+2.50$ OU provided comfortable 14/14 vision. This add represented an increase of $+0.50$ diopter over the patient's present glasses.

Contrast sensitivity testing with the Vistech charts measured 20/20 OD and OS, representing an increased level of acuity over the previous exam. D-15 color vision testing demonstrated a tritan color defect OU. Pressures by applanation tonometry measured 15 mm Hg OD and 17 mm Hg OS. Amsler grid testing showed no distortions or irregularities in either eye.

In the right eye retinal examination showed thickening of the retina greater than 500 µ but at approximately 1 disk diameter from the center of the macula. The hard exudates in the macular area were diminished compared with the previous examination. There were no neovascularizations in the right eye. In the left eye there was thickening of the retina greater than 500 µ and less than 1 disk diameter from the center of the macula. Again there were no neovascularizations.

The maculopathy appeared stable with excellent visual acuity; no laser treatment was initiated. The patient will be followed at 4-month intervals.

Comment

Although the visual acuity measurements are better than 20/20 in each eye and there are no Amsler grid testing changes, it is clear that the retinal changes of diabetic macular edema, although mild, have affected other visual functions, specifically contrast sensitivity and color vision. Clinically, test results for these functions suggest careful following of this patient and even consideration of early focal laser treatment in the presence of what appears to be excellent visual acuity on standard Snellen chart testing. If Amsler grid testing changes were present, we would move even more rapidly to early treatment even in the presence of visual acuity better than 20/20.

In the absence of early treatment, careful follow-up evaluation is indicated at no more than 3- to 4-month intervals. In addition to the description of the physical findings, patient education includes a discussion of the effects of macular edema on visual function. It is possible that certain visual tasks may become compromised by the presence of the pathology in the retina, as indicated by contrast sensitivity and color vision testing, and some visual tasks may be difficult or impossible for this patient.

Case Number 2

Patient AM is a 58-year-old Caucasian man who has had insulin-dependent diabetes mellitus for 18 years. When examined on September 30, 1988, he complained of gradually weakening vision in each eye. Best visual acuity with refraction of $+0.25$ -0.75×110 OD eye and plano -0.75×70 OS was $20/15-4$ and $20/20-2+1$, respectively. Anterior segment evaluation was unremarkable with minor lenticular changes OU consistent with the patient's age. Amsler grid testing showed mild distortion of the grid in the superior temporal quadrant of the right eye and the superior nasal quadrant of the left eye.

Color vision testing with the unsaturated D-15 color vision test as described earlier showed an early tritan defect in the right eye and a more pronounced tritan defect in the left eye. Contrast sensitivity on Vistech acuity charts showed reduction in acuity to the 20/40 level in each eye (Vistech conversion tables).

Retinal examination revealed intraretinal hemorrhages and microaneurysms in each eye. Several soft exudates were also present in each eye. In the right eye there were drusen in the macular area with minimal thickening more than 500 μ but less than 1 disk diameter from the center of the macula. Waxy exudates were present less than 500 μ from the center of the macula. No neovascularization of the retina was present (Fig. 7.3; see Color Plate VIII).

In the left eye there was macular thickening less than 500 μ from the center of the macula with cystoid changes. Waxy exudates were also present less than 500 μ from the center of the macula, but there were no neovascularizations.

A diagnosis of clinically significant diabetic macular edema in the left eye was made and the patient had focal laser treatment in the left eye.

Comment

Although this patient's visual acuity measured 20/20 on Snellen charts, prompt focal laser treatment for clinically significant diabetic macular edema was initiated. The patient reported subjective difficulties and changes in vision related to glare that were reflected in the reduction of the contrast sensitivity curve, particularly at the high spatial frequencies where the effects of maculopathy are most noticeable.[14] The presence of an early tritan color defect, particularly in the left eye, prompted immediate treatment of the left eye.

Case Number 3

WJ is a 43-year-old Caucasian woman with insulin-dependent diabetes of 30 years. The right eye has no light perception and is phthisical with end-stage diabetic retinopathy, leukocoria, long-standing rubeosis iridis, and ectopia uveae. The left eye has vision that has fluctuated from the 20/20+ to 20/50± level by Snellen acuity measurements. The left eye has quiescent diabetic retinopathy status post panretinal photocoagulation more than ten years earlier. Medical history is significant for hypertension, hypothyroidism, left adrenalectomy, and unilateral carotid artery occlusion syndrome. Recent examinations are outlined in the summaries that follow.

On July 6, 1987, WJ complained of awakening with flashing episodes in her vision. These episodes were repeated during the day with postural changes, overactivity, and stress. Left eye acuity with refraction of $-1.50 \; -0.50 \times 120$ was 20/20+. Near acuity without correction was 14/14 slowly. Intraocular pressure by applanation tonometry at 4:20 PM was 12 mm Hg. Anterior segment evaluation was unremarkable, with no rubeosis iridis in the left eye. Retinal examination showed laser scar status post full panretinal photocoagulation, with thin, residual neovascularization on the disk. No neovascularization elsewhere was present. In the macular area there was no thickening or hard exudates but there was mild pigment mottling (Fig. 7.4; see Color Plate VIII).

The diagnosis was mechanical stimulation of the retina of the right eye and/or decreased carotid artery function contributing to the flashing episodes.

On December 28, 1987, the patient was reexamined with history of an automobile accident on September 9, 1987, resulting in a severe concussion. She complained of recurring headaches and decreased vision. Nuclear magnetic resonance imaging of the brain showed no disorder. Visual acuity with unchanged refraction was 20/20+ in the left eye. Intraocular pressure measured 13 mm Hg at 1:40 PM. Peripheral visual field testing showed scattered relative and absolute scotomata more pronounced than on the exams of May and October 1986. Contrast sensitivity testing with Vistech contrast sensitivity charts, as described previously, showed visual acuity reduced to approximately the 20/50 level in the left eye, with reductions particularly in the high-frequency targets. Amsler grid testing showed distortions of the grid pattern inferior to fixation. Color vision testing with the D-15 panel showed definite tritan defect. Retinal examination was similar to the previous exam of July 6, 1987.

The patient was reexamined on April 5, 1988, with a complaint of continued decreased vision OS since September, especially in distance vision. Vision varied with different tasks and lighting situations. Vision at night was also impaired.

Acuity with refraction of -1.50 -0.75 $\times$ 90 was 20/50± in the left eye with searching effort on the Snellen charts; reading vision with a +2.50 D add was 14/24.5. Contrast sensitivity acuity was reduced to lower frequencies compared with the exam of December 1987, and the reduction in the high-frequency targets measured at the 20/50 level. Amsler grid testing revealed several paracentral scotomata. Visual field testing with a threshold-related three-zone screening field showed relative

and absolute scotomata similar to those shown by the field exams of May and October, 1986, but the field was fuller than that in the exam of December, 1987. Pressure by applanation tonometry was 14 mm Hg at 5:00 PM.

Retinal examination showed unchanged neovascularization on the disk. Retinal pigment epithelial defects, as well as an irregular "punched-out" area, were present in the macula. A questionable area of neovascularization inferior to the center of the macula was observed. Diagnosis of decreased function in the center of the macula was made.

On reevaluation August 26, 1988, the patient reported that her Cushing's disease was very active and that her vision remained unchanged since the previous exam of April 5, 1988. Snellen acuity was improved approximately one line to the 20/30+2 level with refraction of -1.50 -0.50 $\times$ 110. Reading vision was improved to the 14/21+ level with a +2.50 D add. Contrast sensitivity acuity was slightly improved, but remained at the 20/50 level in the high-frequency range. Amsler grid testing was unchanged. Pressure by applanation tonometry at 5:15 PM was 11 mm Hg. Retinal examination showed a granular macular area with a small vascular loop inferior to the center of the macula.

Most recent visual function examination was on November 2, 1988. Snellen visual acuity was improved to 20/20−2 with no refractive change OS. Amsler grid testing showed decreased central distortion. Contrast sensitivity testing showed a slight increase in acuity level, to 20/40. Contrast sensitivity acuity level was further enhanced to the 20/30 level using Corning CPF 527 glare-control filtering lenses (see Chapter 6). Intraocular pressure was 10 mm Hg.

Comment

In patients who have had successful panretinal photocoagulation with a decrease in retinal neovascularization and hemorrhagic activity, there is an accompanying alteration in the circulation to the center of the macula secondary to the diabetic vascular disease and the laser photocoagulation itself. Because the alteration of blood flow may vary from time to time, there is accompanying fluctuation in visual acuity level, as well as subnormal results on Amsler grid testing, contrast sensitivity, and color vision testing.

Under certain circumstances the effects of these changes can be lessened or minimized. Clinical experience at the Beetham Eye Research and Treatment Unit suggests that the use of acetazolamide (Diamox) or possibly other intraocular pressure-reducing medications may improve blood flow to the macular area with resulting improvement in visual acuity and widening of the visual field. Glare-control filtering lenses that selectively filter out blue light wavelengths may be helpful for many patients. The filtering out of the blue light is usually not disturbing, since most of these patients have already lost sensitivity to the blue spectrum. The blue cones are functional not only in the macular area but throughout the retina, and damage to them accounts for a decrease in dark adaptation and night vision.

Discussion

The foregoing cases represent patients who have Snellen visual acuity of approximately 20/20 or better in each eye with only minor refractive correction. Testing of the vision with contrast sensitivity charts and the D-15 color vision panel, however, demonstrates that these patients do exhibit deficiencies in visual function as measured by several test parameters. Subjective reduction of vision may or may not be present. Definitive research has not been conducted on the effects of diabetic macular edema, diabetic retinopathy, and laser photocoagulation effects on visual function as measured by contrast sensitivity acuity. Continued studies are needed to establish reliable and reproducible clinical findings about the effects of retinal disease on visual function, to aid in the management of diabetic patients.

One method to attempt to measure the effects of macular edema, diabetic retinopathy, and laser photocoagulation on retinal function is by electroretinogram (ERG) testing. Such testing requires no subjective response from the patient. The response measured by the ERG reflects the rod and cone system but not the ganglion cell layer of the retina.

Lovasik and Spafford[15] examined the neural function of the retina with ERGs and the macular cortical pathways with visual evoked responses in 30 patients with insulin-dependent diabetes and in sex- and age-matched nondiabetic individuals. Their results showed no widespread differences in visual function between the test group and control group, but did show minor changes in the clinical ERG. This study, however, did not evaluate patients on the basis of levels of retinopathy or the presence or absence of macular edema.

Perlman and his study group[16] found that treatment with the argon laser not only reduced electroretinographic responses to areas of the retina directly treated, but also affected the functional integrity of retinal tissue adjacent to these treated areas. Furthermore, it has been demonstrated that ERGs in diabetic patients with microaneurysms and only a few blotch hemorrhages may be normal, but when cotton-wool spots or evidence of capillary nonperfusion is present, the ERG is reduced below the normal value.[17]

Bresnick and co-workers[18,19] used the oscillatory potentials of the ERG in an attempt to predict progression of diabetic retinopathy to severe proliferative diabetic retinopathy. Study results indicate that the summed amplitudes of the oscillatory potentials of the ERG, representing a quantitative measure of the degree of overall inner-layer retinal ischemia, are an independent predictor of progression to severe diabetic retinopathy. Test results based on the summed amplitudes of the oscillatory potentials, it is concluded, can be used to aid and support clinical decisions concerning panretinal laser photocoagulation and follow-up evaluation for patients with less than severe proliferative diabetic retinopathy.

A later study by Bresnick and Palta[20] confirmed original findings relating oscillatory potentials to severity of diabetic retinopathy. This study likewise demonstrated significant correlations between reduced oscillatory potentials and other visual function tests as reflected by lower visual field and visual acuity scores and higher error scores on Fransworth-Munsell 100-hue color tests.

In a study of 30 patients with IDDM, Spafford and Lovasik[21] compared visual resolution, accommodative ability, color discrimination, afferent optic nerve function, and macular photostress recovery times with the same variables in 30 sex- and age-matched nondiabetic individuals. This study revealed that decreased accommodative ability and abnormal recovery time in the photostress test may be early indicators of diabetic retinopathy, although readily detectable differences in visual function between the tested group and control group were not evident.

A study of the relationship between hue discrimination and contrast sensitivity in diabetic patients by Trick and colleagues[22] showed some evidence of visual dysfunction in nearly 38% of patients with no retinopathy and 60% of patients with background retinopathy. Only 5.4% of those with no retinopathy and 10% of those with background retinopathy exhibited both abnormal color vision and contrast sensitivity. Contrast sensitivity abnormalities were more likely to occur than color deficiencies. Bresnick, Condit, and Palta[23] showed that tritan (blue-yellow) defects in color discrimination in diabetic patients correlate with the severity of retinal vascular disease.

Other investigators also have found relationships between diabetic retinopathy and abnormalities of visual resolution as tested by contrast sensitivity.[24-26] Higgins and co-workers[27] have demonstrated a temporary loss of foveal contrast sensitivity in two patients undergoing panretinal photocoagulation, although Snellen visual acuity remained unchanged.

Potentially, any change in refraction or the refractive media of the eye can contribute to glare or to a reduction of contrast sensitivity. Disruption of the retinal surface by either a disease process or by laser treatment can cause decreased contrast sensitivity. Vitreous surgery can result in opacities causing light scatter within the eye and increased glare. The effects of fluctuating blood sugar levels on the refractive state of the eye are well chronicled.[28] While the blurr resulting from this defocusing is readily apparent, clearly an unfocused image is more likely to result in reduced contrast sensitivity.

Another readily identified source of glare is lenticular cataract. There is evidence that cataracts develop at an earlier age and may progress more rapidly in a diabetic than in a nondiabetic population.[29] Frequently these cataracts may be nothing more than peripheral cortical spokes, apparent only after examination of the eye with pupils dilated. These spokes may result in glare sensitivity during night driving or in poorly lit working conditions, both of which are conducive to pupillary dilatation.

Conclusion

Diabetes mellitus is known to affect virtually all ocular structures in some way or another. The refractive media of the eye, including the tear film, the cornea, the aqueous, the crystalline lens, and the vitreous humor—each can be affected to varying degrees, resulting in scattering of light, glare, and potential reduction of contrast sensitivity. Decreased accommodation, diminished pupillary responses, and reduced dark adaptation, resulting from either photocoagulation or direct diabetic effects on ocular structures, also can contribute to an inability to deal with changes in illuminance.

Precise refraction can result in enhanced visual function. Furthermore, appropriate lens filters may assist visual function by reducing glare. Lenses such as Corning CPF glare-control lenses selectively filter out light in the blue spectrum and below, thereby reducing glare. As demonstrated in the third case reported here, these blue filter lenses may improve response on contrast sensitivity testing. Once again, further research is needed to establish the benefit of such lenses in enhancing visual function.

Ocular disease related to diabetes is common, and many Americans suffer from undocumented or untreated visual debilitation. The diabetic effects on visual function need to be addressed in discussion with the patient. Furthermore, visual function parameters may prove helpful in monitoring retinopathy status, particularly in the presence of diabetic macular edema, and may assist in the clinical decision to either treat or withhold focal laser treatment according to the guidelines of the ETDRS. Clearly, more effort needs to be spent in investigating and treating the debilitating effects of impaired contrast sensitivity, glare, and the loss of visual function that may be associated with diabetes.

References

1. U.S. Department of Health and Human Services: *1986 Annual Report: National Diabetes Advisory Board, Public Health Service.* Bethesda, Md., National Institutes of Health, Publication No. 86–1587, April 1986.
2. Aiello LM, Ferris FL: Diabetic macular edema. In Reinecke RD (Ed), *Ophthalmology Annual* (Vol. 3).

Norwalk, Conn., Appleton-Century-Crofts, 1987, p 178.

3. Klein R, Klein B, Moss SE, et al: The Wisconsin epidemiologic study of diabetic retinopathy. 4. Diabetic macular edema. *Ophthalmology* **91**:1461, 1984.

4. Ebert EM, Fine AM, Markowitz J, et al: Functional vision in patients with neovascular maculopathy and poor visual acuity. *Arch Ophthalmol* **104**:109–112, 1986.

5. LeClaire J, Nadler MP, Weiss S, et al: A new glare tester for clinical testing: Results comparing normal subjects and various corrected aphakic patients. *Arch Ophthalmol* **100**:153, 1982.

6. Ginsberg AP: A new contrast sensitivity vision test chart. *Am J Optom Physiol Opt* **61**:403–407, 1984.

7. Pelli DG, Robson JG, Wilkins AJ: The design of a new letter chart for measuring contrast sensitivity. *Clin Vis Sci* **2**:187–199, 1988.

8. The Diabetic Retinopathy Study Research Group: Photocoagulation treatment of proliferative diabetic retinopathy. *Ophthalmology* **85**:82–106, 1978.

9. Early Treatment Diabetic Retinopathy Study Group: Photocoagulation for diabetic macular edema: Early Treatment Diabetic Retinopathy Study Report number 1. *Arch Ophthalmol* **103**:1796–1806, 1985.

10. Russell PW, Sekuler R, Fetkenhour C: Visual function after pan-retinal photocoagulation: A survey. *Diab Care* **8**:57–63, 1985.

11. Early Treatment Diabetic Retinopathy Study Group: Treatment techniques and clinical guidelines for photocoagulation of diabetic macular edema: Early Treatment Diabetic Retinopathy Study Report number 2. *Ophthalmology* **94**:761–774, 1987.

12. Early Treatment Diabetic Retinopathy Study Group: Techniques for scatter and local photocoagulation treatment of diabetic retinopathy: Early Treatment Diabetic Retinopathy Study Report number 3. *Int Ophthalmol Clin* **27**:254–64.

13. Early Treatment Diabetic Retinopathy Study Group: Photocoagulation for diabetic macular edema: Early Treatment Diabetic Retinopathy Study Report number 4. *Int Ophthalmol Clin* **27**:265–272, 1987.

14. Sjostrand J, Frisen L: Contrast sensitivity in macular disease. *Acta Ophthalmol* **55**:507–514, 1977.

15. Lovasik JV, Spafford MM: An electrophysiological investigation of visual function in juvenile insulin-dependent diabetes mellitus. *Am J Optom Physiol Opt* **65**:236–252, 1988.

16. Perlman I, Gdal-on M, Miller B, et al: Retinal function of the diabetic retina after argon laser photocoagulation assessed electroretinographically. *Br J Ophthalmol* **69**:240–246, 1985.

17. Arden GB, Hamilton AMP, Wilson-Holt J, et al: Pattern electroretinograms become abnormal when background retinopathy deteriorates to a preproliferative stage: Possible use as a screening test. *Br J Ophthalmol* **70**:330–335, 1986.

18. Bresnick GH, Korth K, Groo A, et al: Electroretinographic oscillatory potentials predict progression of diabetic retinopathy. *Ophthalmology* **102**:1307–1311, 1984.

19. Bresnick GH, Palta M: Predicting progression to severe diabetic retinopathy. *Arch Ophthalmol* **105**:810–814, 1987.

20. Bresnick GH, Palta M: Oscillatory potential amplitudes: Relation to severity of diabetic retinopathy. *Arch Ophthalmol* **105**:929–933.

21. Spafford MM, Lovasik JV: Clinical evaluation of ocular and visual functions in insulin-dependent juvenile diabetics. *Am J Optom Physiol Opt* **63**: 505–519, 1986.

22. Trick GL, Burde RM, Gordon MO, et al: The relationship between hue discrimination and contrast sensitivity deficits in patients with diabetes mellitus. *Ophthalmology* **95**:693–698, 1988.

23. Bresnick GH, Condit RS, Palta M, et al: Association of hue discrimination loss and diabetic retinopathy. *Arch Ophthalmol* **103**:1317–1324, 1985.

24. Sokol S, Moskowitz A, Skarf B, et al: Contrast sensitivity in diabetics with and without background retinopathy. *Arch Ophthalmol* **103**:51–54, 1985.

25. Sala SD, Bertoni G, Somazzi L, et al: Impaired contrast sensitivity in diabetic patients with and without retinopathy: A new technique for rapid assessment. *Br J Ophthalmol* **69**:136–142, 1985.

26. Ghafour IM, Foulds WS, Allan D: Short-term effect of slit-lamp illumination and argon laser light on visual function of diabetic and non-diabetic subjects. *Br J Ophthalmol* **68**:298–302, 1984.

27. Higgins KE, Meyers SM, Jaffe MJ, et al: Temporary loss of foveal contrast sensitivity associated with panretinal photocoagulation. *Arch Ophthalmol* **104**:997–1003, 1986.

28. Waite JH, Beetham WP: The visual mechanism in diabetes mellitus: A comparative study of 2002 diabetics and 457 non-diabetics for control. *N Engl J Med* **212**:367–379, 429–443, 1935.

29. Varma SD, Richards R: Etiology of cataracts in diabetics. *Int Ophthalmol Clin* **24**:93–110, 1984.

8
New Methods for Diagnosis of Retinal Neural Damage Associated with Primary Open-Angle Glaucoma

Geoffrey B. Arden

Introduction

With the rising age of the population, the number of patients with primary open-angle glaucoma (POAG) is increasing. The consequences of a missed diagnosis or inappropriate treatment also becomes more severe: the condition may progress slowly, but patients live longer and expect to retain good sight. For these reasons it is necessary to monitor retinal functions very carefully in an increasingly large number of elderly persons. Traditionally, field loss has been used for this purpose, but the definition of what constitutes loss of field depends on the equipment used. Recently introduced computer assessment of the results of automated static perimetry have made it possible to spot smaller field losses, and thus to institute treatment earlier.[1,2] However desirable this may be, a price has to be paid. The new equipment is more costly than the systems it has displaced, and the tests are more difficult for the patient and the tester.

Advances have also been made in understanding the pathologic histology of primary open-angle glaucoma; surprisingly, it appears that a majority of the optic nerve fibers may be damaged before any field loss can be detected.[3-5] These findings strongly suggest that more refined testing could disclose damage in a glaucoma patient's eyes at a stage before field losses develop. There has been no lack of claims that various functions are depressed before actual field loss develops.[6-10] Indeed, one criterion of the computer-assisted field test is a global increase of threshold rather than a scotoma. This chapter is concerned with three methods of measurement of visual function. Each is claimed to outperform field tests in the detection of glaucoma.

Luminance Contrast Sensitivity

Visual acuity is lost conspicuously late in POAG, because the initial field losses are frequently in an annulus 15 to 20 degrees from the macula. Measures of extrafoveal function thus might be effective in detecting early changes, and the method of measurement of contrast sensitivity with gratings appeared to be promising. Visual acuity is measured with high-contrast black-on-white objects. Even when the optotype letters are very large, discrimination of the sharp edges is a function of the fovea. By modifying the test objects it is possible to produce tests for extrafoveal retina. It is of course possible to lower the contrast of the optotype letters, so that the letters are gray on a gray background. Campbell and Green[11] introduced the idea of measuring the contrast sensitivity, not of optotypes, but of gratings in which the luminance profile varies sinusoidally. Figure 8.1 shows the method diagrammatically. When the bars of the grating are closely spaced (about 30 repeats, or cycles, per degree of visual angle) the gratings are visible only if the contrast, defined as $(L_{max} - L_{min})/(L_{max} + L_{min})$, equals 1, or 100%. This occurs when the minimum luminance is equal to 0, that is, when the grating is black-on-white like an optotype. Coarser gratings can be seen with lower contrast, and the visibility appears maximal for spacings of 2 to 4 c/degree where the threshold

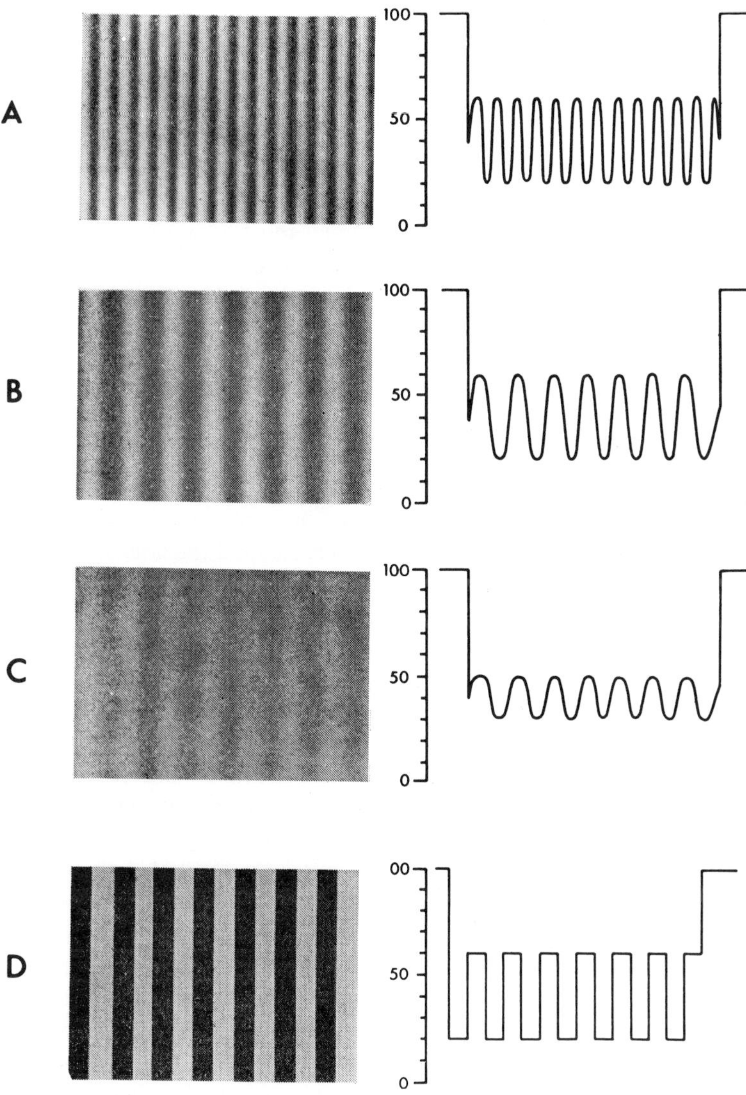

FIGURE 8.1. Schematic gratings and their luminance profile. A, B, and C are sinusoidal; D is a square wave. A and B differ in spatial frequency, B and C in contrast. (From Arden,[12] used with permission.)

contrast is only 0.003 to 0.01. It is usual to express these values as percentages—0.3% to 1%—and to refer to the reciprocal of the threshold contrast as the *contrast sensitivity*. Still coarser gratings are seen with greater difficulty: if there are only two repeats in 10 degrees of visual angle (i.e., 0.2 c/degree), the threshold contrast rises to about 5%. Thus, the function relating contrast sensitivity to spatial frequency is a "bell-shaped curve" with a well-defined maximum. In clinical work, one wishes to know how results depart from the nor-

mal. A graph of the loss of sensitivity as a function of spatial frequency is often called a *visuogram*, in analogy to the audiogram, which charts the loss of hearing. The variation in threshold contrast as a function of spatial frequency has a variety of causes, some neurophysiologic and some optical. Thus, for low spatial frequencies, visibility of a grating remains constant despite a considerable departure from ammetropia. This is a simple consequence of lens optics but is valuable to the clinician, because it means any loss of contrast sensitivity cannot be due to refractive error. For example, at 0.2 c/degree the loss of contrast sensitivity due to 10-D ammetropia is less than one half the interindividual variation in the normal population. Even a person with extreme myopia will therefore have a normal result: very coarse gratings cannot "blur out" with refractive errors because (in a sense) they are already a blur! For finely spaced gratings, the optical properties of the normal eye are important in determining contrast sensitivity. The iron laws of information theory insist that the contrast of any grating is impaired when it is passed through any optical system, and what holds for camera lenses holds for our own crystalline lens. The higher the spatial frequency, the greater the loss of contrast, and it seems that the limiting factor for our eyes is the optical pathway. It is possible to measure the contrast sensitivity of the neural pathway by bypassing the cornea, lens, and vitreous using lasers, and to make an interference pattern on the retina in the form of a grating with a high contrast and a high spatial frequency. Then the perceptual contrast sensitivity improves, but not by a large factor: the neurophysiology of the retina has only evolved to the extent required to handle the information presented to it through the imperfect optics. The details of the neural mechanisms responsible for grating detection have been investigated—in the retina it is supposed that the size of the surround-and-center receptive fields of retinal ganglion cells determine the spatial frequency/contrast sensitivity function. For example, the optimal response of an "on-center" ganglion cell must occur when its central receptive field is covered by the brighter half of a grating period, and the surround (which is of opposite sign) is covered by the darker portions. For off-center cells, the geometry would be reversed. The loss of contrast sensitivity at higher and lower spatial frequencies is due to mismatch between receptive field sizes and the width of the grating bars. This is thought to be especially important for the lower spatial frequencies. Of course there is great variation in the size of the receptive fields of ganglion cells, even at any one retinal locus. It is supposed that the change in the average contrast sensitivity reflects the relative numbers of receptive fields of the appropriate size. However, this simple notion cannot explain all known facts. One additional factor that is of con-

siderable clinical importance is that the eye is much more sensitive if the gratings move, drift, or pattern reverse. Such objects preferentially stimulate the larger (alpha) retinal ganglion cells. Again, the visibility for all gratings, even for the coarsest, increases as the number of cycles (repeats) presented increases. A simple experiment demonstrates this finding. The contrast of a grating on an oscilloscope face is reduced to just above threshold (the grating remains perfectly visible). Next, a card with a circular cutout is placed over the grating so that only part of the screen is visible, and the grating appears to vanish. If contrast is increased, it can once more be seen. Threshold drops as the cutout is made larger, until more than six repeats can be seen. Therefore, for such a grating to be seen optimally, the image on the retina has to be extensive, and the image is the larger, the coarser the grating. This cannot be explained on the basis of the properties of the receptive field of a single ganglion cell. For very coarse gratings, the retinal image for optimal viewing subtends as much as 50 degrees of solid angle. Evidently some form of areal integration must occur, either in the retina itself or in the brain that interprets the retinal messages. Although we normally think of our (foveal) vision in quite different terms—as providing spatial discrimination—spatial integration is known to occur in numerous examples. The central fovea with its close-packed and slender cones is obviously specialized for high acuity, but animal experiments and physiologic experiments in humans have shown that peripheral retina can appreciate small differences between shades of gray. Thus one would expect contrast sensitivity measurements to be particularly helpful in providing information about peripheral retina, and also that when coarse gratings are used, the results of the measurements could provide a "birds eye view" of the average sensitivity of a large retinal area. To a considerable degree these expectations are fulfilled, but the fovea has a very large "cortical magnification factor," and this means that foveal signals are always more important than peripheral ones when the both regions are stimulated at the same time. This limits our ability to detect changes limited to peripheral retina. Nevertheless, the method of measuring the contrast sensitivity of very low spatial frequency gratings appeared to be promising for the detection of peripheral retinal disturbances, and was easy and rapid to carry out. Therefore patients with glaucoma were among the first investigated with this new technique. Since then, a number of papers have appeared, and clinical methods, equipment, and results have been repeatedly reviewed.[12-14] It has been found that in patients with established glaucoma contrast sensitivity to low and mid ranges of spatial frequencies was reduced, even though visual acuity was normal. (Obviously, for the highest spatial frequencies performance had to equal that of normal subjects, because tests were carried out only if acuity was normal.)

These first results were of interest, since they helped to confirm the theory of contrast sensitivity testing. For practical clinical work, however, much more is needed. All the patients investigated were known to have glaucoma, and in most cases were selected so as to have no other disease. The next investigative step was to discover whether any change in contrast sensitivity could be detected in patients with the earliest possible manifestations of glaucoma, that is, those in whom there were clinical signs, such as disk cupping or an elevated intraocular pressure, but in whom there was either no evidence or poor evidence of actual field loss. Such patients are said to have ocular hypertension. In these patients, too, the average contrast threshold is raised. However, this result does not provide evidence that the investigation is useful in discriminating between patients with early glaucomatous damage and those in whom the diagnosis of ocular hypertension is mistaken, and it soon became apparent that early enthusiastic claims were misleading. One reason is that the initial investigations were made on selected patient samples; persons with mild cataracts, systemic disease, or difficulties in comprehension were initially excluded. When such patients were included, the range of normal variation increased considerably, so that results from patient and normal populations overlapped (Fig. 8.2). This is common in many tests, but the questions are, how great is the overlap, and are the number of false-positive and false-negative diagnoses acceptable for the particular condition? In the case of contrast sensitivity used as a single test to screen patients for glaucoma, a significant number of patients with visual impairment would be missed unless normal values were set so that a number of patients without identifiable visual disease of any sort were also considered abnormal.

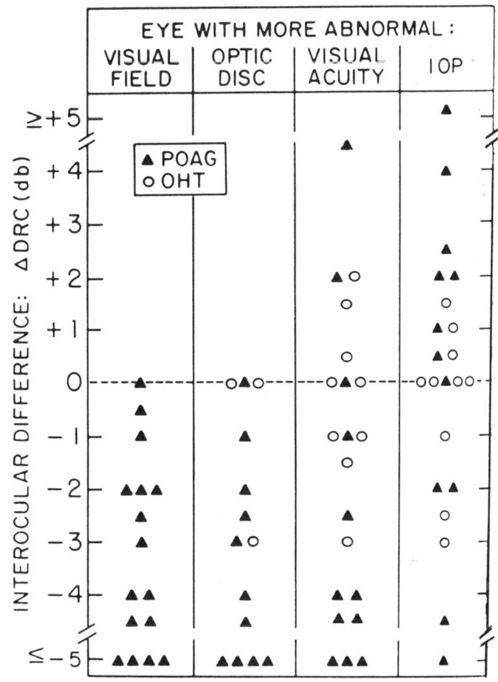

FIGURE 8.2. Relationship between contrast sensitivity in patients with primary open-angle glaucoma (POAG) and with ocular hypertension (OHT). (From Atkin et al,[15] used with permission.)

As a screening test, luminance contrast gratings thus lacked selectivity; indeed, conditions common in the elderly (mild cataract) caused gross changes in contrast thresholds. Some forms of test also lacked sensitivity, for Atkin et al[15] showed that the discrimination among patients with glaucoma, those with ocular hypertension, and normal subjects was much improved if the pattern contrast reversed rapidly. This was not possible with printed sheets of gratings introduced for screening purposes.[15,16] Thus, although such tests can be used to assist in the diagnosis of glaucoma (and are many times more sensitive than the use of optotypes), they cannot by themselves be used to diagnose the condition. Field tests are still required.

Color Vision

Mild defects of color vision have long been known to develop early in glaucoma, and literature on this subject has been reviewed.[8,17,18] Tests for minimal

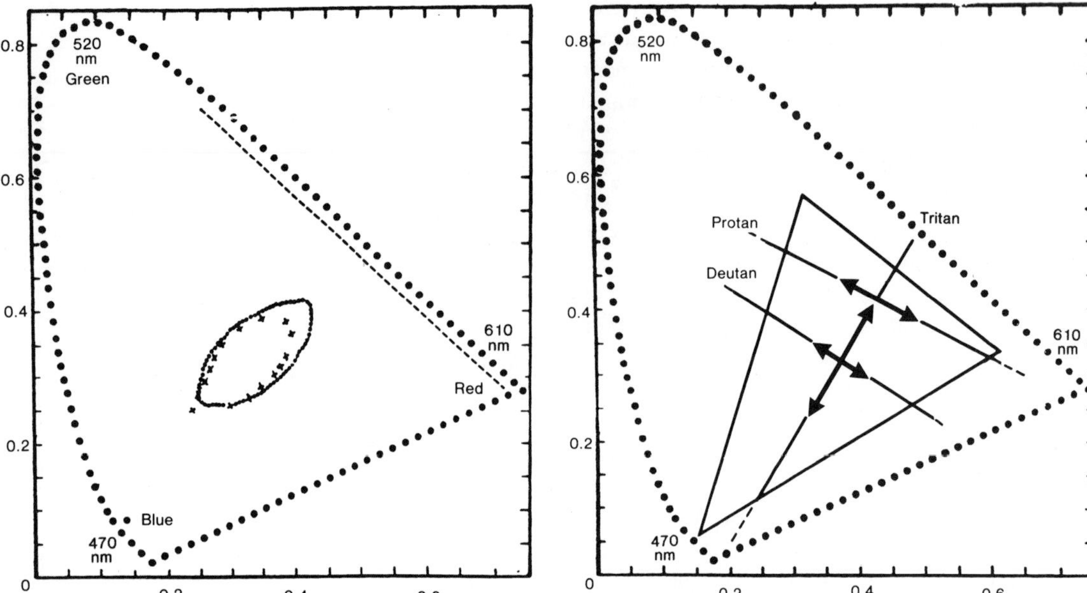

FIGURE 8.3. Color diagram and the relation to TV phosphor colors and the clinical color contrast test. The lines with the arrowheads are ten times longer than the normal mean threshold color contrast modulation. They lie along lines of protan, deutan, and tritan color confusion. See text for further discussion. (From Gunduz et al,[22] used with permission. Copyright 1988, American Medical Association.)

color vision changes have been sought for some time, and in the past the Farnsworth-Munsell 100-hue color test and its variants have proved most sensitive. Recently, however, the notion of color contrast sensitivity has been publicized. It may be that this form of test combines the virtues of gratings with those of a color vision test and will assist in the measurement of neural losses in glaucoma (and other conditions).

In the gratings described in the previous section, the sinusoidal variation in luminance across the grating provides the stimulus. In the newer methods, the luminance remains constant but the *hue* of the grating varies repetitively across the display. The production of such stimuli has been made possible by the development of color television; high-quality computer graphics can now be displayed in color. Several peripherals are available, although the programs to drive them remain complex. The colors displayed are mixtures of three primaries (as in many of the classic experiments on color mixing), but because the light emitted by the TV phosphors is not monochromatic, the region of color space that can be investigated is slightly reduced. However, for any clinical purpose this is of no importance, and the TV systems have several important practical advantages compared with other tests of color vision.[19,20] It is simple to have each patient adjust the relative luminance of the red, green, and blue channels to suit his or her own lens and macular pigmentation (or to compensate for tinted glasses) so that truly equiluminous stimuli can be used. Thus, luminance clues, which bedevil other color vision tests, can be completely eliminated. Again, the minimal color difference that the programs can generate are between one fourth and one seventh of a psychologic "just noticeable difference" (JND); this compares with the 100-hue test, in which adjacent "caps" are separated by about 3 JNDs. In test books like the Ishihara, the differences are of course much greater. Furthermore, the TV system is readily adaptable to provide superior and automated psychophysical routines, so that the color contrast threshold can be obtained with forced-choice methods in an unbiased and objective fashion and the patient's variance can be assessed. Conversely, plates like the Ishihara series cannot easily be used to detect hysterical color blindness, whereas the 100-hue test takes considerable time for the patient to complete

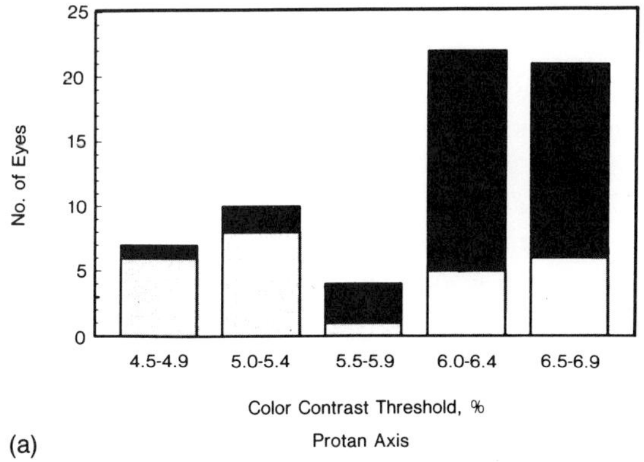

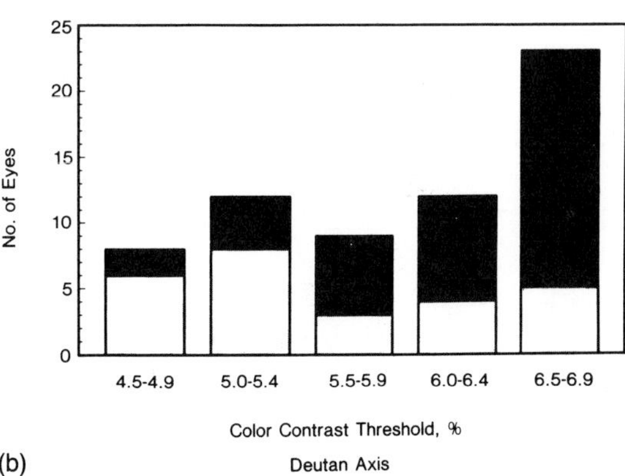

FIGURE 8.4. Comparison between the color contrast thresholds of normal and mildly glaucomatous observers. (a) Along the protan color-confusion axis, and (b) along the deutan color-confusion axis. Black areas represent patients; white, normals. There is obvious loss of sensitivity in the patients, but overlap between normal and patient populations. Compare with Figure 8.5. (From Gunduz et al,[22] used with permission. Copyright 1988, American Medical Association.)

and unless scoring is also automated, working out the test result is very laborious. Even more important is the ability of a TV system to present stimuli that change or appear briefly. In the clinical test, the screen is initially featureless and uniform; the color is midway between the two extreme colors specified and the grating occupies the center of the screen for brief moments only. The average of the grating's colors is also midway between the extreme values specified. For example, a red-green grating appears for 40 msec in the center of a large yellow display. It has been shown that in disease states, loss of color discrimination for such brief flashes is much greater than when the stimulus is presented for longer periods.[21] In addition, when the stimulus is a brief, slowly repeated flash, the stimulus is easily detectable by the retinal periphery. If the same stimulus is steadily presented in the periphery, the colors fade (the Troxler effect) so that color comparisons become impossible. No other test of color vision can easily be used to test the retinal periphery.

These advantages have led to informal and preliminary results in which it appears that for almost all conditions (except, curiously, retrobulbar neuritis), gratings tests of color vision are between three and ten times more sensitive than the 100-hue test. In acquired color vision defects, moreover, the common findings is that color discrimination is unequally affected in the various cardinal directions in color space.[17] This is usually specified in terms of the CIE (Commission Internationale d'Eclairage) primaries, in the color diagram. Figure 8.3 shows the color diagram: the inscribed triangle represents the area of color space that can be investigated by the TV phosphors. The lines represent the directions along which hue is modulated during the test. One line is a protan color confusion line. All colors on this line are confusible by patients with protanopia because, in the absence of the separate red mechanisms, the colors cause equal stimulation of the green and blue primary mechanisms. The tritan color confusion line (blue-yellow discrimination) is nearly orthogonal to this.

Color contrast has been investigated in patients with ocular hypertension and glaucoma, and for colors modulating along protan and deutan color confusion axes, mild defects have been found (Fig. 8.4). However, much greater losses occur along the tritan axis, so much so that nearly all patients who have raised intraocular tension show measurable defects (Fig. 8.5). The increase in threshold is related to the severity of the disease.[22] The reason for such dramatic changes in the tritan axis is not known. However, only about 5% of optic nerve fibers convey information about blue-yellow discrimination, whereas up to 90% of the fibers originate in the small ganglion cells that are concerned with red-green discrimination.[23,24] This suggests that the receptive fields of the blue-yellow ganglion cells may be larger and that there is less overlap

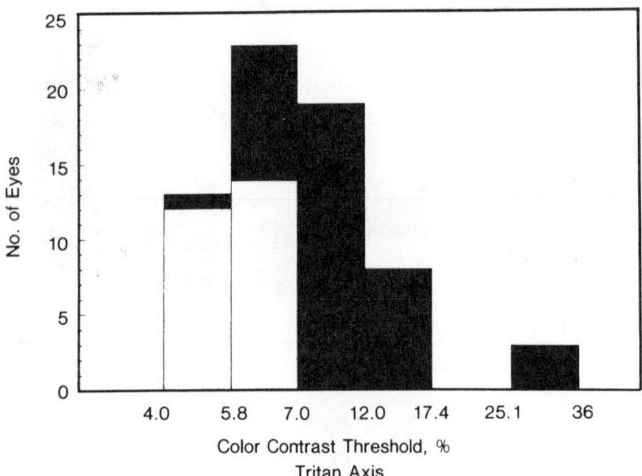

FIGURE 8.5. Comparison between the color contrast thresholds of normal and mildly glaucomatous observers along the tritan color-confusion axis. The loss of sensitivity in the patients is so great that there is scarcely any overlap of the results. Note the different horizontal scales in this figure compared to Figure 8.4. (From Gunduz et al,[22] used with permission. Copyright 1988, American Medical Association.)

between them—the safety factor for blue-yellow may be less—and that when, in early glaucoma, larger optic nerve fibers are preferentially though randomly damaged,[4] "gaps" in the blue-yellow field may develop that selectively raise the color contrast threshold. However that may be, the implication of the results shown is that *all* patients with glaucomatous field defects (and many in whom damage is so mild that absolute scotomata have not yet developed) can be distinguished from the normal population by a *single test* of color vision that is simpler and quicker than any measurement of changes in the visual field.

The use of colored gratings is very new and enthusiasm for them must be tempered: it was also hoped that luminance contrast would uniquely detect patients with glaucoma. A large-scale trial in specialist and general retinal clinics has not yet been undertaken. However, the outlook seems promising. In particular, the fact that there is a specific blue-yellow defect allows the ratio of the increase in tritan to protan thresholds to be used as a very sensitive index of loss. All optical and psychologic factors that might affect the thresholds should apply equally to all colors, and any relative loss of sensitivity to blue (e.g., yellowing lenses) can be compensated for in the initial matching.

Pattern Electroretinography

When the retina is illuminated by flashes of light, the well-known electroretinogram (ERG) is developed as a voltage difference between the cornea and a reference point on the forehead, while cortical evoked responses can be detected from electrodes placed on the occiput. Pattern-reversing checkerboards are most frequently used to evoke the cortical responses, and can also be used as ERG stimulators. They have one great advantage—that as the pattern reverses in contrast, the total quantity of light entering the eye remains constant and the only change occurs in the retinal image of the checkerboard. Hence, any retinal electrical response must be derived from the region where the image falls. Commonly, the macula and paramacula are both stimulated. The ERG evoked by such a stimulus is called the *pattern ERG* (PERG) and is very small, about 3 µV. For many years it was thought that the response had the same characteristics as that of the ERG evoked by flashes of light; it was merely smaller, because with a checkerboard the eye was well light adapted and only a relatively small region of the retina was stimulated. In the last 10 years this view has been challenged. Both clinical experiments and microelectrode recordings in animal retinas have demonstrated that the cellular origin of much of the PERG is from the inner retinal layers. The flash ERG is well known to be derived from the outer retinal layers.[25] Of particular interest is the recent demonstration that loss of the later cornealnegative portion of the PERG occurs in optic nerve disease,[26,27] for this suggests that in a condition such as glaucoma, where ganglion cells and optic nerve fibers are progressively lost, there may be a specific diagnostic change in the waveform of the PERG. There have been many reports of reduction in the amplitude of the PERG in patients with glaucomatous damage. Some of these reports are extremely convincing, and it is reasonable to suppose that in chronic disease, retinal atrophy occurs so that either the PERG current generated is reduced or the spread of current through the eye is affected. In general it has yet to be shown that the reductions in amplitude are diagnostic in an elderly population with an increased incidence of opacities and systemic disease and also a cumulative neuronal loss due to aging itself. Recent reports, however, show that the specific loss of the following negative wave (often

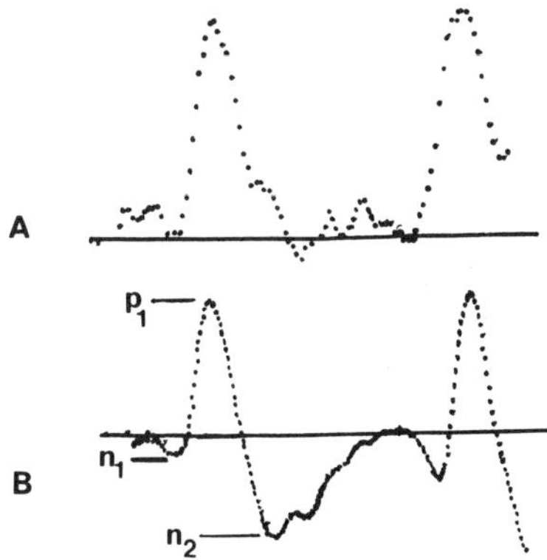

FIGURE 8.6. Normal and affected pattern electroretinograms from a patient with unilateral glaucoma. There is selective loss of the N95 component in the affected eye. (From Weinstein et al,[28] used with permission. Copyright 1988, American Medical Association.)

called N95—the electrical sign of the change at the cornea and trough time are indicated in this nomenclature) is selectively reduced in glaucomatous patients (Fig. 8.6), and it is possible to spot the affected eye in patients with unilateral disease.[28] Indeed, the alteration in waveform has appeared (though unremarked) in several published accounts. The selectivity and sensitivity of one PERG measurement has been found to be about 80% in a series of patients recruited from a family clinic, most with only "soft signs" of glaucoma and without definite field loss. This is better sensitivity and selectivity than has been obtained by automated perimetry in the same population. Thus, the specific reduction in the negative wave may precede the demonstration, by automated perimetry, of changes in visual threshold in parts of the visual field. To achieve a sensitive and reliable statistical evaluation of field loss, it is necessary to do two tests some weeks apart and to obtain a computerized evaluation of the similarities and differences. Thus the PERG test is much easier and quicker for the patient and is simpler and quicker to evaluate than is perimetry. If it can be shown to be more sensitive and less prone to false-positive results, it would have a definite place in evaluation of glaucoma.

Conclusion

Anyone who has taken the casing off a modern automated perimeter must be struck by its enormous complexity; perimetry tests are difficult and time consuming for patients and examiner alike. The question is, is there anything better? An analogy between perimetric field tests and another mechanical marvel springs to mind. The wasteful and complex system of reciprocating pistons in the gasoline engine is evidently a poor engineering solution to the problem of making the automobile run; however, the technology is so highly developed that alternative systems have not supplanted the simple internal combustion device (this may be changing now). Much the same is true of methods of detecting glaucoma. Since field tests are incapable of demonstrating the condition until serious loss has occurred, other methods should be found. But the field tests are reliable and well understood and therefore difficult to supplant. In the last few years some promising prototypes of new clinical tests have been designed. If they succeed in the hurly-burly of the clinical office, our practice may change dramatically.

References

1. Heijl A: The implications of the results of computerized perimetry in normals for the statistical evaluation of glaucomatous visual fields. In Kreiglstein GK (Ed), *Glaucoma Update III*. Berlin, Springer-Verlag, 1986, pp 155–122.

2. Gloor BP, Dimitrakos SA, Rabineau PA: Long-term follow-up of glaucomatous fields by computerized (octopus perimetry). In Kreiglstein GK (Ed), *Glaucoma Update III*. Berlin, Springer-Verlag, 1986, pp 123–138.

3. Quigley HA: Histology of human glaucoma optic nerve damage compared to clinical findings in the same eyes. In Kreiglstein, GK, Leydhecker W (Eds), *Glaucoma Update II*. Berlin, Springer-Verlag, 1986, pp 83–88.

4. Quigley HA: Differences in the amount of 'plaque material' in the outflow system of eyes with chronic simple and exploitation glaucoma. In Kreiglstein GK (Ed), *Glaucoma Update III*. Berlin, Springer-Verlag, 1986, pp 17–22.

5. Hayreh SS: Factors determining the glaucomatous optic nerve head damage. In Kreiglstein GK (Ed), *Glaucoma Update III*. Berlin, Springer-Verlag, 1986, pp 40–46.

6. Quigley HA, Sanchez RM, Dunkleberg GR: chronic glaucoma selectively damages large optic nerve fibers. *Invest Ophthalmol Vis Sci* **28**:913–920, 1987.

7. Iwata K: The earliest finding of primary open-angle

glaucoma (POAG) and the mode of progression. In Kreiglstein GK, Leydhecker W (Eds), *Glaucoma Update II*. Berlin, Springer-Verlag, 1982, pp 133–138.

8. Drance SM, Airaksinen PJ: Signs of early damage in open angle glaucoma. In Weinstein GW (Ed), *Contemporary Issues in Ophthalmology: Open Angle Glaucoma*. New York, Churchill Livingstone, 1986, pp 17–30.

9. Atkin A, Podos SM, Bodis-Wollner I: Abnormalities of the visual system in ocular hypertension and glaucoma: Seeing beyond routine perimetry. In Kreiglstein GK, Leydhecker W (Eds), *Glaucoma Update II*. Berlin, Springer-Verlag, 1982, pp 107–116.

10. Sommer A, Pollack I, Maumenee AE: Optic disc parameters and onset of glaucomatous field loss. *Arch Ophthalmol* **97**:1444–1448, 1979.

11. Campbell FW, Green DG: Optical and retinal factors affecting visual resolution. *J. Physiol Lond 181*: 576–593, 1965.

12. Arden GB: Visual loss in patients with normal visual acuity. *Trans Ophthalmol Soc UK* **98**:219–230, 1978.

13. Arden GB: Advances in diagnostic visual optics. In Breinin GM, Siegel IM (Eds), *Proceedings 2nd International Symposium, 1982*. Berlin, Springer-Verlag, 1983, pp 198–206.

14. Arden GB: Testing contrast sensitivity in clinical practice. *Clin Vis Sci* **2**:213–224, 1988.

15. Atkin A, Wolkstein M, Bodis-Wollner I et al: Interocular comparison of contrast sensitivities in glaucoma patients and subjects. *Br J Ophthalmol* **64**: 858–862, 1980.

16. Atkin A, Bodis-Wollner I, Wolkstein M et al: Abnormalities of central contrast sensitivity in glaucoma. *Am J Ophthalmol* **88**:205–211, 1979.

17. Hart WM: Acquired dyschromatopsias. *Surv Ophthalmol* **32**:10–31, 1987.

18. Drance SM, Lakowski R: Colour vision in glaucoma. In Kreiglstein GK, Leydhecker W (Eds), *Glaucoma Update II*. Berlin, Springer-Verlag, 1982, pp 117–122.

19. Arden GB, Gündüz K, Perry S: Colour vision testing with a computer graphics system. *Clin Vis Sci* **2**: 303–320, 1988.

20. Arden GB, Gündüz K, Perry S: Color vision testing with a computer graphics system: Preliminary results. *Docu Ophthalmol* **69**:167–174, 1988.

21. Scase MO, Foster DH, Honan WP, Heron JR, Gulliford MC, Scarpello JHB: Abnormalities in hue discrimination with very brief stimuli in diabetic patients. *Arch Ophthalmol* (submitted for publication).

22. Gündüz K, Arden GB, Perry S et al: Colour vision defects in ocular hypertension and glaucoma – quantification with a computer-driven color television system. *Arch Ophthalmol* **106**:929–935, 1988.

23. De Monasterio FM: Properties of concentrically organized X and Y ganglion cells of macaque retina. *J Neurophysiol* **41**:1394–1449, 1978.

24. Shapley RM, Perry VH: Cat and monkey retinal ganglion cells and their visual functional roles. *Trends in Neurolog Sci* **9**:229–235, 1986.

25. Berninger TA, Arden GB: The pattern electroretinogram. *Eye* **2**:S257–S283, 1988.

26. Holder GE: Significance of abnormal pattern electroretinography in anterior visual pathway dysfunction. *Br J Ophthalmol* **71**:161–169, 1987.

27. Ryan S, Arden GB: Electrophysiological discrimination between retinal and optic nerve disorders. *Doc Ophthalmol* **68**:247–260, 1988.

28. Weinstein GW, Arden GB, Hitchings RA et al: The pattern electroretinogram (PERG) in ocular hypertension and glaucoma. *Arch Ophthalmol* **106**:923–928, 1988.

9
Overview of Contrast Sensitivity and Neuro-ophthalmic Disease

Rita L. Storch and Ivan Bodis-Wollner

Abbreviations Used in This Chapter

AGP	Arden grating plates
C	Contrast
cpd	Cycle per 1 degree of visual angle. 1 cycle = 1 pair of adjacent dark-bright bars in grating pattern
CS	Contrast sensitivity
CSF	Contrast sensitivity function
GA	Grating acuity (high-frequency cutoff, in cpd)
IOL	Intraocular lens
IOP	Intraocular pressure
L	Mean luminance
L_{max}	Luminance of a light bar in a grating pattern
L_{min}	Luminance of a dark bar in a grating pattern
MS	Multiple sclerosis
OHT	Ocular hypertension
PD	Parkinson's disease
POAG	Primary open-angle glaucoma
PVEP	Pattern visual evoked potential
Sf	Spatial frequency, in cpd
S_{max}	Peak sensitivity of CSF
SMTF	Spatial modulation transfer function
ST-CS	SpatioTemporal CS
Tf	Temporal frequency, in hertz. 1 unit of frequency equals 1 cycle per second.
VA	Snellen visual acuity
VEP	Visual evoked potential

Introduction

Faced with the quantity and quality of recent research in the visual sciences, one might wonder: How does this research affect clinical practice? What benefits do patients derive from the new insights? This chapter is devoted to a diagnostic technique called the contrast sensitivity function (CSF), which is coming into wide clinical use.

For more than a century the tried-and-true Snellen eye chart has been the way to define normal vision. Ophthalmologists have depended on this test, which measures visual performance under conditions of high contrast. However, such testing conditions are not representative of the real world. The functional visual world is not made of small, high-contrast black letters on a bright background but is an ever-changing configuration of objects under viewing conditions as different as the noonday sun and moonless winter night. All of us have been confronted by patients who have 20/20 Snellen visual acuity in the examining room but complain bitterly of having poor vision in the outside world. Many of these patients give imprecise accounts of their difficulties, but a few may tell you that their sight is like having the contrast turned down on the television. And indeed, most are complaining about the loss of a specific visual function, but one that has been recognized only for the past decades—the ability to distinguish variation in luminance of a visual stimulus relative to its background. These patients have disturbed CSF.

Visual Acuity and Contrast Sensitivity

Snellen visual acuity (VA), the traditional index of visual resolution, is a test of the ability to perceive sharp outlines of relatively small objects. It is simple, quick, and of enormous practical importance. With the Snellen chart the observer's VA is

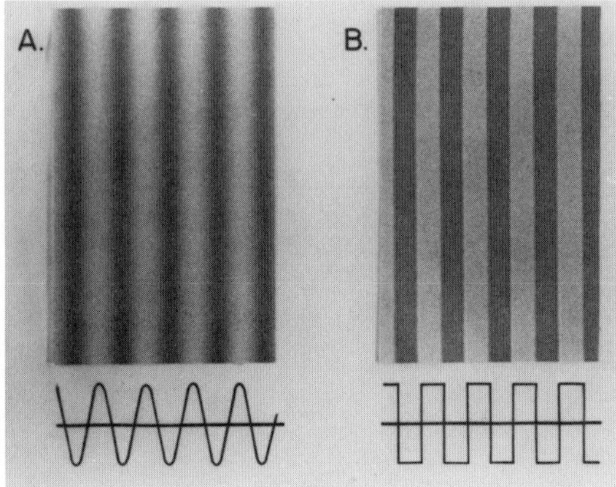

FIGURE 9.1. Photographic reproduction and luminance profile of a sinusoidal (A) and a square wave (B) grating pattern. In the sine wave grating the luminance profile is a sinusoid; in the square wave grating it is a square wave. For spatial contrast sensitivity measurements, sinusoidal gratings, as shown in A, are used. (Reprinted from Bodis-Wollner and Camisa,[1] with permission. Copyright 1980 by Elsevier Science Publishers.)

expressed as a fraction, the denominator being the distance from which the smallest detectable letter subtends 1 minutes of arc at the eye. The value of VA assessment in correcting refractive errors is well proven. However, this method of visual function assessment makes a number of assumptions about the human visual system. One is that quantification of the smallest resolvable letter describes the capacity of the visual system to resolve objects of all sizes. The second is that contrast is not of primary importance in assessing visual competence (Snellen letters have the maximum possible contrast). However, whereas high contrast is required to distinguish small letters, the amount of contrast needed to identify a coarser object or pattern is a function of the object's pattern or size.

Contrast sensitivity (CS) testing assesses the patient's visual sensitivity to large, intermediate, and small objects under circumstances of varying contrast. The contrast sensitivity function (CSF) is a *graphic* representation of the patient's vision for a range of target sizes. The VA score is just one limit of the CSF representing the finest detectable object just at maximum contrast. The CSF allows detection of visual deficits that cannot be detected by testing for the limits of resolution under high-contrast conditions alone. It promises to be an important diagnostic tool that complements the Snellen VA in the early diagnosis of diseases of the eye and visual pathways. Nevertheless, to apply it properly one needs to understand the principles that underlie the human spatial vision.

Sinusoidal Gratings, the Visual Stimuli for CS testing

The CSF is typically measured using sinusoidal grating patterns as the visual stimuli. Black and white bars of equal width have been used since the 18th century as acuity targets.[1] They were first used in clinical CSF studies in patients with cerebral lesions.[2] A sine wave grating pattern is a repeated sequence of dark and light bars with a luminance profile that changes gradually from dark to light without sharp borders, as best described by a sinusoidal waveform (Fig.9.1A). The reason for using sinusoidal gratings is that they offer the simplest configuration for relating stimulus to response.[3] Just as in the field of hearing any sound can be synthesized by combining a number of pure tones (sinusoidal sound waves), so in theory it is possible to construct any complex visual image by combining, in correct proportion, a number of sinusoidal gratings. On the basis of the well-established theory by Fourier,[4] one can describe a square wave pattern (Fig. 9.1B), which contains sharp borders between dark and light bars, as a complex wave that can be considered the sum of a number of sine wave components whose spatial frequencies are odd multiples of a fundamental frequency.[4] Thus, by knowing how an observer detects a number of individual sinusoidal gratings, one would be able to predict how the observer will respond to any complex pattern.

The spatial frequency (Sf) of a grating pattern is expressed in cycles per degree of visual angle (cpd); it defines the width of one bar (W) expressed in minutes of arc by the relation $Sf = 60/2W$. A cycle is a pair of adjacent dark-bright bars. A low Sf pattern contains only a few cycles in 1 degree of visual angle. Therefore it consists of coarse bars. Consequently, a high Sf pattern subtends many cycles in 1 degree of visual angle and the bars are finer (Fig. 9.2). Another advantage of using sine-

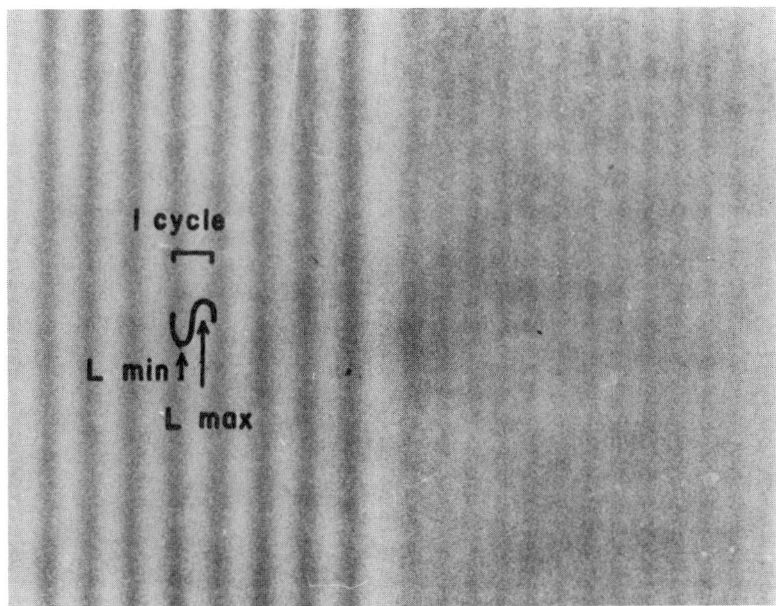

FIGURE 9.2. Two different sinusoidal grating patterns. From a viewing distance of 30 cm, their spatial frequencies will be 1.3 cycles per degree (left) and 2 cpd (right). Spatial frequency is defined as the number of alternating dark and bright bars subtended in 1-degree visual angle. Inset shows sinusoidal luminance changes. Contrast is defined as the luminance difference between bright bars (peak of sinusoid) and dark bars (trough), divided by the sum of their luminance. The pattern on the right is lower in contrast than the one on the left. (Reprinted from Bodis-Wollner and Diamond,[23] with permission. Copyright 1976 by Oxford University Press.)

wave gratings in CS testing is that, since they do not have sharp edges, optical blurring doesn't affect the overall wave shape, but only causes a decrease in contrast.[5]

The CSF of the Normal Observer

For establishing an observer's CSF, both the contrast and the Sf are varied without the average or mean pattern luminance being affected.

The contrast (C) of a pattern is defined as the luminance difference of two adjacent dark-bright bars over the sum of their luminance:

$$C = \frac{(L_{max} - L_{min})}{(L_{max} + L_{min})}$$

The mean luminance of a pattern (L) is defined as half the sum of the luminance of a bright bar (L_{max}) and a dark bar (L_{min}):

$$L = \frac{(L_{max} + L_{min})}{2}$$

The minimum contrast required for an observer to discriminate that there is a pattern on the screen is the contrast threshold of the observer for that pattern. Contrast sensitivity is the reciprocal of the contrast threshold. Thus, the lower the threshold, the higher the sensitivity.

The plot of the CS over a range of spatial frequencies gives the CSF, referred to sometimes as the spatial modulation transfer function. The photopic normal CSF based on data obtained from ten observers (heavy line in Fig. 9.3) shows a bell shape, with a clear optimum (S_{max}) at approximately 5 cpd ($W = 6$ minutes of arc). The CSF shows a rapid falloff in sensitivity at higher Sfs, and a less rapid rolloff in sensitivity at lower spatial frequencies. The intersection point of the CSF with the abscissa is the high-frequency cutoff, or the finest pattern detectable just at the maximum 100% contrast. Any grating of higher Sf will be indistinguishable from a uniform screen. This is equivalent to the definition given for the Snellen VA score. Therefore, the high-frequency

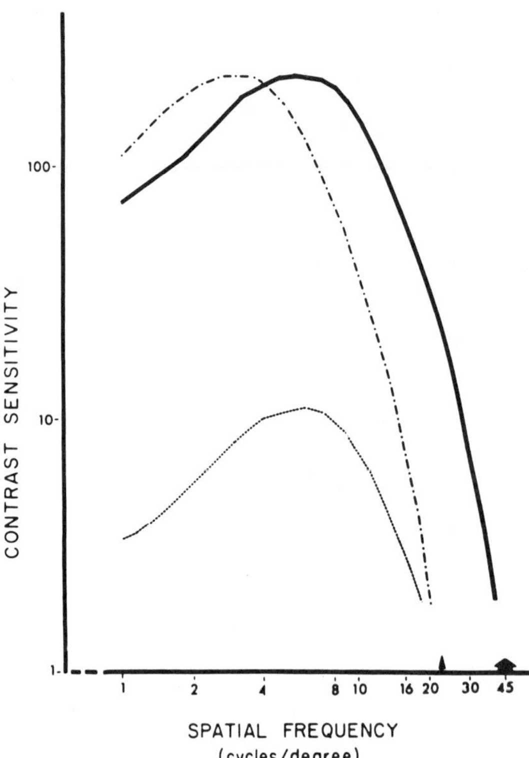

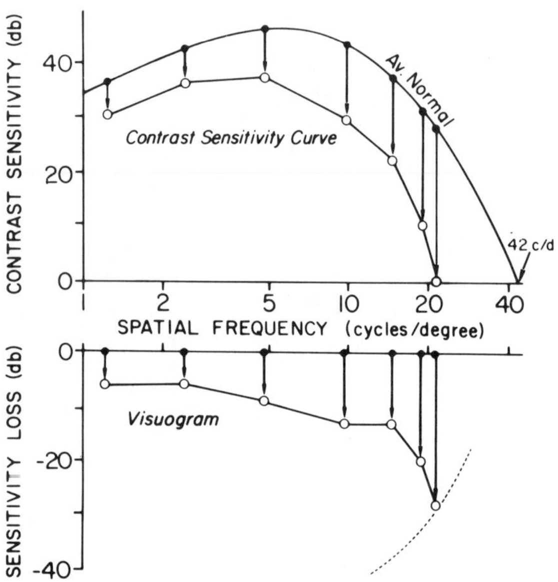

FIGURE 9.4. Contrast sensitivity function (top) and visuogram (bottom). The upper plot shows two contrast sensitivity functions: That of normal subjects with acuity of 1.0 (smooth curve), and that of a patient with visual defects (open circles). Contrast sensitivity (ordinate of upper plot) is specified on a logarithmic scale, in decibels.

The visuogram shows the contrast sensitivity deficit (downward arrow) at each of the tested spatial frequencies for the patient whose contrast sensitivity is given above. A loss of 6 db signifies a twofold reduction of contrast sensitivity; a loss of 20 db signifies a tenfold reduction. The spatial frequency scale (abscissa) of the visuogram is the same as that of the contrast sensitivity function above it. (Published courtesy of *Ophthalmology* **87**:1140–1149, 1980; Ref.8.)

FIGURE 9.3. The normal contrast sensitivity function (heavy lines) based on data from ten observers. The other two curves represent patients having the same visual acuity but vastly different contrast sensitivity functions. (Reprinted from Bodis-Wollner and Diamond,[23] with permission. Copyright 1976 by Oxford University Press.)

cutoff of the CSF, sometimes referred to as the *grating acuity* (GA), is in fact a more precise determination of visual acuity.[6] Since 100% contrast is not realizable physically, the cutoff point is found by extrapolating the CSF to intercept the abscissa. For normal observers the cutoff Sf of 45 cpd is the equivalent of 20/20 VA (Fig. 9.3, broad arrow). The GA for normal observers could range between 35 and 60 cpd, depending on the testing conditions, as will be further discussed.[7] The area under the heavy line in Figure 9.3 represents our window of visibility.

The term *visuogram*, proposed by Bodis-Wollner[2] in analogy to the audiogram and to honor von Bekesy, represents the plot of the loss in CS as the difference in logarithmic units (decibels, db) between a patient's CSF and the average normal CSF, which represents the zero level.[8] Thus a visuogram near the zero level implies a normal CSF, whereas a curve below this level indicates the amount of CS deficit in decibels (Fig. 9.4).

Our Understanding of the CSF

The CSF, which was used by the first researchers to explore the optical qualities of the human eye, turned out to have hidden power for the quantitative description of neural transmission along visual pathways.

Schade[9] in 1956 *created* a photoelectric analog of the eye and made the observation that the high-frequency behavior of the human CSF is a sensitive indicator of various optical factors such as pupil size and refractive power of the eye. Campbell and Green[10] have produced interference sinusoidal fringes directly on the retina. They bypassed the optic media of the eye and were able to distinguish between the modulation transfer function formed by the optics of the eye, which project the image on the retina, and the retinal-neural performance, reflecting the ability of the retina coupled to the brain to resolve the details of that image. They established that the normal human CSF for central vision is determined partly by optic mechanisms of the eye and partly by neural mechanisms, both determining the high Sf falloff. However, as opposed to a purely passive optical filter, the human CSF shows also a low Sf decline, which is the result of neural attenuation alone.

By looking into retinal single-ganglion-cell response one discovers a great deal of similarities to the CSF of the eye. The light-adapted cat retinal ganglion-cell receptive field, described in the pioneering work of Kuffler,[11] consists of two overlapping (excitatory and inhibitory) areas. The two areas are arranged as a circular center (excitatory), surrounded by an annulus of opposite polarity (inhibitory). The signals from the center and surround are additive and may cancel each other. Thus, for each retinal ganglion cell, as in the human CSF, there is an optimum size of stimulus that causes maximum excitation with minimum inhibition. If the stimulus is larger than the optimum it will cause more inhibition than excitation, and the response will decrease. Conversely, if the stimulus is smaller than the optimum the response of the ganglion cell will decrease in a linear fashion. It was therefore concluded[12] that the low Sf attenuation of the human CSF can be attributed to the center and surround organization of ganglion cells' receptive fields. To further investigate this issue, Enroth-Cugell and Robson,[12] using microelectrodes placed directly on cat optic-tract fibers, recorded the response of individual ganglion cells to drifting sinusoidal grating patterns. They were able to define two types of retinal ganglion cells, named X and Y cells, with distinct psychophysical and electrophysiologic proprieties.[12,13]

The dichotomy of the X-Y cell system is maintained up to the parvo and magnocellular layers of the lateral geniculate nucleus.[14] In parallel with the work by Enroth-Cugell and Robson, Hubel and Wiesel[15,16] described single neurons in the visual cortex. They made the distinction between simple and complex cells of the striate cortex, arranged in columns highly selective to orientation and ocular dominance.[16] The most striking characteristic of all the cells in the striate visual cortex, one that distinguishes them from retinal and lateral geniculate nucleus cells, is their linearly oriented receptive fields, compared with the circular organization of receptive fields described above.[15] It is this arrangement that makes the cortical cells respond maximally to slits of light of a specified width and orientation.[16]

These discoveries cast doubt on a simple interpretation of the CSF in terms of single-cell-type function and prepared the ground for psychophysicists to formulate the concept of *tuned pathways* in human spatial vision. In 1968 Campbell and Robson[4] provided an elegant analysis of the human visual spatial response via Fourier theory, and concluded that the nervous system must contain independent operating mechanisms (channels) selectively sensitive to a limited range of Sfs.

However, the assumption that the Fourier theorem would answer all the questions raised by the complex process of human spatial vision, as it does in physics and engineering, was a little simplified, and criticisms were to come. Some evidence for the partial failure of the spatial frequency model came from the same types of experiments that were used earlier to prove its validity.[17,18] Nevertheless, the evidence is still stronger pro than against the existence of Sf channels in the human spatial vision.[19-22] But even if it is eventually determined that our process of spatial vision is far away from Fourier's theorem, Fourier analysis has already proven to be a useful heuristic tool leading us to new experiments and insights.[22]

Can the CSF Be Predicted from the VA Score?

Before we proceed to the more practical part of this chapter, there is one more question we need to ask: Is one able to predict the exact shape of the CSF

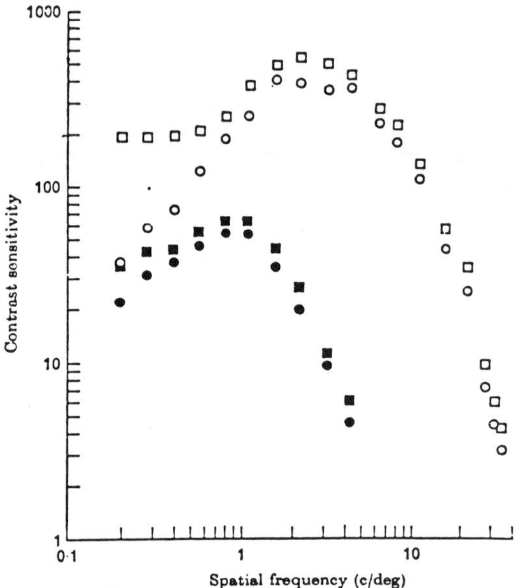

FIGURE 9.5. Contrast sensitivity functions for two different levels of mean luminance. The upper curves were measured with gratings having a mean luminance of 500 cd/m² squared. The lower curves were measured at 0.05 cd/m² squared. (Reprinted from Campbell and Robson,[4] with permission. Copyright 1968 by The Physiological Society.)

from the VA score alone? In other words, is there a specific CSF curve for any given VA? This question was experimentally answered by Bodis-Wollner[2] and by Bodis-Wollner and Diamond,[23] who showed that a decrease in two hypothetical factors of the retinal image, size and contrast, might produce equal high-frequency cutoffs (Fig 9.3, thin arrow) with the same VA and yet markedly different CSFs. Thus it was concluded that from the Snellen VA score alone one cannot predict the shape of the CSF.

With the foregoing information in mind, we are now ready to proceed to the clinical applications of this valuable visual function.

Measuring Contrast Sensitivity

Parameters of Influence

Mean Luminance, Pupil Size, and Refractive Power

The mean luminance (L) of sinusoidal gratings has a profound effect on the CSF. At high photopic levels of mean luminance, the normal CSF has peak sensitivity at about 5 cpd and the high-frequency cutoff at about 45 cpd. As mean luminance is lowered, the peak of the CSF is depressed and shifted, together with the cutoff Sf, toward lower frequencies. At mesopic levels of L, the peak of the CSF has practically disappeared, and the low Sf attenuation is no longer evident (Fig. 9.5). Interestingly, it has been suggested[24] that dopaminergic interplexiform cells of the retina, which are known to exist in humans,[25] might have the function of regulating the center-surround ratio as a function of the adaptation level.[26,27] For a given luminance level with increasing size of the pupil, there is in general an increase in CS at all but the lowest Sfs.[10] Consequently a small pupil is expected to reduce the CSF by reducing retinal illuminance. However, in practice the reduced illuminance caused by a reduced pupil diameter has little effect on the CSF.[28-30] This since a reduction in pupil diameter reduces also geometric aberrations opposing the effect of the reduced retinal illuminance.[28]

Focus is the other major parameter that affects the quality of the retinal image. There is a decrease in contrast sensitivity caused by defocus on either side of a lens power of + 1.5 diopters, with a dramatic effect at high Sfs (9 to 30 cpd) but almost no effect at low Sfs (< 1.5 cpd).[10] Thus, both a decrease in retinal illuminance and optical blur may cause medium to high-frequency loss in the CSF, with almost no effect at low Sfs. These facts should be kept in mind when the CSF is evaluated in various pathologic conditions. Standardizing the ambient luminance, monitoring pupil size, and using the correct refraction for the patient at the test viewing distance are all essential for proper interpretation of the CSF in clinical practice.

Temporal Characteristics

The change, or modulation, of a grating pattern as a function of time is expressed in hertz (Hz) as the temporal frequency (Tf) of the pattern. The Tf plays a crucial role in shaping the CSF.[31] The change in CS as a function of both Sf and Tf is represented by a *three-dimensional CS surface*, (ST-CS)[31-33] (Fig. 9.6). The shape of the ST-CS depends on the mean luminance level and on all other parameters that affect the CSF.[33] The ST-CS improves the accuracy of early diagnosis of glau-

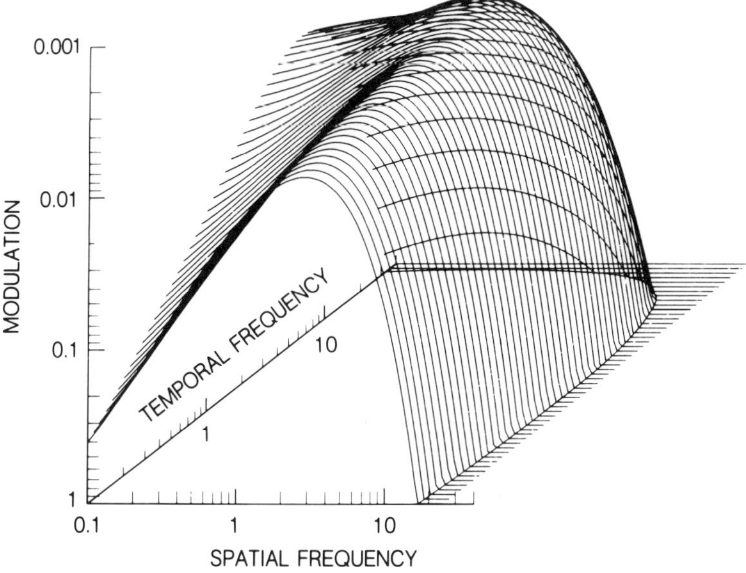

FIGURE 9.6. Spatiotemporal contrast sensitivity surface (ST-CS). It provides a qualitative picture of the combined effect of spatial and temporal frequency on contrast sensitivity. Each curve represents the CSF at a fixed temporal frequency. The neighboring curves are separated by a constant increment of 0.05 log in temporal frequency; modulation in this figure stands for contrast sensitivity since the scale is inversed. (Reprinted from Kelly,[33] with permission. Copyright 1979 by Journal of the Optical Society of America.)

coma[34] of some cases of multiple sclerosis,[35] and could be useful in the follow-up of Parkinson's patients,[36] as will be further discussed.

Retinal Location

The CSF measured at eccentric retinal loci, compared with the CSF measured at the fovea, shows a progressive shift toward lower Sfs of both the peak and the high-frequency cutoff[37-40] (Fig. 9.7). The decreasing CSF with retinal eccentricity could be explained by the retinal inhomogeneity model,[40] which is shown schematically in Figure 9.8. This model proposes a radial increase in the size of the retinal ganglion cells' receptive fields with increasing eccentricity. Each hexagon size in the diagram represents a group of retinal ganglion cells with a relatively narrow range of receptive-field sizes. The cells with the smallest receptive fields are restricted to the macula. When the test gratings are scaled by the magnification factor of the human striate cortex to stimulate equal amounts of visual cortex, the CSF becomes independent of visual field location.[39]

Orientation of Gratings

Our visual system is more sensitive to vertical and horizontal gratings than to other orientations.[41] This was exemplified by the "oblique effect" described by Appelle,[42] who has shown that the CSF for obliquely oriented gratings is reduced, especially at high Sf relative to the CSFs for vertical and horizontal orientation, which are about the same. Orientation selectivity of the CSF will be further discussed in this chapter in some pathologic conditions of the visual system.[43-45]

Sampling Area of Gratings

Visual sensitivity to low Sf depends on the number of gratings included in the field. Sensitivity increases as more cycles are included in the field, up to about 10 complete cycles.[7,46] This effect is of great practical significance, and could explain the low Sf loss observed in patients with macular or optic nerve lesions. Obviously, in these conditions even though many cycles are presented, because of the visual field defect only a few are seen. Reducing gratings length (vertical extent of the

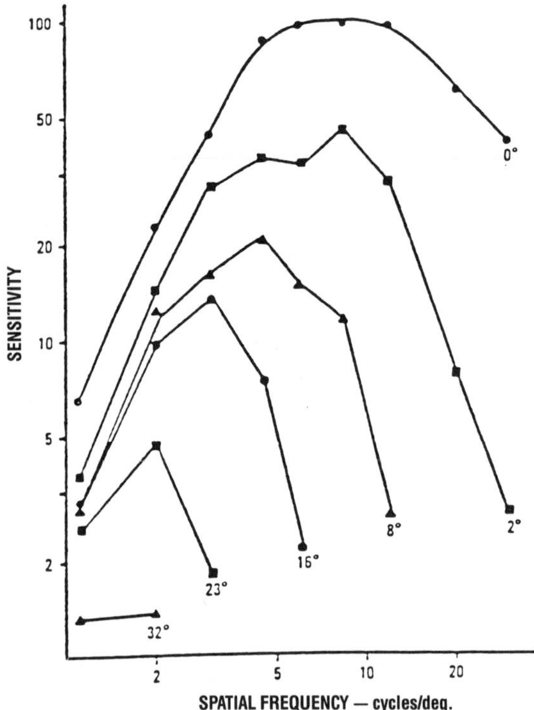

FIGURE 9.7. Contrast sensitivity functions measured at various eccentricities with 2.5-degree targets. (Reprinted from Hilz and Cavonius,[37] with permission. Copyright 1974 by Pergamon Press PLC.)

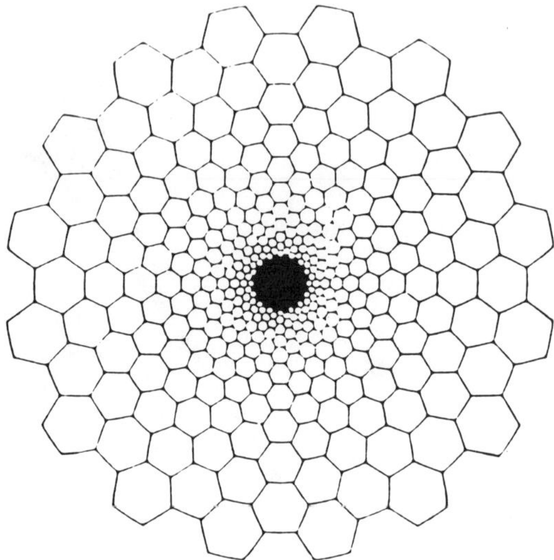

FIGURE 9.8. Schematic diagram of the retinal inhomogeneity model. Retinal structure is symbolized by the size and density of hexagons at each eccentricity. (Reprinted from van Doorn et al.[40] Copyright 1972 by Springer-Verlag, New York.)

bars) was also shown to influence the CSF at low Sf.[47] This finding may be relevant to the CSF obtained in patients with altitudinal visual field defects, although this relationship has never been vigorously examined.

Binocular Contrast Summation

It is generally accepted that in normal observers binocular CSF is higher than monocular sensitivity by some 42%, across all spatial frequencies, as would be predicted by neural summation of the two monocular responses.[10,48,49] Gilchrist and McIver,[49] testing both monocular and binocular CSF at different luminance levels, provided evidence that the reduction in the monocular sensitivity caused by reduced luminance to one eye can in some subjects lower binocular sensitivity to a level below that of the nonaffected eye. This is similar to the paradoxical phenomenon described by Fechner in 1860, and suggests the existence of inhibitory processes in binocular perception.[48,49] Such luminance differences between the eyes arise in practice as a consequence of monocular cataract or other opacities of the ocular media, or as a result of monocular sensitivity differences in macular degenerations and amblyopia.[49]

Effect of Age

Studies done in infants using preferential fixation[50,51] and visual evoked potential (VEP) measurements[52-55] have shown that the infant CSF is depressed at all Sfs compared with the adult CSF. The CSF improves progressively, approaching adult values by the end of the first year of life (Fig. 9.9). The CSF at all Sfs continues to increase steadily with age, to reach maximum levels in the 18- to 29-year age group.[56,57] The CSF begins to decline again after 30 years of age.[58] The reason for the difference in CSF between children and adults is unknown; anatomic and physiologic maturation of receptors, ganglion cells, dendrites, and so on reach adult levels at about 2 years of age or earlier.[57,59] Therefore, it has been speculated that the performance of children in CSF testing might in fact reflect cognitive rather than sensory factors.[57] Further support to the possible influence of cognitive factors on the CSF of children was given by Kirzner,[60] who showed a significant correlation between a child's CSF and his or her scholastic achievement.

Studies regarding the influence of aging on the CSF have shown widely disparate results.[29,30,61-66] Some of the contradictions can be explained by methodologic differences,[61] small sample, age-related criteria differences,[64] or concurrent undisclosed ocular pathologies.[29] The general view is that the CS declines with age for medium and high Sfs, but that little change occurs at low Sfs.[63-66] Owsley, Sekuler, and Siemsen[66] have implied an impairment in *temporal processing* of vision in the elderly. Since optical and neural characteristics of the visual system change throughout adulthood, both may account for the CSF of aging. Weale[67] estimated that as a result of the optical changes of aging, namely the reduction in pupil size, or senile miosis, and the increased density of the crystalline lens, the average 60- year-old eye transmits approximately one third of the light transmitted by the average 20-year-old eye. As already pointed out in this chapter, the reduction in retinal illuminance caused by a small pupil has only little effect on the CSF and cannot account alone for the decreased CS of aging. The role of the lens changes was evaluated by Owsley et al.,[68] who showed a similar loss in CS in older adults in good ocular health and in a group of age-matched patients who had undergone cataract extraction and intraocular lens (IOL) insertion. Moreover, the optical factors reviewed here cannot explain the temporal visual deficit of aging.[66] Morrison and McGrath[30] have shown that the optical modulation transfer function does not vary systematically with age, while the laser interference fringe-obtained CSF shows a continuous decline with age. Devaney and Johnson[69] have found an absolute fall with aging in the *number of neurons* in the macular projection area of the human visual cortex. In addition there is a loss in the *quality of the surviving neurons*, which show significant decrease in the number of dendritic spines. Similar neuronal loss has been identified at other levels of the visual pathways.[30] Therefore, Morrison and McGrath[30] were able to conclude that the age-related deterioration of the CSF is primarily of neural origin. Nevertheless, in the presence of a central cataractous change, a small pupil may have a dramatic effect on the CSF.

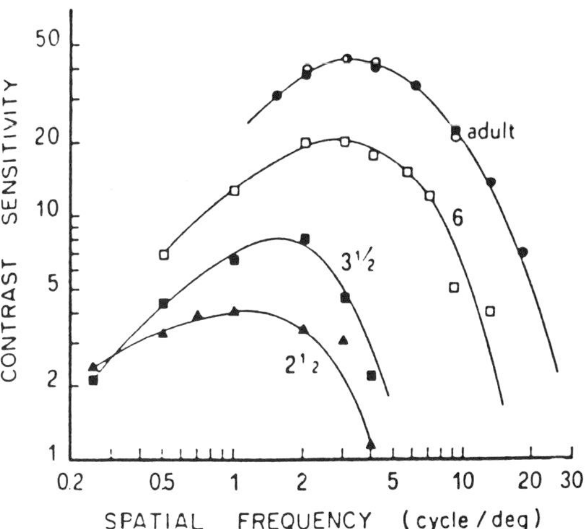

FIGURE 9.9. Amplitudes of VEP for an infant aged 2½ months (triangles), 3½ months (full squares), and 6 months (open squares) at various spatial frequencies. Each point is the mean of several records. Data from an adult subject are reported for comparison. (Reprinted from Pirchio et al.,[52] with permission. Copyright 1978 by Elsevier Science Publishers B.V.)

Miscellaneous Factors

Chromatic gratings

In a psychophysical study in humans using sinusoidal gratings, Mullen[70] found that the CS for chromatic gratings consisting of two monochromatic gratings added in antiphase (red-green or blue-yellow), was lower than the CS for either monochromatic gratings alone, for Sf above 0.5 cpd. At lower Sfs the CS was greater for the chromatic gratings. Thus, Mullen concluded that the sensitivity of the visual system to chromatic and luminance contrast depends on spatial frequency.[70] Besides providing insight into human color vision,[71] measurement of chromatic CSF could play a valuable role in the early detection of glaucoma and optic nerve diseases.[72]

Dopaminergic effects

Administration of dopaminergic drugs to healthy volunteers[73] has induced in all cases an increase in the CS at medium and high Sfs. This is to be expected according to previous studies, which have demonstrated the presence of dopaminergic cells in the retina.[24,25] It has been shown that the application of dopaminergic agents modifies the center-surround balance of ganglion cells' receptive fields.[24,74] The above findings have broad implications in Parkinson's disease, a pathologic condition characterized by a deficiency of the dopaminergic system, including the visual pathways.[36]

Cholinergic effects

Cholinergic influences have been found at various stages of visual processing. Harding, Wiley, and Kirby,[75] in an electrophysiologic study, demonstrated the existence of a cholinergic-sensitive channel tuned to low Sfs in the cat visual system. Since cholinergic neurons in the basal forebrain are affected in patients with Alzheimer's disease,[76] this finding could be relevant to the recently described visual deficits of the disease which will be further discussed.

Effect of anoxia

In one of the earliest studies done on contrast discrimination of letters, Hecht et al.[77] were able to show a deterioration in contrast discrimination in normal observers as a result of anoxia at altitudes of 15,000 ft or above. Fine and Korbrick[78] have recently studied the CSF of 25 military civilian volunteers, to evaluate the effect of smoking. According to their findings, habitual smoking causes an approximately 10% decrease in CS at medium and high Sfs. It could be postulated that this small depression in CS caused by habitual cigarette smoking is related to the effect of anoxia previously mentioned.

Effects of learning and cognitive factors

The effects of repeated testing are relevant to the clinical applications of the CSF, such as monitoring the progression of pathology. From the few studies available[79,80] there is no evidence for a major practice effect in the CSF of an adult. As pointed out previously, cognitive factors could play an important role in the CSF of children.

Gender differences

Brabyn and McGuinness[81] reported gender differences in the CSF, more pronounced at the outer regions of the curve, where females were significantly more sensitive to low Sfs and males were more sensitive to high Sfs. No sex differences in CS were observed in the mid range of Sfs. The origin of these differences is obscure, and their magnitude is negligible compared with the effect of pathology or aging.

Methods of Testing

There are two main approaches for obtaining a CSF. The first is the subjective psychophysical approach, further divided into printed and electronically generated patterns. The second is the more objective approach that makes use of electrophysiologic means, applied mostly in research and in testing infants or uncooperative patients. Some of the advantages and disadvantages of each method will be discussed below.

The prototypes of the printed tests, the Arden grating plates (AGP),[82] consist of six photographic prints. Each print changes in contrast in a direction parallel to the gratings, which appear to fade out down the page. The tester and the patient sit facing each other. The tester uncovers each print from bottom to top at a constant rate, so that regions of higher contrast are revealed. The patient is asked to indicate when the gratings first become visible. The measurement of CSF with the AGP covers just the low range of Sf (0.2–6.4 cpd), does not restrict the viewing area to a constant visual angle, does not ensure an equal rate of presentation for all the gratings, and lacks temporal and orientation parameters. With the AGP, the length of the gratings becomes a variable in addition to contrast as more of the print is disclosed. Furthermore, the appearance of the gratings might change with aging of the paper, and with ambient luminance. These factors can all cause significant variability in the scores obtained.

Since the AGP method was proposed, a variety of other printed and photographic systems for CSF testing have been developed. To mention just a few, there are a set of three to five Snellen-type letter charts, each of a different contrast (between 4% and 96%), but otherwise alike.[83] The main advantages of these charts are that the test procedure is familiar to the patient and clinician, being similar to the well-known Snellen chart. These charts contain some information related to orientation, since letter recognition is degraded by sensitivity loss along any orientation. This method appears to be more accurate than the AGP, but it also lacks temporal parameters.

Last for this group of tests are three simple and ingenious tests, providing a great amount of information. The Vistech acuity chart, the principle of which was first described by Bodis-Wollner,[84] further developed by Ginsburg,[85] and evaluated recently by Corwin and Richman,[86] is designed to be viewed at a distance of 3.05 m (10 ft) with a luminance of 100 cd/m². The chart consists of five rows of circular grating targets of four possible orientations. Each target subtends 3 degrees of visual angle at the viewing distance. Each row is of a single Sf (between 1.5 and 18 cpd) and of a variable orientation. The contrast of each row fades left to right. Proceeding from left to right, the patient is asked to identify the orientation of each target. The last correctly identified target in each row is scored as the contrast threshold for that Sf. Thus, the CSF may be plotted directly by darkening in the corresponding patches preprinted on an evaluation form. The main advantages of this chart are the rapidity of testing and the information regarding orientation provided. Its disadvantages are the small target area and the lack of temporal parameters.

On the basis of a theory developed by Howell,* Verbaken and Johnston[87] developed the Melbourne edge test. Howell's theory states that the detection of large objects with sharp edges is mediated by the same channels that detect the peak spatial frequencies of the CSF. This test is designed as a single chart containing 20 test patches, each 25 mm in diameter and of decreasing contrast and variable orientation of the edge (vertical, horizontal, oblique-right, oblique-left). The observer is required to indicate the orientation of the edge for each patch.

Finally, the most promising is the recently developed Pelli-Robson[88] single-size letter chart. This is a variable contrast chart having all letters of the same size, each subtending 0.5 degree at a viewing distance of 3 m. This is presumed to measure a subject's CS at a Sf between 3 and 5 cpd, corresponding to the peak of the normal CSF (S_{max}). With

both the Melbourne edge test and the Pelli-Robson chart, only S_{max} is tested; in common with all other printed charts these also lack temporal parameters. Whether the peak of the CSF is the best screening range for disclosing a loss in visual function remains still to be proven. Abrahamsson, Frisen, and Sjöstrand[89] in a recent study have shown that the $S_{max}/\sqrt{VA}$ (quotient between S_{max}, peak sensitivity of the CSF, and $\sqrt{VA}$, square root of the VA), based on both the CSF and VA data, could be a powerful clinical parameter. This also needs further evaluation.

The second group of subjective tests makes use of electronically generated grating patterns. These tests, compared with the printed tests, allow for more precise monitoring of stimulus parameters. Most important, they permit the control of temporal factors (modulation or change in time) as well. These advantages of the electronically generated tests requires a precise calibration of the stimulus at the expense of more time and money. The *method of constant stimuli*[23] used in our laboratory since 1972 is, in our opinion, superior to other methods. By this method patients are presented a pattern at various contrast levels but at the same Sf. The patient is asked to indicate "yes" or "no" to the presence of the gratings. Both false-positive and false-negative responses are recorded and a full psychometric function is generated. An estimation of the 75% detectability of the pattern is usually derived as the threshold level, offering some control over the observer visibility criteria. After the threshold is established, a pattern of a different Sf is presented in the same fashion. Since the same stimuli are used throughout the experiment, the method is called *constant stimuli*.

With the *method of limits*,[90,91] the principle employed is that the subject or the examiner varies the pattern, adjusting it in different manners (ascending, descending, or both) to meet the patient threshold. The important point is that ultimately it is the patient who decides what the threshold level is, and this depends largely on subjective criteria.[92] This drawback is more accentuated in children, and in elderly or confused patients. The employment of a forced-choice paradigm with the method of limits was suggested to minimize observer bias.[93] Typically this method consists of simultaneously presenting two alternatives, one with the pattern and one without it, and

---

*Howell ER: Visual mechanisms for the detection and perception of the contrast of large objects. Unpublished PhD dissertation, University of Melbourne, Australia, 1980.

the subject is "forced" to choose between the two. The patient's judgment for the visibility of the gratings is therefore comparative and not absolute.[92,93] From our experience, for most patients the method of constant stimuli is more easily understood and performed than a forced-choice method of limits. The latter also gives considerably lower threshold values.[94]

One limitation of all of the psychophysical tests, printed or electronically generated, is that they permit only threshold data to be obtained, providing no information about valuable suprathreshold functions.

The second approach for obtaining a CSF is by electrophysiologic means, which requires no judgment and only minimal cooperation from the patient. This offers obvious advantages. The term *spatial modulation transfer function* (SMTF) will be used in this chapter for these tests, to distinguish them from the psychophysically obtained CSF. One such technique, making use of the pattern visual evoked potential (PVEP), was proved possible by the initial work of Campbell and Kulikowski.[95] Several subsequent investigators[96-100] have demonstrated good correlation between the so-called *electrophysiological zero amplitude response* and the psychophysical threshold to temporally modulated sinusoidal gratings. The main disadvantage of the PVEP-SMTF test is that the acquisition of data for establishing a complete CSF is usually long and exhausting. This makes the technique unattractive to the clinician and unsuitable as a screening procedure. The sweep technique, first used by Regan[101] for rapid objective refraction by the PVEP and further developed by several investigators,[98-100] shortens the time required for obtaining a PVEP-SMTF. This method consists of one-trial, real-time retrieval of visual responses to continuously changing stimuli. The contrast changes from 0 toward suprathreshold levels over a brief period.

Regardless of their faults, the printed tests have the great merit of making the clinical use of CS testing a reality. By being simple and quick, they have brought CS testing out of the research laboratory and made it appealing to clinicians. As has been pointed out, the automated systems, despite their evident advantages in controlling stimulus parameters, are not free from observer bias and are largely dependent on observer cooperation. The PVEP-SMTF is an alternative, objective way of

assessing the CSF. It requires less patient cooperation, giving the bonus of suprathreshold information. However, the major problem with all of the aforementioned tests, which prevents the potential of the CSF from being fully exploited, is the lack of a single standardized procedure both universally available and acceptable by all.

Clinical Applications

In reviewing the clinical applications of the CSF, we have chosen an anatomic approach, moving from the anterior to the posterior segments of the eye through the optic nerve and up to the cerebral cortex.

Within-the-Eye Pathology

Corneal Pathology

As a result of intraocular light scattering, part of the light reaching the retina does not participate in image formation. Instead of converging to a focal point in the eye, some rays are dispersed to other areas by optical imperfections, such as corneal abnormalities, cataract, floating particles in the chambers, or macular diseases.[102] The relationship between visual disability and pathologic intraocular light scatter was recently explored by Van den Berg.[102] His remarkable finding was that VA correlates rather weakly with the amount of scatter, which causes considerable loss of visual function as can be shown by the loss in CS at low and medium Sfs (a drop in peak CS by a factor of 10 against a factor of only 1.8 decrease in VA). The decrease in CS for low Sfs can be explained by a decrease in the "sampling area of gratings" as a result of the intraocular light scatter.

Hess and Carney[103] reported that experimentally induced corneal distortion and edema in normal human subjects produce two distinct types of contrast attenuation. Distortion produces contrast attenuation, which is restricted to high and medium Sfs, whereas edema produces a decrease in CS, also at low Sfs.[103,104] The CSF of patients with keratoconus follows the prediction of experimentally induced corneal distortion, with diminished CS at high and medium Sfs but sparing at low Sfs.[102] An interesting finding is that sometimes CS at medium Sfs is more affected than at high Sfs. Whether this is a true bandpass effect or merely spurious resolution was not established.[103] A "notch" type of CS loss, selective for medium Sf, was recently associated with monocular diplopia of optical origin.[105] It could serve as a plausible explanation in patients with keratoconus with CS loss at medium-Sf only. Since monocular diplopia can also be of neurologic origin,[23,43] an important characteristic favoring an optical etiology is that the diplopia can be altered by placing a pinhole before the eye. Pinhole viewing restricts the area of incoming light, thereby reducing or eliminating the doubling image in case of an optical etiology.[105] In cases of keratoconus, where opacities are present, a severe decrease in CS of approximately 50%, at low Sfs (< 1 cpd), has been noted. The presence of the low-Sf loss depends only partially on the severity of the medium- to high-Sf degradation.[104] This low-Sf loss in CS has an important role in everyday visual performance,[106] and emphasizes the need for CSF testing in the evaluation of visual function in corneal diseases.

Effect of Contact Lenses

CS is lowered with soft contact lenses for only the highest Sfs (> 22 cpd). This loss, usually caused by lens deposits, is minor and well tolerated by most patients.[107] However, the complaints of some contact lens wearers truly reflect a debilitating impairment of vision at low and medium Sfs. In most of these cases the CS loss is caused by both the optical quality of the lens and damage to the cornea due to hypoxia and edema. For these patients the CSF provides a useful means for identifying the nature of the visual loss at an early and reversible stage and for monitoring the course of remedial action.[108,109]

Cataract

As senile cataract develops, optical aberrations and intraocular light scattering are the major factors in the visual deficit. Hess and Woo[110] have reported two distinct types of CS abnormalities in ten subjects with uniocular senile cataract, similar to what has been described already for corneal pathology. The visual deficit is either restricted to the high-medium Sf domain, or, as cataract develops and scattering of light becomes the major factor in the visual loss, a low-Sf CS loss (below 1 cpd) appears.

No correlation between the CS loss and the type of cataract was found. Unfortunately the sample of this study was small. Nevertheless the results add to our present appreciation of the nature of the visual function cataract patients might have. Establishing the CSF could have important implications in determining the timing for removal of a cataract, since a patient might still have reasonably good VA but suffer from a debilitating loss of visual function. Therefore, it is suggested that the assessment of CS for low- and medium Sf gratings (large objects), should supplement the present evaluation of vision in every cataract patient.

Cataract patients usually show a great difference between the VA measured in a darkened room and VA obtained in daylight. This occurs because a bright light within a cataract patient's visual field acts as a veiling luminance source, causing more scattering of light within the eye. The increased scattering of light superimposes on the retinal image with a contrast-lowering effect, causing additional impairment of visual ability. This phenomenon is called *disability glare* and it is discussed in more detail elsewhere in this book. Abrahamsson and Sjöstrand[111] have described a useful method for measuring disability glare in clinical practice. On the background developed by Paulsson and Sjöstrand,[112] they determined the glare score as the discrepancy in CS obtained with and without a circular fluorescent surrounding glare light. The visual stimulus used, was vertical sinusoidal gratings electronically generated on a TV monitor. Their data show that the density of the cataract is strongly related to the glare score whereas correlation to VA is rather weak. Thus the glare score gives important clinical information in patients with developing cataract and may validate a patient's complaints at a time when VA is still good. The glare score could be valuable also in the postoperative follow-up of patients with intraocular lenses,[113] radial keratotomy (surgical correction of myopia),[114] and penetrating keratoplasty (corneal transplantation).[115] In these patients 20/20 VA may not tell the whole story in the presence of debilitating intraocular scattering of light. The glare score could be useful also in evaluating vision for driving and in industry for developing optimal working routines in conditions that may enhance intraocular scattering of light.[116]

Kerstein, Hess, and Plant[117] have recently described a promising psychophysical method for the assessment of visual function behind cloudy media. They measured the CS for gratings in the presence and absence of visual noise as a function of Sf and noise level. Given certain assumptions,[117] it appears that when noise is added to the stimulus, if the CS loss is purely optical the visual deficit tends to normalize (becomes equal to the deficit of a normal observer in the same condition), whereas if the loss is neural in origin the deficit will become further depressed. Although more studies are needed, this method could provide a clinical tool for separating the optical and neural components of a visual deficit in the presence of cloudy media.

A more established technique for detection of neural deficits in the presence of a cataract is measurement of the CSF with a He-Ne laser interference device.[10,118] Widespread clinical use of interference fringes is presently limited by the amount of time and money needed for this test. In addition the technique needs much cooperation from the patient and is ineffective in the presence of a dense cataract.

Aphakia and High Refractive Errors

In high refractive errors in general and in aphakia in particular, the size of the retinal image is altered by the power and vertex distance of the lens and by optical parameters of the eye (axial and focal length). Thus, for a given object Sf, a different retinal image Sf will be formed.[119] In aphakia the corrective lenses cause an approximately 25% to 30% magnification of the retinal image and a reduction in the viewed Sf.[119] The examiner may assume that a given Sf is being tested when in fact a much coarser pattern forms on the retina. The overall CSF will be shifted toward higher Sfs with an apparent falloff in CS at low Sf. With aphakic contact lens correction, the image magnification effect is smaller and the CSF is closer to normal.[119] Since concurrent pathology is quite frequent in aphakia, it is of particular importance to recognize a shift in CSF, as just described, from a true pathologic loss.

In high myopia the minus spectacle correction is expected to cause just the inverse of that described, namely, a reduction in retinal image size with an increase in the effective Sf. This will cause a shift of the CSF toward lower Sfs, with an apparent worse performance at high Sf.[119] The effect of high myopia is, however, much more complex. Many cases of high myopia are axial, caused by a longer than normal eye, which brings an increase in retinal image size and counteracts the effect of the corrective minus lenses.[119] This could explain why the CSF obtained in high myopia is not different from the normal CSF.[120,121]

Pseudophakia

Intraocular lens (IOL) implants have been associated with different types of CSF abnormalities, from a loss at high Sf only[122] to a loss at medium Sf only,[122,123] or a loss at high and low Sfs and sparing at medium Sfs.[122] Weatherill and Yap[124] found no differences in CSF between patients with anterior chamber-iris-supported IOL implants and posterior chamber IOL implants. Some factors that could affect CSF in pseudophakic patients are the contrast-filtering properties and manufacturing quality of the IOL, the traumatized cornea, and in some cases the remaining posterior capsule and the miotic pupil.[123,124] The loss restricted to medium Sfs described in some IOL cases[122] could represent a "diplopic notch," a result of monocular diplopia caused by a malposition of the IOL.

Macular and Retinal Diseases

Most macular and retinal diseases affect mainly the medium-high Sf domain of the CSF.[8,125-130] Dissociation between VA score and the GA (high-frequency cutoff of the CSF) is another common finding of retinal diseases. A patient with VA of 20/20 may have a GA below expected, as reported in cases of retinitis pigmentosa, central serous retinopathy, and diabetic retinopathy[8,129,130] (Fig. 9.10). It could be that in these cases the fovea is still intact, allowing preserved VA but decreased CSF, which requires a broader retinal area. Surprisingly, in age-related macular degeneration, a "reverse VA-GA dissociation" has been described, with the GA being better than predicted from the VA[8] (Fig. 9.11). The reason for this kind of VA-GA dissociation is uncertain, but it may be assumed that the fovea is affected more than the surrounding area. A similar "reverse" VA-GA dissociation was also reported in some cases of amblyopia.[131] Brown and Garner[132] obtained a shift in the peak of the CSF toward lower SFs in patients with age-related macular degeneration, similar to the effect

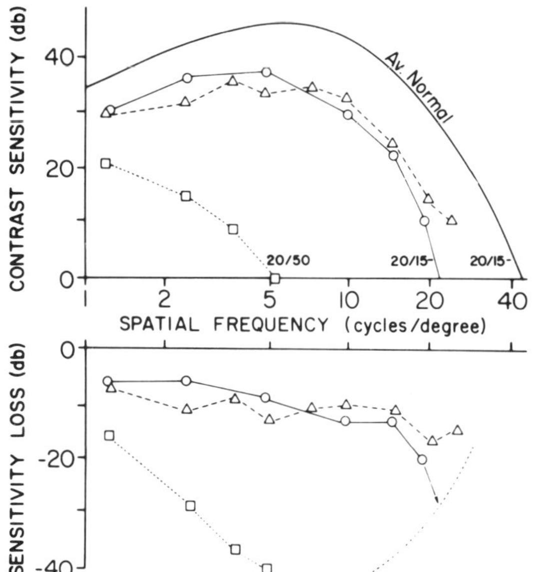

FIGURE 9.10. Grating detection of patients with central serous retinopathy. Contrast sensitivity losses were noted throughout the spatial frequency spectrum in spite of only moderately reduced Snellen acuities. The cutoff frequencies were less than would have been expected from the patients' Snellen acuities. (Published courtesy of *Ophthalmology* **87**:1140–1149, 1980, Ref. 8.)

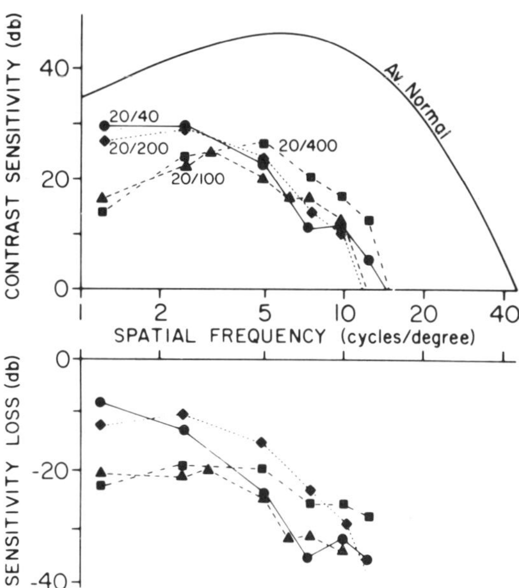

FIGURE 9.11. Grating detection of patients with age related macular degeneration. All curves show both low frequency and high frequency losses. All cut-off frequencies were reduced. In three of the four patients tested, however, the cut-off frequency was better than would have been predicted from the patient's Snellen acuity. (Published courtesy of *Ophthalmology* **87**:1140–1149, 1980, Ref. 8.)

of a low luminance level on the normal CSF. Thus it has been speculated that in these patients the normal mechanism of adaptation could be disrupted.[24,26,27,132]

A promising finding by several investigators[126-128] is that the CSF may be a valuable index of central visual dysfunction at the stage when macular changes are too subtle to be visible. Moreover, since the CSF is a noninvasive functional test, it has obvious advantages over fluorescein angiography. Measurement of the CSF with various visual field sizes (between 2.5 and 20 degrees) in patients with central scotoma due to macular or optic nerve pathology showed that the CS at low Sfs depends on the size of the visual field employed.[126,127] The size of the smallest visual field that is needed to reach normal CS values at low Sfs in these patients gives an estimation of the size of the central scotoma.[126,127,133]

Bodis-Wollner et al.[134] have reported recently that a pathologic condition confined to the retina does not cause orientation asymmetry of the PVEP. Thus, CS testing of more than one orientation could aid in the differential diagnosis of macu-

lar from demyelinating diseases of the optic pathways, in which orientation selectivity has been described both psychophysically[135] and by PVEP testing.[136-138]

Glaucoma and Ocular Hypertension (OHT)

One present aim of the diagnosis and treatment of primary open-angle glaucoma (POAG) is the search for noninvasive tests that will detect the visual deficit prior to the development of a functional and often irreversible visual field defect. The need for new and sensitive tests in the early diagnosis of glaucoma is best stressed by the finding that *close to half of the optic nerve fibers may be lost before a scotoma can be detected in the visual field* by routine perimetry.[139] CS studies in glaucoma and OHT (elevated intraocular pressure, IOP, with no evidence of optic nerve damage) have shown a specific CSF loss limited to low Sf (below the peak Sf).[82,140,141] Electrophysiologic studies[142-145] have shown also tuning for high Tf in glaucoma and OHT. By extending the CS measurement to eccentric retinal area, Lundh and Lennerstrand[146] have found a strong correlation between the visual field defects and the CSF of glaucoma patients. The finding that the CS loss in glaucoma and OHT is tuned for both low Sf and high Tf could be relevant to the mechanisms of the disease and not just be a "sampling area" effect. A grating of low Sf (1–4 cpd), which is modulated at high Tf (about 8 Hz), is a near-optimal stimulus for many neurons in the magnocellular layers of the primate lateral geniculate nucleus but not for the parvocellular layer neurons.[147] It follows that the specific spatiotemporal loss of glaucoma could be attributed to selective damage to the magnocellular "stream." A selective magnocellular loss was confirmed in primates with experimentally induced glaucoma.[148] The electrophysiology of these monkeys is consistent with the data summarized above.[149] Gunduz et al.[72] have shown in a recent study that *chromatic CS testing*, obtained with a computer-driven color TV system, is most effective in detecting OHT patients at risk of developing POAG, compared with other color vision tests and the achromatic CSF test. These findings support previous studies showing an early foveal (central) vision depression in glaucoma.[150,151]

The investigation of CS employing low Sf high Tf and/or chromatic visual stimuli promises to become an important clinical tool in the evaluation of OHT and early detection of POAG. The role of Arden plates in mass screening for glaucoma has been investigated in several studies.[152-156] High false-negative[152,156] and high false-positive scores[153] have been reported especially in elderly subjects.

Retro-orbital Pathology

Anterior Visual Pathways

The CSF is a sensitive index for the diagnosis and follow-up of compressive lesions of optic nerve or chiasm, at the stage when VA, color vision, and perimetry are still intact or show minimal changes. Tytla and Bunic[157] recently reported a loss of 10 db in CS restricted to the low Sf domain (0.33–3 cpd) in 72% of the 22 patients with papilledema (optic disk edema) tested. The test was performed by the method of limits using vertical sinusoidal gratings presented on an oscilloscope. Once the edema had resolved, little or no CS loss was detected. In a previous study[158] done in patients with compressive lesions of the anterior visual pathways but only

subtle disturbance of vision and no papilledema, the CS loss was also reported in the low Sf domain. However, since Arden plates were used in this study, high Sfs were not tested.

These studies raise the possibility that increased intracranial pressure and increased IOP may have similar effects on the anterior optic nerve.[148,157]

Toxic Optic Neuropathy

Ethambutol (antituberculosis drug) optic neuropathy

Ethambutol therapy for tuberculosis has the serious side effect of dose-related retrobulbar optic neuropathy.[159] It has been suggested that the neuritis is reversible if the drug is stopped, and that the speed of recovery depends on early recognition. Routine visual tests are not optimal for early diagnosis of this condition, since VA, color perception, visual fields, and optic disks may be normal in the presence of subjective visual disturbances. Salmon, Carmichael, and Welsh[160] have reported abnormal Arden scores in 38.2% of 100 patients receiving ethambutol therapy for 3 months. Five patients also had disturbed color perception; one had reduced VA. No abnormalities of the optic disk were observed. Electrophysiologic studies[161-163] have shown that the PVEP is also disturbed in subclinical ethambutol-toxic neuropathy, with peak latency recovering faster than the amplitude, following the discontinuation of the drug.

Acrylamide toxicity

Exposure to acrylamide monomer, an industrial and experimental chemical hazard,[164] causes dramatic changes in the visual function of monkeys. These changes are only partially reversible.[165] CS loss was reported for medium and high Sfs.[166] Acrylamide exposure produces an early latency increase and a subsequent amplitude reduction of the major positive wave of the PVEP, which is obtained at high contrast. Both the latency and amplitude of the PVEP recover before the CSF.[166]

Multiple sclerosis (MS)

MS may cause highly variable loss of visual functions.[43] The visual loss may occur in an eye with clinical evidence of optic or retrobulbar neuritis, but also in a clinically unaffected eye. Psychophysical and electrophysiologic studies have demonstrated CS deficits specific to stimulus Sf[43,138] and/or orientation.[45,135-138,167] The CSF loss in MS is selective to a narrow Sf band and/or a particular orientation in an individual patient. It is not always the same for both eyes, and it sometimes fluctuates from day to day. No particular orientation or Sf is more affected than another in all MS patients as a group.[43] The existence of an orientation-selective CS loss strongly suggests cortical involvement in MS.[167] An eye movement disorder could be another explanation for an orientation-specific loss, however in this case the deficit is unlikely to be restricted to a narrow Sf band. In addition, since the major eye movement disorder in MS is horizontal, the orientation deficit will cluster for vertical gratings. The combined value of CSF and PVEP testing in the diagnosis of MS and optic nerve diseases has received attention in the literature.[167,168] Delayed PVEPs are found in about 70% to 80% of patients with MS.[167] Bodis-Wollner et al.[167] have reported no concordance between prolonged PVEP latency and CS for sinusoidal gratings of the same Sf in 24 MS patients. However, considering the difference in contrast between the PVEP and the CS setting, this result is not surprising. Lorance et al.[168] have found the CSF to be more reliable than the PVEP in the early diagnosis of optic nerve disease. However, since they used sine wave gratings for CSF testing but checkerboards for PVEP, this comparison is also not fully interpretable. Sekular, Onsely, and Berenberg[169] have shown deterioration in CS induced by a short exercise period, with no effect on VA, in a patient with MS having subjective visual complaints that were intensified by exercise (Uthoff sign). Various deficits in temporal processing of vision in patients with demyelinating lesions of the visual pathways have been described.[35,170-172]

These data emphasize the importance of CSF testing in MS patients, using a temporally modulated sine wave visual stimulus rather than a complex stimulus such as a checkerboard.[5] A checkerboard pattern will stimulate simultaneously several Sfs, and several orientations, failing to uncover the selective and unpredictable pathology of the demyelinating process.

Cerebral Diseases

In clinical practice, patients with cerebral lesions often complain of blurred vision, while their VA is only mildly impaired. Bodis-Wollner and Diamond[23] have shown that in patients with cerebral (including retrochiasmatic) lesions, central (foveal) vision is affected as measured by CSF tests. These investigators have suggested that the "macular sparing" demonstrated by VA testing and by most forms of perimetry might be a stimulus artifact, requiring further verification with the CSF. Using the method of constant stimuli they have described three types of CSF losses in these patients: most often a high Sf loss, but also a level loss (for all Sfs), or a notch loss (selective for medium Sfs) (Fig. 9.12). An additional finding reported in cases of cerebral blindness[173] is that

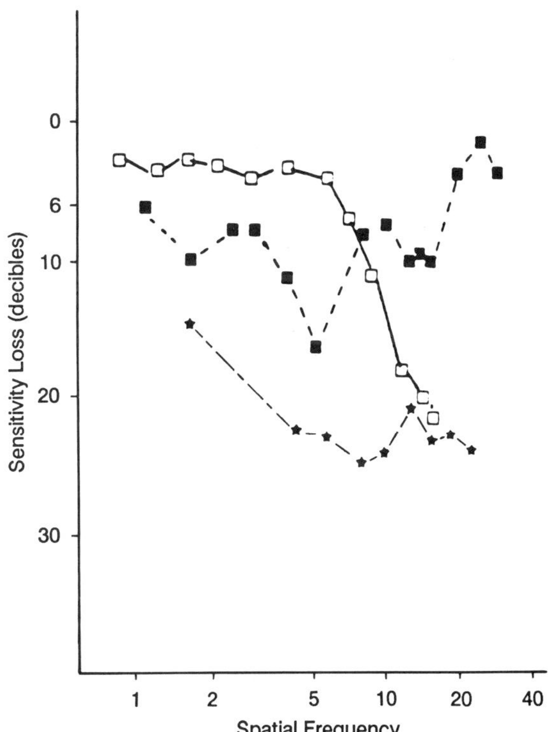

FIGURE 9.12. Visuograms of three patients. Empty squares: high-frequency loss (OD) of a 60-year-old patient with 20/30 Snellen acuity and a diagnosis of occlusion of the left posterior cerebral artery. Filled squares: selective frequency loss (OS) of a 63-year-old patient with occipital pole metastasis and 20/30 visual acuity. Stars: level loss (OD) of a 19-year-old patient with 20/40 visual acuity and granulomatous infection of the brain. (Reprinted from Bodis-Wollner,[6] with permission.)

the recovery of vision proceeds in a definite pattern, with low Sfs recovering first, then medium Sfs, and last and incompletely the high Sfs. Kobayashi et al.[174] have determined the CS with Arden plates in 23 patients following cerebral infarction involving the primary visual cortex, or the visual-associated cortex. Their data imply that the CSF is more affected when the lesion has an influence on the non-dominant lateral parieto-occipital area. While a lesion on the dominant lateral parieto-occipital area causes only a slight reduction in CS. Their findings are at variance with Bodis-Wollner and Diamond previous study,[23] which didn't disclose hemispheric asymmetry. It could be that the discrepancy is associated with Kobayashi et al. using AGP, which have as variables not only the contrast, but also the length of the gratings as more of the print is uncovered. Soso et al.[175] made the interesting observation that pattern sensitivity epilepsy, which is a pattern induced epileptic seizure, was Sf selective. The CSF of these patients tested with vertical sinusoidal gratings by a 2-alternative forced-choice method was essentially normal.

These findings as well as the narrow-band deficits found in patients with MS and some cerebral lesions,[43,23] and the specific pattern of recovery described in cortical blindness,[173] give clinical support to the existence of grouped neurons with similar receptive field sizes, termed *spatial frequency channels* in human spatial vision.

The CSF was found useful in detecting visual loss and in the follow-up of patients with pseudotumor cerebri (idiopathic intracranial hypertension.[176] Since the decision of therapy in pseudotumor cerebri is based largely on changes of visual function, the assessment of the CSF in these patients is strongly advocated.[168,176]

Miscellaneous

Amblyopia

Amblyopia is defined as impaired foveal vision, unilateral or bilateral, in the absence of organic disease.[177] CSF measurement in children with amblyopia has attracted much interest over the past years. The known etiologies of amblyopia are anisometropia, strabismus, and sensory deprivation. Although all three types of amblyopia are characterized by decreased VA, there might be substantial differences among the groups in spatial processing of vision. According to psychophysical and electrophysiologic studies, two distinct patterns of CS loss are found in amblyopia. In strabismic amblyopia the CSF is depressed only for a limited band of high Sfs, whereas in anisometropic amblyopia the depression is spread over the entire frequency range.[177-179] This difference in CS loss might reflect different amblyogenic mechanisms.[177-183] It has been shown that the spatial deficit manifested by humans with strabismic amblyopia tends to normalize at low background luminance,[180] whereas in the lens-reared monkey model of anisometropic amblyopia,[181] the deficits in the spatial resolving capacity of the defocused eyes were observed over a large range of background luminance. More recent evidence does, however, support the hypothesis that amblyopia is in fact one single mechanism and the recognized types represent different degrees on a single continuum.[184,185] Hess, Campbell, and Greenbalgh[186] have investigated the contrast threshold measurement compared with suprathreshold perception in humans with amblyopia. They found a spatial distortion component in amblyopia as well as a CS loss. The distortion was present at all orientations and over a range of retinal illuminance, especially at high Sf. This could imply an anatomic anomalous projection within the amblyopic visual system, which would explain also the dissociation between letter and grating acuity sometimes seen in amblyopia (VA < GA); letters are more distorted than gratings.[131] These findings add an extra dimension to our appreciation of the visual dysfunction of amblyopia in humans.

Meridional amblyopia

Subjects with substantial amounts of astigmatism (2.75 D or more) are described as having *meridional amblyopia*. They have reduced resolution for details on a given orientation, with no apparent organic cause to the condition. Freeman and Thibos[44] have found reduced CS for gratings coinciding in orientation to the amblyopic meridian at all Sfs, with prominent orientation difference in the cutoff Sf.

Parkinson's disease (PD)

Parkinson's disease (PD) is primarily defined as a motor disorder resulting from a deficiency of striatal dopamine.[36] The possible existence of primary

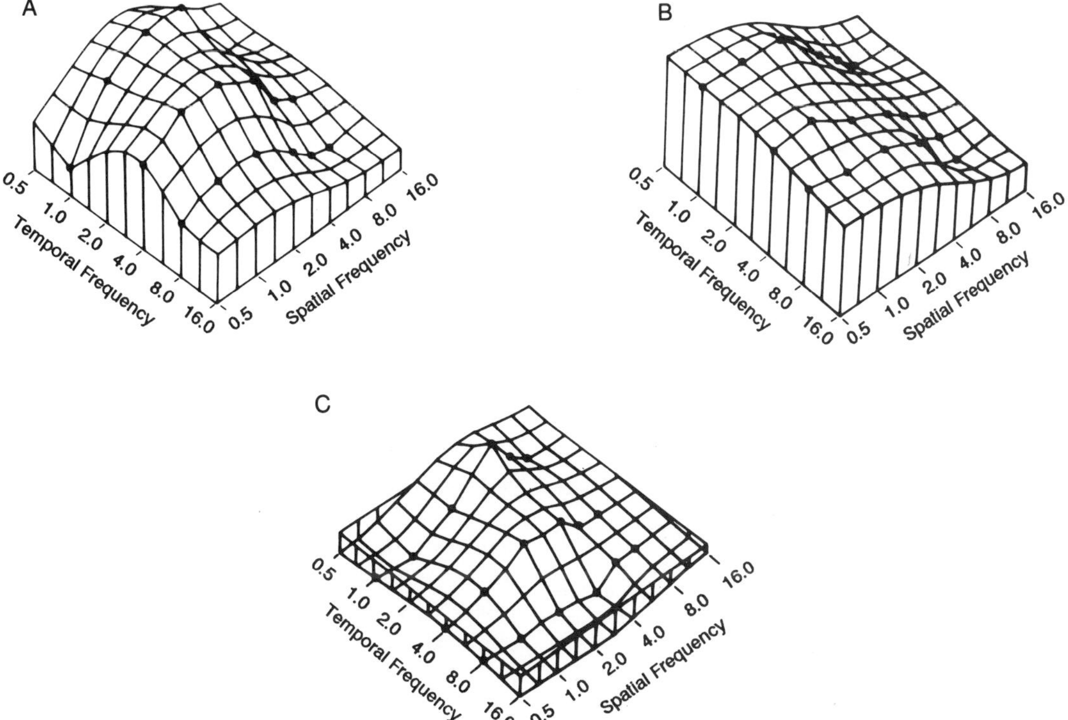

FIGURE 9.13. Spatiotemporal contrast sensitivity to a 9-degree field is shown for six spatial frequencies and six temporal frequencies in a three-dimensional *surface plot* for a 46-year-old man with Parkinson's disease who shows the "on-off" syndrome. Snellen visual acuity was 20/20 and 20/30. A, The three-dimensional surface measured when the patient was in the "on" phase. B, the surface measured when the patient was in the "off" phase. C, the "difference" three-dimensional surface resulting when the "off" phase responses are subtracted from the "on" phase responses. The shape of the "difference" surface suggests that dopamine enhances sensitivity at the peak of the spatiotemporal surface and attenuates sensitivity at the lower spatial frequencies. (Reprinted from Bodis-Wollner et al.,[36] with permission. Copyright 1987 Oxford University Press.)

sensory alterations in PD has been suggested by several authors.[187,188] However, only recently was visual dysfunction described in these patients and correlated with clinical evidence of low dopaminergic striatal activity.[36] The study by Bodis-Wollner et al.[36] was based on the configuration of the spatiotemporal CS surface obtained in six PD patients affected by the "on-off" syndrome.[189] This syndrome is found in patients receiving regular doses of levodopa. In the "on" stage patients show practically no symptoms of disease for several hours, after which disabling rigidity, akinesia, or tremor sets in ("off" stage). It is thought that the on and off stages are caused by high and low dopamine responsiveness of postsynaptic dopamine receptors, respectively.[189] The ST-CS was studied in both phases and was found to switch in parallel to the motor symptoms of the disease (Fig. 9.13).

Configuration of the ST-CS surface of the off stage was remarkable; there was not simply CS loss but an overall change in the shape of the spatiotemporal interaction. The peak of the ST-CS surface was flattened and the low-frequency attenuation was less apparent, compared with results in normal observers (Fig. 9.13B). There was no evidence of eccentric viewing or miosis in these patients, which could cause similar results.[36] Changes in CSF similar to those reported in the off stage were found in many patients affected by PD[36,190] (Fig. 9.14). It is known that dopamine neurons exist in the retina in several species including humans, mainly among the "interplexiform" cells.[24,25] These cells may modulate in a feedback loop the center-surround interaction of ganglion cells receptive fields.[24,74] Thus it is conceivable that the lack of dopamine in the retina in PD leads to a

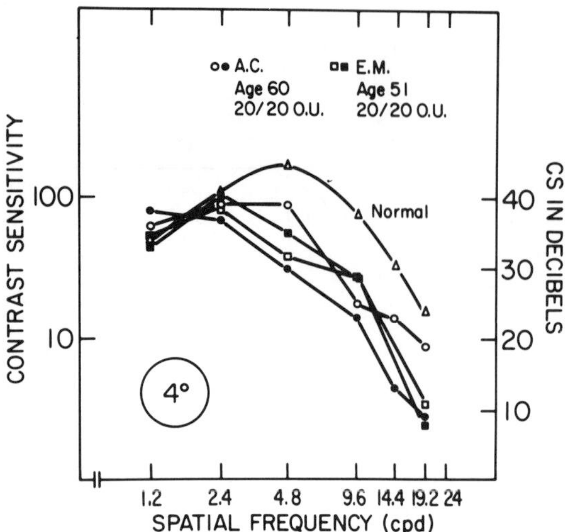

FIGURE 9.14. Contrast sensitivity to a 4-degree field is presented for the mean normal curve (open triangles), for each eye of a 60-year-old patient with Parkinson's disease (right eye, open circle; left eye, closed circle), and for each eye of a 51-year-old patient with Parkinson's disease (right eye, open square; left eye, closed square). The peak of the CSF is flattened and the low Sf attenuation is less apparent in the patients compared with the normal curve. Spatial contrast sensitivity is also shown in terms of decibels (db) on the right vertical axis. (Reprinted from Bodis-Wollner et al.,[36] with permission. Copyright 1987 by Oxford University Press.)

loss of CS that is a characteristic of reduced mean luminance.[26,27]

Several questions regarding the role of dopamine in human spatial vision and identification of the precise site and type of dopamine receptors involved (D1, D2, or both) are still to be answered by histochemical studies. Nevertheless, the data reviewed here imply that the CSF could play an important role in monitoring the effectiveness of therapy in PD patients.[36]

Regan and Maxner[45] recently made an interesting observation of orientation-selective CS loss to horizontal gratings, in ten patients with PD.

Alzheimer's Disease

Alzheimer's disease is a dementing disorder of unknown cause in which there is degeneration of neuronal subpopulation in the central nervous system.[76] Patients may have difficulty with a variety of complex visual tasks, reflecting impairment of cognitive skills. However, it is possible that basic visual processes are also compromised in this disorder. There are only a few studies on the CSF of Alzheimer's patients. Nissen et al.[191] have reported that the CSF was depressed in 14 patients compared with their age-matched spouses at all Sfs tested (from 0.5–8 cpd). One patient had a markedly reduced CS at low Sfs in relation to other patients. This patient had an impairment in object and face recognition. Schlotterer, Moscovitch, and Crapper-McLachlan,[192] on the other hand, could find no difference between the CSF of patients with Alzheimer's disease and that of normal controls. Optic nerve axonal degeneration[193] and delayed PVEP[194] have been recently reported in patients with Alzheimer's disease.

Further studies on the spatial vision of Alzheimer's patients are needed. One of the questions still to be answered is whether the low-Sf CS loss observed in some Alzheimer's patients[191] could reflect a disturbed cholinergic channel, as was pointed out earlier in this chapter.

Chronic Renal Failure

Patients with chronic renal failure have complaints about vision that may be attributed to changes in refraction after dialysis treatment[195] and to ocular pathology, including calcium deposits in the conjunctiva and cornea, cataracts, retinal vascular abnormalities, and fluctuations of IOP during dialysis.[196] In addition, the uremic state in humans is characterized by a wide variety of mental and neurologic aberrations, with many factors implicated but no definite etiology found.[197,198]

To our knowledge there are only two psychophysical studies in dialysis patients.[199,200] Russell et al.[199] have reported a deficit in CS of approximately 30% at medium-high Sfs and 13% at low Sfs, and no deficit at the lowest Sf (0.5 cpd), in 14 patients undergoing hemodialysis for chronic renal failure, compared with controls. The CS losses could not be explained by the ocular status of the patients. Woo et al.[200] also reported subtle changes in the CSF obtained before and after hemodialysis, without detectable VA or refractive changes. Both studies used the method of limits with electronically generated sinusoidal gratings to determine the CSF. The CSF changes of patients receiving chronic hemodialysis resemble the changes reported by some[191] for Alzheimer's disease, and differ from those reported for Parkinson's disease,[36,190] since the normal overall shape of the CSF was preserved.[199,200]

Although further studies are required, CSF testing may become a useful clinical tool in the early detection of central nervous system damage in uremia.

Latent Nystagmus

Latent nystagmus is a condition of unclear etiology manifested by involuntary oscillations of both eyes when either eye is occluded. Characteristically the nystagmus is horizontal and jerky, with the fast phase directed toward the open eye. This disorder appears to be part of an oculomotor syndrome, with some genetic influences.[201] Abadi[202] has measured the CSF in three patients with latent nystagmus. All three had a dominant eye that displayed a lesser intensity (amplitude $\times$ frequency) of nystagmus than the fellow eye, when each eye viewed the target monocularly. The CSF for the dominant eye was higher than that of the fellow eye at all Sfs, whereas in normal observers both eyes have approximately equivalent CSF. In addition, the CSF of the patients showed no low-Sf attenuation, probably due to the temporal movements induced on the retinal image by the nystagmus.[203]

Final Comments

The Snellen chart has, for more than 200 years, provided a simple, rapid, and easy to perform test. It is perfectly suitable for the evaluation of patients with refractive errors. This test is unlikely to be superseded. Nevertheless, in view of the overwhelming information that has accumulated during the last decades, it certainly requires augmentation.

The CSF, as we hope this chapter emphasized, represents one possible augmentation. The CSF offers a way to detect visual deficits in the central visual field that will escape detection when one tests for the limits of resolution alone. Evidence show that the VA score is just one extreme value on the scale of the complex function of human spatial vision. Although the VA can be estimated from the CSF as the GA, the reverse is not true. Furthermore, we have summarized evidence of VA-GA dissociation. Therefore, the *CSF and the VA should complement each other* in the evaluation of the visual performance. Recent studies suggest that the $S_{max}/\sqrt{VA}$ (quotient of S_{max}, the peak sensitivity of CSF, and $\sqrt{VA}$, the square root of VA), making use of both CSF and VA data, may become a useful clinical index of visual function. The purpose for the anatomic approach in reviewing the clinical applications of the CSF in this chapter is to emphasize that the CSF can be altered by pathology at various levels of the visual pathways, and its use as a mass screening test should be with caution.[204] Nevertheless, by utilizing recent physiologic knowledge it is becoming possible to use the CSF to answer certain questions in specific disorders. In glaucoma, the physiologic principle of separating magno from parvo cellular neurons makes the CSF a promising clinical tool for early detection of visual deficits. In Parkinson's disease, a dopaminergic deficiency at the retinal level correlates with a specific ST-CS surface deficit.

CSF testing at a specific orientation or with chromatic gratings has proven to be of great value. It could be more reliable than the PVEP in the early diagnosis of optic nerve diseases. With a specific spatiotemporal combination, and various field sizes or eccentric fixation, the CSF may become a valuable clinical tool in the evaluation of ocular hypertension and early diagnosis of glaucoma and macular diseases. Supplemented by a glare source or a superimposed visual noise, the CSF appears useful in the evaluation and follow-up of conditions with increased intraocular scattering of light. The measurement of CSF in diseases of uncertain etiology has given us important insights regarding their pathophysiology and has suggested future research directions. All of the foregoing are impressive reminders that the CSF is a functional, noninvasive test.

In summary, the vast literature that has accumulated over the past 40 years has established without a doubt that the CSF should become an integral part of every routine ophthalmologic examination. However, the variety of tests available now makes its clinical use confusing, preventing its potential from being fully exploited. Thus, as a future aim there is need to standardize these tests to one single procedure universally acceptable and available to all. The importance of using a simple sinusoidal grating pattern, with control of spatial, temporal, and orientation parameters, has been stressed throughout this chapter. The questions, (1) for which Sfs the CS should be routinely tested and (2) whether the peak sensitivity of the normal curve is the best screening range, remain as the major future determinants in the clinical application of the CSF.

Acknowledgments. We thank Dr. Julie R. Brannan for her critical reading of an earlier version of this manuscript and for her invaluable suggestions. The preparation of this chapter and research described herein were supported in part by grants EY01708 and EY01867 from the National Eye Institute, Bethesda, MD, and by Fight For Sight, Inc., New York City postdoctoral fellowship 88001, in memory of Mary E. and Alexander P. Hirsch.

References

1. Bodis-Wollner I, Camisa JM: Contrast sensitivity in clinical diagnosis. Lessell S, Van Dalen JTW (Eds), *Neuro-ophthalmology*, Amsterdam, Elsevier Science Publishers, 1980, pp 373–401.
2. Bodis-Wollner I: Visual acuity and contrast sensitivity in patients with cerebral lesions. *Science* **178**:769, 1972.
3. Andrews BW, Pollen DA: Relationship between spatial frequency selectivity and receptive field profile of simple cells. *J Physiol* **287**:163, 1979.
4. Campbell FW, Robson JG: Application of Fourier analysis to the visibility of gratings. *J Physiol (Lon)* **197**:551, 1968.
5. Bobak P, Bodis-Wollner I, Guillory S: The effect of blur and contrast on VEP latency: Comparison between check and sinusoidal patterns. *Electroencephalog Clin Neurophysiol* **68**:247, 1987.
6. Bodis-Wollner I: Visual acuity measurements with grating patterns. *Lancet* **2**:503, 1975.
7. Committee on Vision, Commission on Behavioral and Social Science and Education, National Research Council: *Emergent Techniques for Assessment of Visual Performance*. Washington, D.C., National Academy Press, 1985.
8. Wolkstein M, Atkin A, Bodis-Wollner I: Contrast sensitivity in retinal disease. *Ophthalmology* **87**(11):1140, 1980.
9. Schade OH: Optical and photoelectric analog of the eye. *J Opt Soc Am* **46**:721, 1956.
10. Campbell FW, Green DC: Optical and retinal factors affecting visual resolution. *J Physiol (Lond)* **181**:576, 1965.
11. Kuffler SW: Discharge patterns and functional organization of mammalian retina. *J Neurophysiol* **40**:37, 1952.
12. Enroth-Cugell C, Robson JG: The contrast sensitivity of retinal ganglion cell of the cat. *J Physiol (Lond)* **187**:517, 1966.
13. Kaplan E, Shapley RM: The primate retina contains two types of ganglion cells, with high and low contrast sensitivity. *Proc Natl Acad Sci USA* **83**:2755, 1986.
14. Kaplan E, Shapley RM: X and Y cells in the lateral geniculate nucleus of Macaque monkeys. *J Physiol (Lond)* **330**:125, 1982.
15. Hubel DH, Wiesel TN: Receptive fields and functional architecture of monkey striate cortex. *J Physiol* **195**:215, 1968.
16. Hubel DH, Wiesel TN: Sequence regularity and geometry of orientation columns in the monkey striate cortex. *J Comp Neurol* **158**:267, 1974.
17. Tolhurst OJ: Adaptation to square-wave gratings: Inhibition between spatial frequency channels in the human visual system. *J Physiol (Lond)* **226**:231, 1972.
18. Nachmias J, Sansbury R, Vassilev A, et al: Adaptation to square wave gratings: In search of the elusive third harmonic. *Vis Res* **13**:1335, 1973.
19. Blakemore C, Campbell FN: On the existence of neurons in the human visual system selectively sensitive to the orientation and size of retinal images. *J Physiol* **203**:237, 1969.
20. Campbell FN, Maffei L: Electrophysiological evidence of orientation and size detectors in the human visual system. *J Physiol (Lond)* **207**:635, 1970.
21. Tootell RB, Silverman MS, Switkes E, et al: Deoxyglucose analysis of retinotopic organization in primate striate cortex. *Science* **218**:902, 1982.
22. Weisstein N, Harris CS: Masking and unmasking of distributed representations in the visual system. In Harris CS (Ed), *Visual Coding and Adaptability*. Hillsdale, N.J., Lawrence Erlbaum, 1980, pp 317–361.
23. Bodis-Wollner I, Diamond SP: The measurement of spatial contrast sensitivity in cases of blurred vision associated with cerebral lesions. *Brain* **99**:695, 1976.
24. Cohen JL, Dowling JE: The role of the retinal interplexiform cell: Effects of 6-hydroxydopamine on the spatial properties of carp horizontal cells. *Brain Res (Amster)* **264**:307, 1983.
25. Frederick JM, Rayborn ME, Laties AM, et al: Dopaminergic neurons in the human retina. *J Comp Neurol* **210**:65, 1982.

26. Barlow HB: Temporal and spatial summation in human vision at different background intensities. *J Physiol* **141**:337, 1958.

27. Enroth-Cugell C, Lennie P: The control of retinal ganglion cell discharge by receptive field surround. *J Physiol (Lond)* **247**:551, 1975.

28. Woodhouse JM: The effect of pupil size on grating detection at various contrast levels. *Vis Res* **15**:645, 1975.

29. Sekuler R, Hutman LP: Spatial vision and aging. I. Contrast sensitivity. *J Gerontol* **35**(5):692, 1980.

30. Morrison JD, McGrath C: Assessment of the optical contributions to the age-related deterioration in vision. *Q J Exp Physiol* **70**:249, 1985.

31. Robson JG: Spatial and temporal contrast sensitivity functions of the visual system. *J Opt Soc Am* **56**:1141, 1966.

32. Kelly DH: Visual contrast sensitivity. *Optica Acta* **24**(2):107, 1977.

33. Kelly DH: Motion and vision. II. Stabilized spatiotemporal threshold surface. *J Opt Soc Am* **69**:1340, 1979.

34. Atkin A, Bodis-Wollner I, Wolkstein M, et al: Abnormalities of central contrast sensitivity in glaucoma. *Am J Ophthalmol* **88**:205, 1979.

35. Medjbeur S, Tulunay-Keesey U: Spatiotemporal responses of the visual system in demyelinating diseases. *Brain* **108**:123, 1985.

36. Bodis-Wollner I, Marx MS, Mitra S, et al: Visual dysfunction in Parkinson's disease: Loss in spatiotemporal contrast sensitivity. *Brain* **110**:1675, 1987.

37. Hilz R, Cavonius CR: Functional organization of the peripheral retina: Sensitivity to periodic stimuli. *Vis Res* **14**:1333, 1974.

38. Rijsdijk JP, Kroon JN, Van der Wildt GJ: Contrast sensitivity as a function of position on the retina. *Vis Res* **20**:235, 1980.

39. Rovamo J, Virsu V: An estimation and application of the human cortical magnification factor. *Exp Brain Res* **37**:495, 1979.

40. Van Doorn AJ, Koenderink JJ, Bouman MA: The influence of retinal inhomogeneity on the perception of spatial patterns. *Kybernetik* **10**:223, 1972.

41. Campbell FW, Kulikowski JJ, Levinson J: The effect of orientation on the visual resolution of gratings. *J Physiol* **187**:427, 1966.

42. Appelle S: Perception and discrimination as a function of stimulus orientation: The "oblique effect" in man and animals. *Psychol Bull* **78**:266, 1972.

43. Regan D, Silver R, Murray TJ: Visual acuity and contrast sensitivity in multiple sclerosis: Hidden visual loss. *Brain* **100**:563, 1977.

44. Freeman RD, Thibos LN: Contrast sensitivity in humans with abnormal visual experience. *J Physiol* **247**:687, 1975.

45. Regan D, Maxner C: Orientation-selective visual loss in patients with Parkinson's disease. *Brain* **110**:415, 1987.

46. McCann JJ, Savoy RL, Hall JA Jr: Visibility of low frequency sine wave targets: Dependence on number of cycle and surround parameters. *Vis Res* **18**:891, 1978.

47. Wright MJ: Contrast sensitivity and adaptation as a function of grating length. *Vis Res* **22**:139, 1982.

48. Leege GE: Binocular contrast summation. 1. Detection and discrimination. *Vis Res* **24**(4):373, 1984.

49. Gilchrist J, McIver C: Fechner's paradox in binocular contrast sensitivity. *Vis Res* **25**(4):609, 1985.

50. Banks MS, Salapatek P: Contrast sensitivity function of the infant visual system. *Vis Res* **16**:867, 1976.

51. Banks MS, Stephens BR: The contrast sensitivity of human infants to gratings differing in duty cycle. *Vis Res* **22**(7):739, 1982.

52. Pirchio M, Sinelli D, Fiorentini A, et al: Infant contrast sensitivity evaluated by evoked potentials. *Brain Res* **141**(1):179, 1978.

53. Fiorentini A, Pirchio M, Spinelli D: Electrophysiological evidence for spatial frequency selective mechanisms in adults and infants. *Vis Res* **23**(2):119, 1983.

54. Norcia AM, Tyler CW, Allen D: Electrophysiological assessment of contrast sensitivity in human infants. *Am J Optom Physiol Opt* **63**(1):12, 1986.

55. Norcia AM, Tyler CW, Hamer RD: High visual contrast sensitivity in the young human infant. *Invest Ophthalmol Vis Sci* **29**:44, 1988.

56. Beazley LD, Illingworth DJ, Jahn A, et al: Contrast sensitivity in children and adults. *Br J Ophthalmol* **64**:863, 1980.

57. Atkinson J, French J, Braddick O: Contrast sensitivity function of preschool children. *Br J Ophthalmol* **65**:525, 1981.

58. Ross JE, Clarke DD, Bron AJ: Effect of age on contrast sensitivity function: Uniocular and binocular findings. *Br J Ophthalmol* **69**:51, 1985.

59. Hickey TL: Postnatal development of the human lateral geniculate nucleus: Relationship to a critical period for the visual system. *Science* **198**:836, 1977.

60. Kirzner SL: The effect of scholastic achievement and age on contrast sensitivity testing in school children. *Am J Ophthalmol* **92**(5):739, 1981.

61. Arden GB: The importance of measuring contrast sensitivity in cases of visual disturbances. *Br J Ophthalmol* **62**:198, 1978.

62. Skalka HW: Effect of age on Arden grating acuity. *Br J Ophthalmol* **64**:21, 1980.

63. Morrison J, Reilly J: An assessment of decision-

making as a possible factor in the age-related loss of contrast sensitivity. *Perception* **15**:541, 1986.

64. Arundale K: An investigation into the variation of human contrast sensitivity with age and ocular pathology. *Br J Ophthalmol* **62**:213, 1978.

65. Derefeldt G, Lennerstrand G, Lundh B: Age variations in normal human contrast sensitivity. *Acta Ophthalmol* **57**:679, 1979.

66. Owsley C, Sekuler R, Siemsen D: Contrast sensitivity throughout adulthood. *Vis Res* **23**(7):689, 1983.

67. Weale RA: Senile changes in visual acuity. *Trans Ophthalmolog Soc UK* **95**:36, 1975.

68. Owsley C, Garoner T, Sekuler R, et al: Role of crystalline lens in the spatial vision loss of elderly. *Invest Ophthalmol Vis Sci* **26**:1165, 1985.

69. Devaney KD, Johnson HA: Neuron loss in the aging visual cortex of man. *J Gerontol* **35**(6):836, 1980.

70. Mullen KT: The contrast sensitivity of human colour vision to red-green and blue-yellow chromatic gratings. *J Physiol* **359**:481, 1985.

71. Petry HM, Donovan NJ, Moore RK, et al: Changes in the human visually evoked cortical potential in response to chromatic modulation of a sinusoidal grating. *Vis Res* **22**:745, 1982.

72. Gunduz K, Arden GB, Perry S, et al: Color vision defects in ocular hypertension and glaucoma: Quantification with a computer-driven color television system. *Arch Ophthalmol* **106**:929, 1988.

73. Domenici L, Trimarchi C, Piccolino M, et al: Dopaminergic drugs improve human visual contrast sensitivity. *Hum Neurobiol* **4**:195, 1985.

74. Piccolino M, Neyton J, Gerschenfeld HM: Decrease of gap junction permeability induced by dopamine and cyclic AMP in horizontal cells of turtle retina. *J Neurosci* **4**:2477, 1984.

75. Harding TH, Wiley RW, Kirby AW: A cholinergic sensitive channel in the cat visual system tuned to low spatial frequencies. *Science* **221**:1076, 1983.

76. Ruberg M, Villageois A, Bonnet AM, et al: Acetylcholinesterase and butyrylcholinesterase activity in the cerebrospinal fluid of patients with neurodegenerative diseases involving cholinergic systems. *J Neurol Neurosurg Psychiat* **50**:538, 1987.

77. Hecht S, Hendley LD, Frank S, et al: contrast discrimination charts for demonstrating the effect of anoxia on vision. *J Opt Soc Am* **39**(11):922, 1949.

78. Fine BJ, Kobrick JL: Cigarette smoking, field dependence and contrast sensitivity. *Aviat Space Environ Med*, August 1987, p 777.

79. Kelly SA, Tomlinson A: Effect of repeated testing on contrast sensitivity. *Am J Optom Physiol Opt* **64**:241, 1987.

80. Long GM, Penn DL: Normative contrast sensitivity functions: The problem of comparison. *Am J Optom Physiol Opt* **64**(2):131, 1987.

81. Brabyn LB, McGuinness D: Gender differences in response to spatial frequency and stimulus orientation. *Percep Psychophy* **26**(4):319, 1979.

82. Arden GB, Jacobson JJ: A simple grating test for contrast sensitivity: Preliminary results indicate value in screening for glaucoma. *Invest Ophthalmol Vis Sci* **17**(1):23, 1978.

83. Regan D, Neima D: Low-contrast letter charts as a test of visual function. *Ophthalmology* **90**:1192, 1983.

84. Bodis-Wollner I: Test your eyes in 7 minutes. *Am Health* **1**(5):52, 1982.

85. Ginsburg AP: A new contrast sensitivity vision test chart. *Am J Optom Physiol Opt* **61**(6):403, 1984.

86. Corwin TR, Richman JE: Three clinical tests of the spatial contrast sensitivity function: A comparison. *Am J Optom Physiol Opt* **63**(6):413, 1986.

87. Verbaken JH, Johnston AW: Population norms for edge contrast sensitivity. *Am J Optom Physiol Opt* **63**(9):724, 1986.

88. Pelli DG, Robson JG, Wilkins AJ: The design of a new letter chart for measuring contrast sensitivity. *Clin Vis Sci* **2**(3):187, 1988.

89. Abrahamsson M, Frisen M, Sjöstrand J: Statistical evaluation of contrast sensitivity function (CSF) In visual disorders: Can diagnostic indices of CSF and acuity data be clinically useful? *Clin Vis Sci* **2**(3):159, 1988.

90. Sekuler R, Tynan P: Rapid measurement of contrast sensitivity functions. *Am J Optom Physiol Opt* **54**:573, 1977.

91. Ginsburg AP, Cannon MW: Comparison of three methods for rapid determination of threshold contrast sensitivity. *Invest Ophthalmol Vis Sci* **24**:798, 1983.

92. Higgins KE, Jaffe MJ, Coletta NJ, et al: Spatial contrast sensitivity: Importance of controlling the patient's visibility criterion. *Arch Ophthalmol* **102**:1035, 1984.

93. Vaegan, Halliday BL: A forced-choice test improves clinical contrast sensitivity testing. *Br J Ophthalmol* **66**:477, 1982.

94. Kelly DH, Savoie RE: A study of sine-wave contrast sensitivity by two psychophysical methods. *Percept Psychophys* **14**:313, 1973.

95. Campbell FW, Kulikowski JJ: The visual evoked potential as a function of contrast of a grating pattern. *J Physiol (Lond)* **222**:345, 1972.

96. Howe JW, Mitchell KW: The objective assessment of contrast sensitivity function by electrophysiological means. *Br J Ophthalmol* **68**:626, 1984.

97. Allen D, Norcia AM, Tyler CW: Comparative study of electrophysiological and psychophysical

measurement of the contrast sensitivity function in humans. *Am J Optom Physiol Opt* **63**(6):442, 1986.

98. Seiple WH, Kupersmith MJ, Nelson JI, et al: The assessment of evoked potential contrast thresholds using real-time retrieval. *Invest Ophthalmol Vis Sci* **25**:627, 1984.

99. Tyler CW, Apkarian P, Levi DM, et al: Rapid assessment of visual function: An electronic sweep technique for the pattern visual evoked potential. *Invest Ophthalmol Vis Sci* **18**:703, 1979.

100. Spileers W, Orban GA, Maes H, et al: CMSS-VEPs: Contrast modulated steady visual evoked potentials: Its neuronal origin and clinical use. *Docu Ophthalmol* **68**(3–4):363, 1988.

101. Regan D: Rapid objective refraction using evoked brain potentials. *Invest Ophthalmol Vis Sci* **12**:669, 1973.

102. Van den Berg TJTP: Importance of pathological intraocular light scatter for visual disability. *Codu Ophthalmol* **61**:327, 1986.

103. Hess RF, Carney LG: Vision through an abnormal cornea: A pilot study of the relationship between visual loss from corneal distortion, corneal edema, keratoconus and some allied corneal pathology. *Invest Ophthalmol Vis Sci* **16**:5, 1977.

104. Hess RF, Garner LF: The effect of corneal edema on visual function. *Invest Ophthalmol Vis Sci* **16**:5, 1977.

105. Apkarian P, Tijssen R, Spekreije H, et al: Origin of notches in the CSF: Optical or neural? *Invest Ophthalmol Vis Sci* **28**:607, 1987.

106. Yates JT, Harrison JM, O'Connor PS, et al: Contrast sensitivity: Characteristics of a large, young, adult population. *Am J Optom Physiol Opt* **64**(7):519, 1987.

107. Kirkpatrick CDL, Roggenkamp JR: Effects of soft contact lenses on contrast sensitivity. *Am J Optom Physiol Opt* **62**(6):407, 1985.

108. Woo G, Hess R: Contrast sensitivity and contact lenses. *Int Contact Lens Clin* **6**:37, 1979.

109. Mitra S, Lamberts DN: Contrast sensitivity in soft lens wearers. *Contact Intrao Lens Med J* **7**:315, 1981.

110. Hess R, Woo G: Vision through cataracts. *Invest Ophthalmol Vis Sci* **17**(5):428, 1978.

111. Abrahamsson M, Sjöstrand J: Impairment of contrast sensitivity (CSF) as a measure of disability glare. *Invest Ophthalmol Vis Sci* **27**:1131, 1986.

112. Paulsson LE, Sjöstrand J: Contrast sensitivity in the presence of glare light. *Invest Ophthalmol Vis Sci* **19**:401, 1980.

113. Nadler DJ, Jaffe NS, Clayman HM, et al: Glare disability in eyes with intraocular lenses. *Am J Ophthalmol* **97**:43, 1984.

114. Atkin A, Asbell P, Justin N, et al: Radial keratot-omy and glare effects on contrast sensitivity. *Docu Ophthalmol* **62**:129, 1986.

115. Mannis MJ, Zaonik K, Johnson CA, et al: Contrast sensitivity after penetrating keratoplasty. *Arch Ophthalmol* **105**:1220, 1987.

116. Carlsson L, Knave B, Lennerstrand G, et al: Glare from outdoor high mast lighting: Effects on visual acuity and contrast sensitivity in comparative studies of different floodlighting systems. *Acta Ophthalmol (Suppl)* **164**:84, 1984.

117. Kerstein D, Hess RF, Plant GT: Assessing contrast sensitivity behind cloudy media. *Clin Vis Sci* (3):143, 1988.

118. Dressler M, Rasson B: Neural contrast sensitivity measurements with laser interference system for clinical screening application. *Invest Ophthal Vis Sci* **21**:737, 1981.

119. Enoch JM, Yamade S, Namba A: Contrast (modulation) sensitivity functions measured in patients with high refractive error with emphasis on aphakia. I. Theoretical consideration. II. Determinations in patients. *Docu Ophthalmol* **47**(1):139, 147, 1979.

120. Fiorentini A, Maffei L: Spatial contrast sensitivity of myopic subjects. *Vis Res* **16**:437, 1976.

121. Thorn F, Corwin TR, Comerford JP: High myopia does not affect contrast sensitivity. *Curr Eye Res* **4**(9):635, 1986.

122. Hess RT, Woo G, White P: Contrast attenuation characteristics of iris clipped intraocular lens implants in situ. *Br J Ophthalmol* **68**:129, 1985.

123. Howe JW, Mitchell KW, Mahabaleswara M, et al: Visual evoked potential latency and contrast sensitivity in patients with posterior chamber intraocular lens implants. *Br J Ophthalmol* **70**:890, 1986.

124. Weatherill J, Yap M: Contrast sensitivity in pseudophakia and aphakia. *Ophthalmol Physiol Opt* **6**(3):297, 1986.

125. Anderson C, Sjöstrand J: Contrast sensitivity and central vision in reattached macula. *Acta Ophthalmolog* **59**:161, 1981.

126. Hyvarinen L, Laurinen P, Rovama J: Contrast sensitivity in evaluation of visual impairment due to macular degeneration and optic nerve lesions. *Acta Ophthalmolog* **61**:161, 1983.

127. Mitra S: Spatial contrast sensitivity in macular disorders. *Docu Ophthalmol* **59**:247, 1985.

128. Vaegan, Billson FA: Macular electroretinogram and contrast sensitivity detectors of early maculopathy. *Docu Ophthalmol* **63**:399, 1986.

129. Kayazawa F, Toshio Yamamoto, Motokazu Itoi: Contrast sensitivity measurement in retinal diseases by laser generated sinusoidal grating. *Acta Ophthalmolog* **60**:511, 1982.

130. Sokol S, Moskowitz A, Skarf B, et al: Contrast

sensitivity in diabetes with and without background retinopathy. *Arch Ophthalmol* **103**:51, 1985.

131. Volkers ACW, Hagemans KH, Van Der Wildt GJ, et al: Spatial contrast sensitivity and the diagnosis of amblyopia. *Br J Ophthalmol* **71**:58, 1987.

132. Brown B, Garner LF: Effects of luminance on contrast sensitivity in senile macular degeneration. *Am J Optom Physiol Opt* **60**(9):788, 1983.

133. Higgins KE: Clinical spatial contrast sensitivity measurement: Implications of artificial scotoma experiments. *Am J Optom Physiol Opt* **63**(2):266, 1972.

134. Bodis-Wollner I, Feldman RB, Guillory SL, et al: Delayed visual evoked potentials are independent of pattern orientation in macular disease. *Electroencephalog clin Neurophysiol* **68**:172, 1987.

135. Regan D, Whitlock JA, Murray TJ, et al: Orientation-specific losses of contrast sensitivity in multiple sclerosis. *Invest Ophthalmol Vis Sci* **19**(3):324, 1980.

136. Camisa J, Mylin LH, Bodis-Wollner I: The effect of stimulus orientation on the visual evoked potential in multiple sclerosis. *Ann Neurol* **10**:532, 1981.

137. Coupland SG, Kirkham TH: Orientation-specific visual evoked potential deficits in multiple sclerosis. *Can J Neurol Sci* **9**:331, 1982.

138. Kupersmith MJ, Seiple WH, Nelson JI, et al: Contrast sensitivity loss in multiple sclerosis: Selectivity by eye, orientation, and spatial frequency measured with the evoked potential. *Invest Ophthalmol Vis Sci* **25**:632, 1984.

139. Quigley HA, Addicks EM, Green NR: Optic nerve damage in human glaucoma. III. Quantitative correlation of nerve fiber loss and visual field defect in glaucoma, ischemic neuropathy, papilledema and toxic neuropathy. *Arch Ophthalmol* **100**:135, 1982.

140. Atkin A, Wolkstein M, Bodis-Wollner I, et al: Interocular comparison of contrast sensitivities in glaucoma patients and suspects. *Br J Ophthalmol* **64**(11):858, 1980.

141. Bodis-Wollner I: Differences in low and high spatial frequency vulnerabilities in ocular and cerebral lesions. In Maffei L (Ed), Pathophysiology of the visual system, Doc Ophthalmol Proc Series Vol. 30. The Hague, Dr. W. Junk Publishers, 1981, pp 195–204.

142. Towle VL, Moskowitz A, Sokol S, et al: The visual evoked potential in glaucoma and ocular hypertension: Effects of check size, field size, and stimulation rate. *Invest Ophthalmol Vis Sci* **24**:175, 1983.

143. Trick G: Retinal potentials in patients with primary open-angle glaucoma: Physiological evidence for temporal frequency tuning defects. *Invest Ophthalmol Vis Sci* **26**:1750, 1985.

144. Howe JW, Mitchell KW: Visual evoked potential changes in chronic glaucoma and ocular hypertension. *Trans Ophthalmol Soc UK* **105**(4):457, 1986.

145. Porciati V, Falsini B, Brunori S, et al: Pattern electroretinogram as a function of spatial frequency in ocular hypertension and early glaucoma. *Docu Ophthalmol* **65**:349, 1987.

146. Lundh BL, Lennerstrand G: Eccentric contrast sensitivity loss in glaucoma. *Acta Ophthalmology* **50**:21, 1981.

147. Derrington AM, Lennie P: Spatial and temporal contrast sensitivities of neurons in the lateral geniculate nucleus of Macaque. *J Physiol (Lond)* **357**:219, 1984.

148. Quigley HA, Dunkelberger GR, Sanchez RM: Chronic experimental glaucoma causes selectively greater loss of larger optic nerve fibers. *Invest Ophthalmol Vis Sci (Suppl)* **27**:42, 1986.

149. Marx MM, Podos SM, Bodis-Wollner I, et al: Signs of early damage in glaucomatous monkey eyes: Low spatial frequency losses in the pattern ERG and VEP. *Exp Eye Res* **46**:173, 1988.

150. Adam AJ, Heron G, Husted R: Clinical measures of central vision function in glaucoma and ocular hypertension. *Arch Ophthalmol* **105**(6):782, 1987.

151. Marx M, Bodis-Wollner I, Lustgarten JS, et al: Electrophysiological evidence that early glaucoma affects foveal vision. *Docu Ophthalmol* **67**:281, 1988.

152. Cooper RL, Constable IJ, Terrell A: Mass screening for glaucoma and other eye diseases using the Arden grating test. *Aust J Ophthalmol* **8**:131, 1980.

153. Sokol S, Domar A, Moscowitz A: Utility of Arden grating test in glaucoma screening: High false-positive rate in normals over **50 years of age.** *Invest Ophthalmol Vis Sci* **19**(12):1529, 1980.

154. Weatherhead RG: Use of the Arden grating test for screening. *Br J Ophthalmol* **64**:591, 1980.

155. Hitchings RA, Powell DJ, Arden GB, et al: Contrast sensitivity gratings in glaucoma family screening. *Br J Ophthalmol* **65**:615, 1981.

156. Singh H, Cooper RL, Alder VA, et al: The Arden grading acuity: Effect of age and optical factors in the normal patient, with prediction of the false negative rate in screening for glaucoma. *Br J Ophthalmol* **65**:518, 1981.

157. Tytla M, Buncic JR: Optic nerve compression impairs low spatial frequency vision in man. *Clin Vis Sci* **2**(3):179, 1988.

158. Kupersmith M, Siegel IM, Carr RE: Subtle disturbances of vision with compressive lesions of the anterior visual pathway measured by contrast sensitivity. *Ophthalmology* **89**:68, 1982.

159. Carr RE, Henkind P: Ocular manifestations of ethambutol. *Arch Ophthalmol* **67**:566, 1962.

160. Salmon JF, Carmichael TR, Welsh NH: Use of contrast sensitivity measurement in the detection of subclinical ethambutol toxic optic neuropathy. *Br J Ophthalmol* **71**:192, 1987.

161. Yiannikas C, Walsh JC, McLeod JC: Visual evoked potentials in the detection of subclinical optic toxic effects secondary to ethambutol. *Arch Neurol* **40**:645, 1983.

162. Kakisu Y, Adachi-Usami E, Mizota A: Pattern electroretinogram and visual evoked potential in ethambutol optic neuropathy. *Docu Ophthalmol* **67**:327, 1987.

163. Petrera JE, Fledelius HC, Trojaborg W: Serial pattern evoked potential recording in a case of toxic optic neuropathy due to ethambutol. *Electroencephalog Clin Neurophysiol* **71**:146, 1988.

164. Tilson HA: The neurotoxicity of acrylamide: An overview. *Neurobehav Toxicol Teratol* **3**:445, 1981.

165. Eskin TA, Lapham LW, Maurissen JPJ, et al: Acrylamide effects on the Macaque visual system. II. Retinogeniculate morphology. *Invest Ophthalmol Vis Sci* **26**:317, 1985.

166. Merigan WH, Barkdoll E, Maurissen JPJ, et al: Acrylamide effects on the Macaque visual system. I. Psychophysics and electrophysiology. *Invest Ophthalmol Vis Sci* **26**:309, 1985.

167. Bodis-Wollner I, Hendley CD, Mylin LH, et al: Visual evoked potentials and the visuogram in multiple sclerosis. *Ann Neurol* **5**:40, 1979.

168. Lorance RW, Kaufman D, Wray SH, et al: Contrast visual testing in neurovisual diagnosis. *Neurology* **37**:923, 1987.

169. Sekuler R, Onsley C, Berenberg R: Contrast sensitivity during provoked visual impairment in multiple sclerosis. *Ophthal Physiol Opt* **6**(2):229, 1986.

170. Hess RF, Plant GT: The effect of temporal frequency variation on threshold contrast sensitivity deficits in optic neuritis. *J Neurol Neurosurg Psychiat* **46**:322, 1983.

171. Marx MS, May JG, Reed JL, et al: Spatio-temporal processing in multiple sclerosis. *Docu Ophthalmol* **56**:243, 1984.

172. Wright CE, Drasdo N, Harding GFA: Pathology of the optic nerve and visual association areas: Information given by the flash and pattern visual evoked potential and the temporal and spatial contrast sensitivity function. *Brain* **110**:107, 1987.

173. Bodis-Wollner I: Recovery from cerebral blindness: Evoked potential and psychophysical measurements. *Electroencephology Clin Neurophysiol* **42**:178, 1977.

174. Kobayashi S, Mukuno K, Ishikawa S, et al: Hemispheric lateralization of spatial contrast sensitivity. *Ann Neurol* **17**:141, 1985.

175. Soso MJ, Lettich E, Belgum JH: Pattern-sensitive epilepsy. I. Demonstration of a spatial frequency selective epileptic response to gratings. *Epilepsia* **21**:301, 1980.

176. Wall M: Contrast sensitivity testing in pseudotumor cerebri. *Ophthalmology* **93**:4, 1986.

177. Levi DM, Harwerth RS: Contrast sensitivity in amblyopia due to stimulus deprivation. *Br J Ophthalmol* **64**:15, 1980.

178. Sjöstrand J: Contrast sensitivity in children with strabismic and anisometropic amblyopia: A study of the effect of treatment. *Acta Ophthalmol* **59**:25, 1981.

179. Campos C, Prampolini ML, Gulli R: Contrast sensitivity difference between strabismic and anisometropic amblyopia: Objective correlate by means of visual evoked responses. *Docu Ophthalmol* **58**:45, 1984.

180. Hess R, Campbell FN, Zimmern R: Differences in the neural basis of human amblyopia: The effect of mean luminance. *Vis Res* **20**:295, 1980.

181. Smith EL III, Harwerth RS, Crawford MLJ: Spatial contrast sensitivity deficits in monkeys produced by optically induced anisometropia. *Invest Opthalmol Vis Sci* **26**:330, 1985.

182. Norton TT, Casagrande VA, Sherman MS: Loss of Y cells in the lateral geniculate nucleus of monocularly deprived tree shrews. *Science* **197**:784, 1977.

183. Jones KR, Kalil RE, Spear D: Effects of strabismus on responsivity, spatial resolution and contrast sensitivity of cat lateral geniculate neurons. *J Neurosci* **52**(3):538, 1984.

184. Katz LM, Levi DM, Bedell HE: Central and peripheral contrast sensitivity in amblyopia with varying field size. *Docu Ophthalmol* **58**:351, 1984.

185. Rogers GL, Bremer DL, Leguire LE: The contrast sensitivity function and childhood amblyopia. *Am J Ophthalmol* **104**:64, 1987.

186. Hess RF, Campbell FW, Greenbalgh T: On the nature of the neural abnormality in human amblyopia: Neural aberrations and neural sensitivity loss. *Pflug Arch* **377**:201, 1978.

187. Snider SR, Fahn S, Isgreen WP, et al: Primary sensory symptoms in Parkinsonism. *Neurology* **26**:423, 1976.

188. Bodis-Wollner I, Yahr MD: Measurements of visual evoked potentials in Parkinson's disease. *Brain* **101**:661, 1978.

189. Marsden CD, Parkes JD: "On-off" effects in patients with Parkinson's disease on chronic levodopa therapy. *Lancet* **i**:292, 1984.

190. Domenici L, Trimarchi C, Marconi F, et al: Modificazioni visive in Parkinsoniani ed in soggetti tratamento con dopemino-agonisti. In Agnoli A, Battistin L (Eds), *Semeiologiae Terapia della Malattie Extrapiramidali, le Nuove Frontiere.* Rome, D. Guanella, 1985, pp 362–369.

191. Nissen MJ, Corkin S, Buonanno FS, et al: Spatial vision in Alzheimer's disease: General findings and a case report. *Arch Neurol* **42**:667, 1985.

192. Schlotterer G, Moscovitch M, Crapper-McLachlan D: Visual processing deficits as assessed by spatial frequency contrast sensitivity and backward masking in normal aging and Alzheimer's disease. *Brain* **107**:309, 1983.

193. Hinton DR, Sadun AA, Blanks JC, et al: Optic nerve degeneration in Alzheimer's disease. *N Engl J Med* **315**(8):485, 1986.

194. Sadun AA, Borchert M, DeVita E, et al: Assessment of visual impairment in patients with Alzheimer's disease. *Am J Ophthalmol* **104**:113, 1987.

195. Kollaritis CR, Shapiro RS, Swann ER, et al: Effect of hemodialysis on selected physical ocular parameters. *Metab Pediat Syst Ophthalmol* **5**:73, 1981.

196. La Piana FG: Renal Disease: Ocular complications. In Duane TD (Ed), *Clinical Ophthalmology.* New York, Harper and Row, 1979, pp 1–6

197. Arieff AC: Central nervous system. Medical aspects of hemodialysis. In Brenner BM, Rector FC (Eds.), *The Kidney.* Philadelphia, W.B. Saunders, 1986, pp 1731–1756.

198. Alfrey AC, Hegg A, Craswell P: Aluminum metabolism and toxicity in uremia. *Sangyo Ika Daigaku Zasshi* **20**(suppl 9):123, 1987.

199. Russell P, Sekuler R, Roxe D, et al: Contrast sensitivity of hemodialysis patients. *Met Pediat Syst Ophthalmol* **7**:201m, 1984.

200. Woo GC, Mandelman T, Liu TT, et al: Effect of hemodialysis on contrast sensitivity in renal failure. *Am J Optom Physiol Opt* **63**(5):356, 1986.

201. Anderson JR: Latent nystagmus and alternating hyperphoria. *Br J Ophthalmol* **38**:217, 1954.

202. Abadi RV: Pattern contrast thresholds in latent nystagmus. *Acta Ophthalmol* **58**(2):210, 1980.

203. Kulikowski JJ: Effect of eye movements on the contrast sensitivity of spatio-temporal patterns. *Vis Res* **11**:261, 1971.

204. Legge GE, Rubin GS: Contrast sensitivity function as a screening test: A critique. *J Optom Physiol Opt* **64**(4):265, 1986.

10
Standards for Contrast Acuity/Sensitivity and Glare Testing

Philip Lempert

standard

:a definite level or degree of quality that is proper and adequate for a specific purpose
:something that is set up and established by authority as a rule for the measure of quantity, weight, extent, value, or quality.

Webster's Third New International Dictionary, 1971.

Introduction

The central element of contrast sensitivity and glare testing is edge detection at specific contrast and brightness levels. Discernment of luminance gradients is a delicate task that is significantly affected by alterations in test procedures. Differences in display area, luminance, test object design, statistical validation procedures, and contrast often generate inconsistent and/or contradictory test results.[1-7] Future difficulties will inevitably occur because of the inability to transfer, correlate, or confirm laboratory and clinical information. There is an immediate need for general agreement on the critical design criteria of these devices and on uniform test procedures.

Many of the currently available devices embody compromises of ideal psychophysical test procedures because of their technical limitation.[8,9] For example, oscilloscopes can generate gratings but are unable to display shapes such as Sloan optotypes. Printed and projected charts are vulnerable to memorization and are limited to static displays. Early versions of computer graphics equipment lack adequate screen resolution, uniformity, and luminance control.

Contrast Acuity/Sensitivity Testing

Prior to 1968, when the British Standard, BS 4274, was published there were so many versions of the Snellen chart that it became extremely difficult to equate acuity measurements.[10] In 1980, comprehensive standards for the assessment of visual acuity were developed by the National Academy of Sciences/National Research Council (NAS/NRC).[11] They specified test parameters that include optimal screen luminance, test object design, and the number of test objects for statistically adequate testing. The International Council of Ophthalmology, in 1984, published a similar set of standards.[12] An analogous evolutionary process is proceeding in regard to contrast sensitivity and glare.

Contrast acuity/sensitivity test results are determined by the detection of edges that are characterized by a luminance gradient. The threshold for

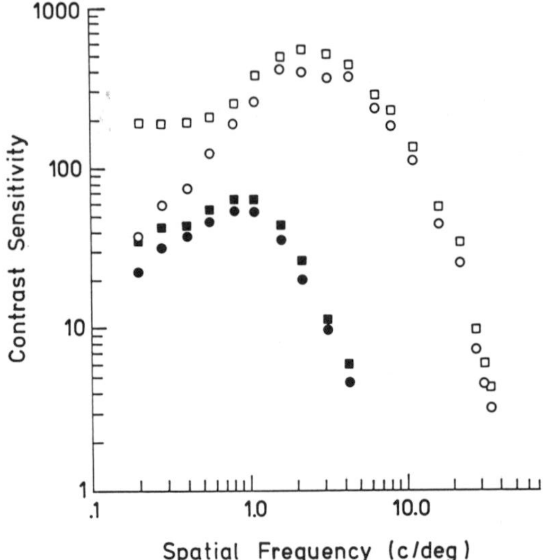

FIGURE 10.1. Contrast sensitivity functions for different levels of mean luminance. The upper curves were measured with gratings having a mean luminance of 500 cd/m². The lower curves were measured at 0.05 cd/m². (From Campbell FW, Robson JG: Application of Fourier analysis to the visibility of gratings. *J Physiol* **197**:557, 1968; used with permission.)

detection or identification at several different spatial frequencies and contrast is usually measured. A plot of these measurements constitutes a profile of the subject's spatial vision.

A basic requirement for contrast acuity/sensitivity testing is that the background luminance must remain constant at all levels of contrast. This is essential because the contrast sensitivity function correlates to mean luminance. (Fig. 10.1) In normal eyes, at high luminance the peak sensitivity is about 5 cycles per degree, and high-frequency cutoff occurs at approximately 60 cpd. As the luminance drops, and peak sensitivity and the high-frequency cutoff both move toward lower frequencies. The amplitude of the contrast sensitivity curve decreases markedly in the mesopic range.[13] In addition, since background luminance is a critical factor in determination of the contrast, any variation in background luminance will alter the contrast of the test image.

Contrast is sometimes defined as the maximum deviation from the background luminance divided by the background luminance[11]:

$$\text{Contrast} = \frac{\text{lum}_{\text{background}} - \text{lum}_{\text{letters}}}{\text{lum}_{\text{background}}}$$

This definition is usually applied to eye charts using optotypes. A difficulty with this format is that the mean luminance decreases with optotypes that occupy a large proportion of the total screen.

A more rigorous definition of contrast, which is used for luminance-corrected optotype displays[14,15] and sine wave gratings, is as follows:

$$\text{Modulation} = \frac{\text{lum}_{\text{max}} - \text{lum}_{\text{min}}}{\text{lum}_{\text{max}} + \text{lum}_{\text{min}}}$$

where lum_{max} is the luminance at the peak of the sine wave and lum_{min} is the luminance at the trough of the sine wave. In this instance *contrast* is regarded as *modulation*, which is the ratio of the maximum change in luminance from its mean value.[16]

Determinations of contrast levels made with these two formulas are not directly comparable. The modulation transfer function is concerned with perception at the peaks and troughs around a mean level of luminance. The image contrast changes as the dark areas gain illumination and the light areas lose illumination. The simpler contrast formula relates solely to the relationship of the background luminance and the dark component of the image.

The display brightness recommendations of the NAS/NRC and the BS 4274 are 85 cd/m² and 150 cd/m², respectively. High-contrast acuity can be decreased by either high or low luminance.[16,17] Although visual acuity increases slightly with excessive light levels, the concurrent effects on pupillary size and adaptation state limit the improvement.[16] Projected charts with reflective screens are compromised because of inconsistent contrast and luminance. Increasing the surround luminance by turning on room lights lowers the screen contrast.[18] The type of reflective surface and the wattage and age of the bulb can induce as much as a threefold difference in surround brightness.[19] Screen luminance varies exponentially with changes in lane length, so that a reduction in the viewing distance from 20 to 12 ft will more than double screen brightness.

Evaluating vision accurately depends on using reliable test objects with consistent recognizability.

The initial studies of contrast sensitivity were conducted with sinusoidal gratings.[20,21] The protocols for sine wave grating presentations share a common definition of spatial frequency but differ from each other in all other features. There is no accord on the size of the image, number of lines in the presentation, orientation of the lines, edge interactions, luminance,[22-24] adaptation state,[23] image dynamics, testing distance,[22] display or test duration,[11,25] or method for determining the detection threshold.[3,4]

Control of field size is a crucial factor in the perception of gratings.[26] Basic concepts in contrast acuity testing are that low-frequency images are detected outside the fovea and contrast measurement describes visual functions relating to objects larger than the resolution limit.[26] Images that are larger than the fovea are perceived by summation of signals from extrafoveal photoreceptors.

The relationship between the size of the presentation field and sensitivity to low-frequency images has been demonstrated repeatedly. Field size in scientific and clinical studies has ranged from 1.5 to 24 degrees. Estimations of low-frequency sensitivity with small field devices have been shown to differ significantly from determinations made with equipment that has a presentation area of greater than 6 degrees[2,5,6,25-28] (Fig. 10.2). Small fields—less than 6 degrees/of visual angle—introduce artefactual sensitivity depressions at low spatial frequencies.[21,26] Truncation— the masking of a grating field by a small, often circular mask—reduces the contrast sensitivity compared with the larger field. This phenomenon has particular importance in neurologic[5] and low vision testing.[26]

The threshold for sinusoidal gratings is also a function of the length of the bars[21,26] and the number of bars in the grating display. Summation is reduced with short lines or when the number of cycles is fewer than 6 or 7.

Round displays of gratings produce irregular edge interactions because of variable-length curved terminators. In addition, lines at the center of the target are longer than those at the edges. These factors limit the usefulness of circular displays for contrast and conventional vision testing.[11,13] The irregular boundaries created by lines in round targets, when used for contrast sensitivity, introduce

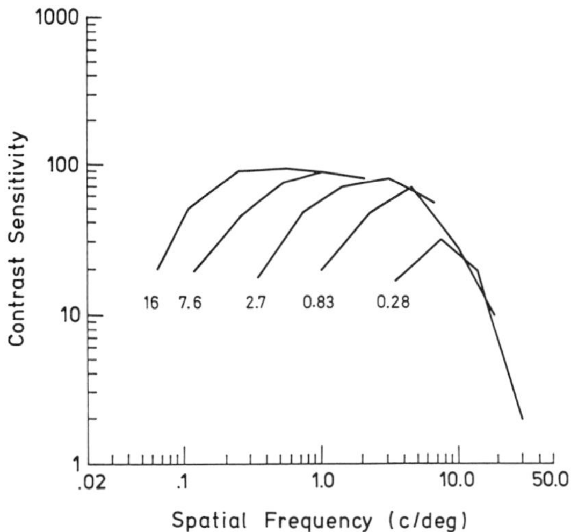

FIGURE 10.2. Contrast sensitivity as a function of the test field size in degrees of visual angle. (Reprinted with permission from McCann JJ, Savoy RL, Hall JA Jr: Visibility of low frequency sine wave targets. *Vis Res* **18**:892, 1978. Copyright 1978, Pergamon Press PLC.)

yet another confounding factor. Contrast gradients between the ends of the lines and the edge of the target are more abrupt than the gradient across the sinusoidal grating. The presence of different contrast boundaries in the same target is a source of confusion (personal communication, M. Jackowski, March, 1988.)

Uncorrected refractive errors or refractive effects induced by intermediate testing distance in presbyopia have a significant effect on the CSF. The perception of high-frequency gratings and small optotypes is more sensitive to defocus.[9,16] A focusing error of 0.5 D can make gratings finer than 15 cpd imperceptible while still permitting coarser gratings to be seen.[16] The minimum testing distance recommended by the Committee on Vision, NAS/NRC, is 4 m. Testing distances used by some instruments range from less than 1 to 3 m. This variation can generate a spurious change in the slope of the CSF. Orientation- and frequency-specific impairments of perception in persons with astigmatism have raised additional concerns about the use of gratings[22] (Fig. 10.3). These findings require that optical factors be considered before changes in the contrast sensitivity function curve can be attributed to pathology.[29]

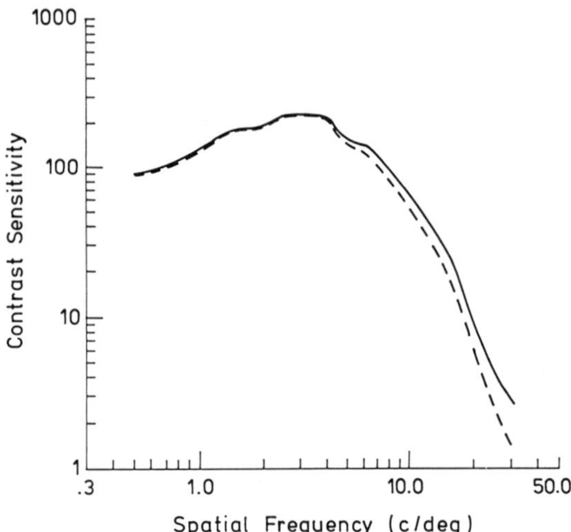

FIGURE 10.3. Contrast sensitivity function for vertical (solid line) and oblique (dashes) orientations. Note the lower sensitivity at oblique orientations. (From Campbell FW, Kulikowski JJ, Levinson J: The effect of orientation on the visual resolution of gratings. *J Physiol* **187**:434, 1966; used with permission.)

Recent developments that enhance the clinical usefulness of contrast testing employ optotypes. Some advantage of optotypes, such as the Landolt *C* ring and the ten Sloan letters, are that they are familiar to patients, incorporate proven design parameters, and have defined equivalences.[11,12,24] Optotype displays usually measure contrast perception. However, high-resolution computer graphics equipment can measure the modulation transfer function with optotypes.[14]

Dynamic presentations can help to detect degradation of retinal summation mechanisms. This may have particular application in the management of glaucoma patients and in selection of candidates for complex visual tasks. Current dynamic vision testing methods include continuous horizontal movement of vertical gratings, reversal of black and white at relatively low temporal frequency, detection of a disk moving over a grating background field,[31] and flicker of low contrast peripheral stimuli.[32] It is appropriate that modern standards include criteria for dynamic testing.

End point determination is an inherent problem in the standardization of testing procedures. There are at least four different methods for determining the detection threshold of sine wave grating. They

are methods that increase contrast, Bekesy tracking, methods of adjustment,[4] and forced choice.[30] Tracking methods are associated with a high degree of subject variability because the observer must establish and maintain a fixed criterion for target appearance to produce an accurate threshold measure.[3,33] Proficiency in this task will vary more among untrained observers. These variations in procedural conditions and training can markedly affect a subject's CSF as determined with sine wave gratings.

Printed targets on paper panels encourage forced-choice determination but have major disadvantages—they permit the subject to become familiar with the display and there are too few targets for the test to be statistically reliable.[3,6,11] When there are ten possible responses, as with the Sloan letters, a minimum of six correct identifications of at least eight choices is needed to determine the acuity level. If a protocol is used in which guesses have a 1 in 3 chance of being correct, then the standard deviation rises disastrously with even 1% misreporting.[3] An inadequate number of targets, as in a letter chart using only three letters at each contrast or with only one optotype of each size and contrast, seriously undermines test validity.[3,7,11]

Designers attempting to increase the number of choices on a paper chart of finite size may limit the size of the test objects.[3,30] This results in either too short a testing distance or an insufficient display area.

It is therefore not surprising, given the physiologic parameters, that a test consisting of a single, truncated, circular presentation at each contrast and acuity step has the poorest test-retest reliability when compared with letter charts or cathode-ray-tube based procedures.[6,7] The reliability is particularly poor at low spatial frequencies.[5] Charts of this type are also most likely to produce anomalous CSFs, with notches or low-frequency loss on one chart that does not appear on a second trial.[7] Letter charts, on the other hand, have higher reliability.[1,2,7,24,34] Variable-contrast letters are reliable and sensitive indicators of visual function.[5,14,35,36] Proper comparisons require that the optotypes have essentially equal recognizability. The Sloan letters—*C*, *D*, *H*, *K*, *N*, *O*, *R*, *S*, *V*, and *Z*—and the Landolt *C* ring meet that criterion.[11,12,24] Letter targets can be designed so that thresholds for detection and recognition are almost identical.[33]

Glare Testing

Glare is broadly defined as representing those effects of light that impair visual efficiency. It has the following subgroups:

1. Dazzling glare. A form of disability glare associated with bright lights in the field of view which form images upon the peripheral portions of the retina off the line of sight and which ...reduce sensitivity of the eye for seeing objects imaged upon the central or foveal region of the retina. (L.L. Holladay, 1926)
2. Veiling glare. "Stray light is uniformly distributed across the retinal image of interest, thus resulting in reduced brightness contrast between the image and its background."[35]
3. Scotomatic glare. Light overloads the retinal photoreceptors and produces functional neural and/or photochemical changes that culminate in significantly reduced retinal sensitivity.

Veiling glare testing is a variant of contrast acuity/sensitivity testing in which the background luminance is very high. In the following examples, A is conducted at the recommended standard screen luminance of 85 cd/m² and (B) is conducted at 1000 cd/m²:

$$(A)\ Contrast\ at\ 85\ cd/m^2 = (85 - 3)/85 = 96\%$$

$$(B)\ Contrast\ at\ 1000\ cd/m^2 =$$
$$(1085\text{-}1003)/1085 = 7\%$$

Since contrast is based on a luminance gradient, an increase in ambient luminance reduced the relative difference between the background and the test object. The contrast is therefore reduced. Increasing the room light, for example, is a simple but imprecise method for veiling glare testing.[37] A germane comment in the National Research Council's Standards for the Assessment of Distance Visual Acuity is that a back-lit screen should be used for high-luminance testing. Only two of the commercially available devices—the EyeCon 5[14] and the Miller-Nadler glare tester[38]—comply with that recommendation.

Glare testing methods and concepts continue to defy standardization because, in part, there is no consensus on which of the listed glare effects is representative of "real world" disability nor which glare source provides an adequate stimulus.[39]

Conclusions

Scientifically based and clinically proven criteria must form the foundation of standards. In that regard, the Recommended Standards for the Measurement of Distance Visual Acuity is the most objective, authoritative, and comprehensive. It addresses important variables in vision testing—luminance, optotype spacing, statistical validity, contrast, and optotype design. The validity and reliability of Sloan letter optotypes in contrast sensitivity/acuity testing has been proven.[3,35,36,40,41] The existing NAS/NRC standards could be supplemented with the inclusion of specified contrast levels, for example, 90%, 30%, 20%, 10%, 3%.[35,36,40]

In many instances clinical concepts are limited by the available technology. Clinical instruments often reflect the selective application of physiologic rules as dictated by the limits of the devices. However, it is neither desirable nor practical to discover repeatedly the relevance of physiologic principles in vision testing through technically deficient instruments. Modern technology can provide instruments without these compromises. Instruments can be engineered in an orderly and rational manner by first determining the function to be measured and the paramount factors in the testing environment. The recommendations of the Committee on Vision for the Assessment of Distance Visual Acuity and the Committee's observations on contrast testing should be the basis for new clinical contrast acuity/sensitivity systems.

References

1. Long GM, Penn DL: Normative contrast sensitivity functions: The problem of comparison. *Am J Optom Physiol Opt* **64**:131–135, 1987.
2. Trick GL, Burde RM, Gordon MO, et al: The relationship between hue discrimination and contrast sensitivity deficits in patients with diabetes mellitus. *Ophthalmology* **95**:693–698, 1988.
3. Pelli DG, Robson JG, Wilkins AJ: The design of a new letter chart for measuring contrast sensitivity. *Clin Vis Sci* **2**:187–199, 1988.
4. Ginsburg AP, Cannon NW: Comparison of three methods for rapid determination of threshold contrast sensitivity. *Invest Ophthal Vis Sci* **24**:798–802, 1983.
5. Corwin TR, Richman JE: Three clinical tests of the

spatial contrast sensitivity function: A comparison. *Am J Optom Physiol Opt* **63**:413–418, 1986.

6. Long GM, Tuck JP: Reliabilities of alternate measures of contrast sensitivity functions. *Am J Optom Physiol Opt* **65**:37–48, 1988.

7. Rubin GS: Reliability and sensitivity of clinical contrast sensitivity tests. *Clin Vis Sci* **2**(3):169–177, 1988.

8. Wolkins AJ, Della Sala S, Somazzi L, et al: Age-related norms for the Cambridge low contrast gratings, including details concerning their design and use. *Clin Vis Sci* **2**:201–212, 1988.

9. Arden GB: Testing contrast sensitivity in clinical practice. *Clin Vis Sci* **2**:213–224, 1988.

10. Marg E: *Computer Assisted Eye Examination*. San Francisco, The San Francisco Press, 1980, p 23.

11. National Academy of Sciences-National Research Council: Recommended standard procedures for the clinical measurement and specification of visual acuity: Report of Working Group 39. *Adv Ophthalmol* **41**:103–148, 1980.

12. Visual Functions Committee, Consilium Ophthalmologicum Universale: *Visual Acuity Measurement Standard*. San Francisco, International Council of Ophthalmology, 1984.

13. Committee on Vision, Commission on Behavioral and Social Sciences and Education, National Research Council: *Emergent Techniques for Assessment of Visual Performance*. Washington, D.C., National Academy Press, 1985, pp 47–48.

14. Lempert P, Hopcroft M, Lempert Y: Evaluation of posterior subcapsular cataracts with spatial contrast acuity. *Ophthalmology* **94**(S):14–18, 1987.

15. Howland H, Lempert P: A comparison of contrast acuity measurements in individuals with amblyopia due to anisometropia or strabismus. *ARVO Abstr* **28**:37, 1987.

16. Bennett A, Rabbetts RB: *Clinical Visual Optics*. London, Butterworths, 1984, pp 21–59.

17. Sheedy JE, Baily IL, Raasch TW: Visual acuity and chart luminance. *Am J Optom Physiol Opt* **61**:595–600, 1984.

18. Lempert P: Correspondence—An analysis of the effect of intravitreal blood on visual acuity. *Am J Ophthalmol* **105**:218–219, 1988.

19. Augsburger AM, Sheedy JE, Schoessler JP: Reflectance of visual acuity screens. *Am J Optom Physiol Opt* **56**:531–537, 1979.

20. Bodis-Wollner I: Application to lesions of the retina and visual pathways. In Sekular R, Kekion D, Dismukes K. (Eds), *Aging and Human Visual Function*. New York, Alan R.Liss, 1982, p 54.

21. Arden GB: The importance of measuring contrast sensitivity in cases of visual disturbance. *Br J Ophthalmol* **62**:198–209, 1978.

22. Proenza LM, Enoch J, Jamplosky A: *Clinical Application of Visual Psychophysics*. New York, Harvard University Press, 1981.

23. Hess RF, Howell ER: The threshold contrast sensitivity function in strabismic amblyopia. *Vis Res* **17**:1059–1055, 1977.

24. Sloan L: New test charts of the measurement of visual acuity at far and near distances. *Am J Ophthalmol* **48**:807–813, 1959.

25. Heijl A: Time changes of contrast thresholds during automatic perimetry. *Acta Ophthalmol* **55**:696–708, 1977.

26. Sjostrand J: Contrast sensitivity in macular disease using a small-field and a large-field TV system. *Acta Ophthalmol* **57**:832–846, 1979.

27. Kruk R, Regan D: Visual test results compared with flying performance in telemetry tracked aircraft. *Aviat Space Environ Med* **54**(10):906–911, 1983.

28. Kruk R, Regan D, Beverley KI, et al: Correlations between visual test results and flying performance on the advanced simulator for pilot training (ASPT). *Avait Space Environ Med* **52**(8):455–460, 1981.

29. Apkarian P, Tijssen R, Spekreijse H, et al: Origin of notches in CSF: Optical or neural. *Invest Ophthal Vis Sci* **28**:607–612, 1987.

30. Ginsburg AP: A new contrast sensitivity test chart. *Am J Optom Physiol Opt* **61**:403–407, 1984.

31. Barbur JL: Spatial frequency specific measurements and their use in clinical psychophysics. *Clin Vis Sci* **2**: 225–233 1988.

32. Stellmach LB, Drance SM, Di Lillo V: Tow-pulse temporal resolution in patients with glaucoma, suspected glaucoma, and in normal observers. *Am J Ophthalmol* **102**:617–620, 1986.

33. Howland B, Ginsburg A, Campbell F: High-pass spatial frequency letters as clinical optotypes. *Vis Res* **18**:1963–1066, 1977.

34. Coren S: Reporting the visual acuity of groups: The relation among alternate measures. *Am J Optom Physiol Opt* **64**:897–900, 1987.

35. Strobel J, Jacobi F, Jacobi KW: *Evaluation of Cataract Under Different Contrast and Glare Conditions—A New Computerized Concept*. Jerusalem, Israel, European Intraocular Implant Lens Council, 1987.

36. Mainster MA, Timberlake GT, Schepens CL: Automated variable contrast acuity testing. *Ophthalmology* **88**:1045–1053, 1981.

37. Thompson JT, Stoessel K: An analysis of the effect of intravitreal blood on visual acuity. *Am J Ophthalmol* **104**:353–357, 1987.

38. Hirsch RP, Nadler P, Miller D: Clinical performance of a disability glare tester. *Arch Ophthalmol* **102**:1633–1636, 1984.

39. Neumann AC, McCarty GR, Locke J, et al: Glare

disability devices for cataractous eyes: A consumer's guide. *J Catar Refract Surg* **14**:212–216, 1988.

40. Carter JH: The effects of aging upon selected visual functions: Color vision, glare sensitivity, field of vision, and accommodation. In Sekular R, Kelion D, Dismukes, K. (Eds), *Aging and Human Visual Function*. New York, Alan R. Liss, 1982, pp 131–161.

11
Some Basic Concepts and Field Applications for Lighting, Color, and Vision

Mark S. Rea

Introduction

The field of illuminating engineering is closely allied to the fields of ophthalmology and optometry. All are concerned with providing adequate conditions for seeing. In fact, the Illuminating Engineering Society of North America was founded on the premise that the lighting engineer shares a joint responsibility with ophthalmologists and optometrists to provide "good visual hygiene"; ophthalmologists and optometrists should provide proper ocular health and refraction and the illuminating engineer should provide adequate lighting.[1]

Both illuminating engineers and ocular clinicians draw upon a common base in visual science for technical information important to their respective professions. Quite naturally, different aspects of visual science are emphasized by these two areas. Consequently, some of the concerns and information important to illuminating engineers are less well known by professionals in allied fields, and vice versa.

Perhaps one of the largest differences between illuminating engineers and professional ocular clinicians are their tools. Clinicians are blessed with a large array of sophisticated instrumentation to diagnose and treat patients in their offices. Illuminating engineers are obliged to work in the field. Until very recently only crude tools have been available for this field work. Further, no matter how much knowledge is available to the illuminating engineer, without satisfactory measurement tools it is difficult or impossible to assess lighting quality and quantity accurately in the field.

The purpose of this chapter is to describe some of the visual science that forms the bases for illuminating engineering. Since the foundations for illuminating engineering and ocular clinicians are so similar, it is hoped that this chapter will be instructive to members of both professional areas. The last section of the chapter discusses some of the tools now becoming available to the illuminating engineer.

Key Aspects of the Visual Stimulus

Although lighting can affect human physiology in a variety of ways, the foremost is through the eye and visual system. Therefore, when one describes the quantity or quality of lighting, it is always necessary to define how lighting has affected the stimulus for vision. Fortunately, considerable effort has been given to elucidating human responses to the key aspects of visual stimuli. Consequently, illumination engineers have gained a better understanding of what constitutes good lighting.

The key aspects of visual stimuli may be conveniently labeled as absolute level, spectral composition, contrast, size, and temporal modulation and movement. To describe the stimulus for vision they must all be considered. Lighting affects the visual stimulus either directly (e.g., the illuminance level will affect the absolute level of adaptation) or indirectly (e.g., the illuminance level can induce people to move closer or further from a visual task, thus increasing or decreasing the apparent size of the task). It is helpful, therefore, to describe human responses to these key aspects of visual stimuli and how lighting can affect them.

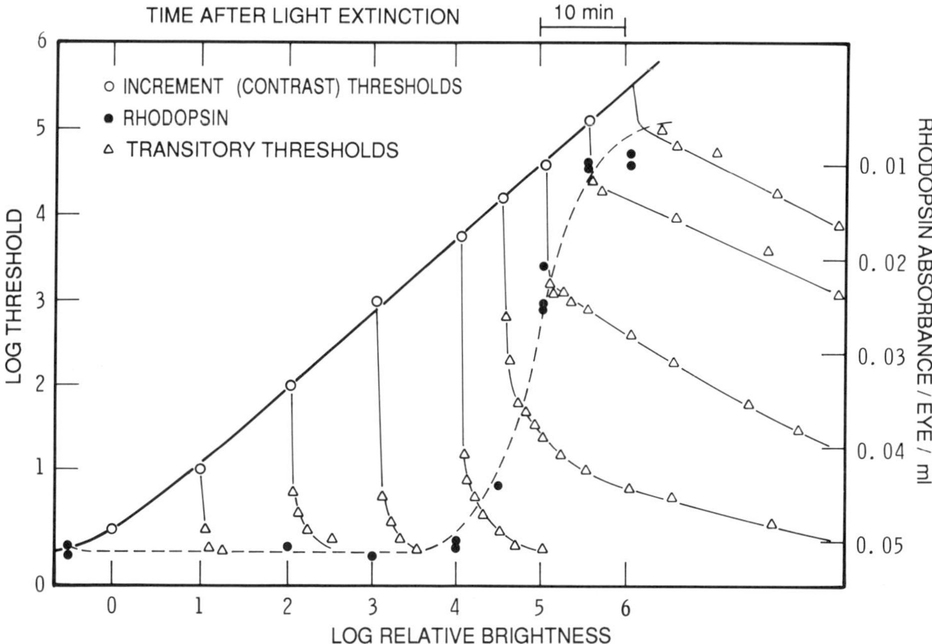

FIGURE 11.1. Rod behavior in rat retinas. The heavy solid line represents the steady-state adaptation level of the visual system to the log relative brightness level of the visual field scaled on the bottom abscissa. Adaptation level is measured by the increment threshold values (open circles) scaled on the left ordinate. The dashed line represents the amount of bleached photopigment in the rods for these same brightness levels. Photopigment bleaching is characterized by the rhodopsin absorbance values (closed circles) scaled on the right ordinate. The thin solid line represents the "transient" dark adaptation level, again characterized by increment threshold values (triangles) scaled on the left ordinate, after extinction of the steady-state brightness level. The time following light extinction is shown on the top abscissa. Dark adaptation shows two distinct phases, rapid and slow recovery, which are demarcated by the amount of bleached photopigment in the rods. The slow recovery phase, to the right of the dashed lines, represents regeneration of photopigment in the dark by the rods. The rapid recovery phase to the left of the dashed line represents neural adjustments in the retina to the dark. Data and curves are from Figure 1 in Dowling[5] (copyright 1967 by AAAS).

Absolute Level

The visual system operates in a range between the light of stars and the light of sunshine on snow. This represents a dynamic range of about 10^{13} to 1. The visual system "adapts" to a given level of stimulation within this very large range by changing its operating characteristics. Muscular, photochemical, and neural changes take place during adaptation, and these processes influence the effectiveness of the visual stimulus. For example, the iris dilates and constricts in response to lower and higher levels of luminous stimulation, respectively. Frowning, squinting, and shading the eyes can also limit the amount of light entering the eye.[2] Such muscular changes do not, however, account for the largest changes in adaptation. For example, variations in the size of the iris account for less than 1 log unit change in adaptation.[3]

Photochemical reactions in the two classes of receptors, rods and cones, account for the largest variations in adaptation level.[4] At very low levels of stimulation the rods are active. As the level of luminous stimulation increases the rods bleach, their response saturates, and cones begin to dominate the visual response. As the level of stimulation continues to increase, the cones also begin to bleach. Photochemical reactions are relatively slow, and sometimes an hour or more is needed for the eye to readapt from high to low light levels. Rapid changes can take place, however, through neural interactions in the retina.[5] Under optimal conditions neural changes occur very quickly (within 100 ms), handling luminous variations of about 1000 to 1. Under very dim or very bright conditions this range may be only about 3 to 1 (Fig. 11.1).

Not only does the absolute level of stimulation affect the dynamic range of the visual system, it also influences visual responses to other key aspects of the stimulus. These interactions can either improve or degrade visibility, but generally our ability to see objects will be better at higher absolute levels of stimulation. For example, acuity, or the ability to resolve small spatial detail, becomes better as the absolute level of stimulation increases.[6,7] Further, the speed and accuracy with which people can process visual information improves with increasing light level.[8]* Of course there are important exceptions to this rule. Most notably perhaps, the luminous uniformity of the visual scene must be considered; luminous nonuniformity will degrade acuity[6] and contrast sensitivity, or the ability to resolve small differences in luminance[10]; this is discussed in more detail in a later section. Under extremely nonuniform conditions, the same light source that increases the absolute level of stimulation may also degrade visibility if it shines into the eyes directly (known as *glare*) or by reflection (known as *veiling reflections*). Therefore, while higher levels of stimulation generally improve visual functioning, this may not necessarily be the case when the higher levels also produce nonuniform luminous conditions.

Lighting can obviously influence the absolute level of stimulation. The visual system will change in response to higher or lower brightness levels. In most indoor environments illuminated by electric lights, variations in the absolute level of stimulation rarely exceeds 10^4 to 1; more typically they are on the order of 10 to 1. Consequently, variations in the operating characteristics of the visual system will be small relative to the total range possible.

The absolute level of stimulation in electrically illuminated environments will usually be in the photopic range but rarely high enough to produce cone bleaching (although the rods are usually saturated). At these levels the visual system can handle rather abrupt changes in luminous stimulation through rapid neural adaptation. Thus the visual system can adapt quickly and completely to a wide range of luminances in the electrically illuminated environment. Again, there are exceptions. Light from uncovered windows or bare lamps can be bright enough to produce cone bleaching. These sources of light may or may not produce after-images which are perceptible when one views the darker room interior. Nevertheless, the bleached portion of the retina will have reduced sensitivity and, therefore, darker areas in the room may be less perceptible until photochemical readaption has taken place. Further, these bright sources of illumination may be deleterious to vision because the illumination is not uniform, producing either veiling reflections or glare. Glare is particularly noticeable at low absolute levels as, for example, occurs with viewing headlights from approaching automobiles at night. These interactive effects with the absolute level of stimulation are discussed in more detail in subsequent sections.

Spectral Composition

Brightness and Luminance

As already noted, there are two classes of photoreceptors in the eye. Each has a different selective sensitivity to radiant energy. Generally the rods operate at very low to medium absolute levels of stimulation; the cones, of which there are three types, operate at medium to high levels of stimulation. Functionally, the rods are sensitive to wavelengths between 380 and 650 nm and have a peak sensitivity at 507 nm (Fig. 11.2). The envelope that defines the spectral response of rods is known as the *scotopic spectral sensitivity function*. The overall spectral response of the cones is less defi-

---

*The effect of absolute level of stimulation on visual response time can be readily demonstrated with the Pulfrich effect.[9] If a filter is placed over one eye and a moving pendulum is viewed binocularly, the pendulum will appear to traverse an elliptical path. Without the filter, the pendulum will appear to move normally; that is, it will appear to be moving in one plane only. The speed of visual processing is greater in the eye adapted to the higher absolute level. Thus, the information from the eye adapted to the higher level of stimulation reaches the brain before that from the other eye. Apparently the brain "resolves" this problem by seeing the pendulum swinging in an ellipse. The size of the ellipse can be made larger by using a darker filter. If the filter is too dark, however, the visual system can no longer "resolve" the latency difference and will, effectively, shut down the information coming from the eye adapted to the lower level of stimulation.

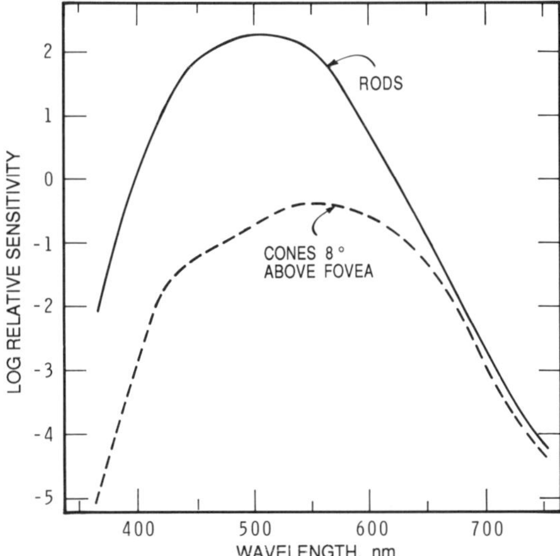

FIGURE 11.2. Spectral sensitivities of rods (solid line) and cones (dashed line) as determined by the minimum energy required for the detection of a 1° test flash of various monochromatic wavelengths. (From G Wald: Human vision and the spectrum. *Science* **101**:653, 1945. Copyright 1945 by the AAAS.)

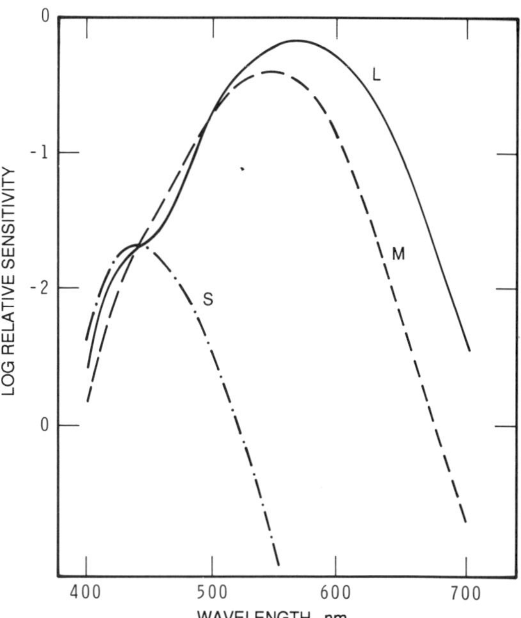

FIGURE 11.3. Spectral sensitivity functions for the three types of cones: long (L), middle (M), and short (S), sometimes referred to as the red, green, and blue cones, respectively. (From Boynton RM, MacLeod DIA: *Human Color Vision.* Copyright © 1979, by Holt, Rinehart and Winston, Inc., reprinted by permission of the publisher.)

nite, since the three types of cones, each with a different spectral sensitivity, operate in several ways to evoke visual perceptions (Fig. 11.3). One combination of these cone spectral sensitivities has been defined as the *photopic spectral sensitivity function* (or V-lambda), and it forms the basis of what is normally called light. The photopic spectral sensitivity function includes wavelengths primarily between 400 and 720 nm, with a peak sensitivity at 555 nm (Fig. 11.2).

Light can be regarded as a physical quantity, like mass or volume, and is measured in standard internationally agreed on units. Without going into the details of photometry, which are well explained in other texts[11] it is useful to describe two photometric measurements of importance for lighting appli-

cations. The first, illuminance, is the amount of light falling on a surface and is measured in lumens per square meter (lm m⁻²), or lux. The second, luminance, corresponds to the photometric brightness of objects and is measured in candelas per square meter (cd m⁻²), or nits. There are readily available commercial products that measure illuminance or luminance.*

Unless otherwise specified, luminance (and illuminance) is defined in terms of the photopic spectral sensitivity function. Thus, light measurements are only appropriate at absolute levels where the cones are functioning. Traditionally, rods are

---

*When concerned with the stimulus for vision, the amount of light actually reaching the retina should be considered. Thus, pupil area and light transmission through the optical media of the eye should also be defined. Although there are no orthodox specifications of light transmission through the optical media, there is a conventional unit of retinal illuminance, known as the *troland*, which takes into account pupil area. Retinal illuminance, in trolands, is simply the product of luminance in candelas per square meter and pupil area in millimeters squared. Thus, a unit troland is defined as

the retinal illuminance associated with viewing a surface of 1 cd m² when seen through a pupil area of 1 mm². Retinal illuminance is a slight misnomer since, again, light transmission through the various optical media of the eye is not considered and can vary considerably among individuals (as can pupil area). Although trolands are a more appropriate measure of brightness than luminance, there are no commercially available instruments that measure trolands directly. Thus, luminance, a well-defined physical quantity, is used most frequently in specifying the stimulus for vision.

taken to be inactive above about 3 cd m², but it is well documented that above this level rods still contribute to color vision[11] and pupil size.[12] Nevertheless, 3 cd m² is a practical, convenient lower limit in absolute level for making luminance measurements.

Often there is interest in light measurements below 3 cd m² (e.g., roadways at night). When photometric measurements are made below about 10^{-3} cd m², the scotopic spectral sensitivity function should weight the electromagnetic spectrum. For photometric measurements below this level and weighted by the rod spectral sensitivity, the adjective *scotopic* should always precede the term *luminance* (or trolands). Between 10^{-3} and 3 cd m² both rods and cones contribute to the visual response. A family of so-called *mesopic spectral sensitivity functions* is used to weight the electromagnetic spectrum.[13,14] At the lower end of this range sensitivity is dominated by rods; at the upper end it is dominated by cones. Between these extremes there is a smooth transition between the scotopic and the photopic spectral sensitivity functions.* As yet there are very few measurement devices and no formal guidelines for evaluating light at mesopic levels.

As previously noted, luminance is the physical quantity most closely correlated with brightness perception. However, its definition is based on a particular psychophysical technique known as *flicker photometry*. Typically with this technique a person views a circular disk that is illuminated alternately by two different-colored lights (e.g., red and yellow). As the substitution rate is increased the two lights "fuse" to become one color (e.g., a rapid substitution of red and yellow produces orange), but the disk still appears to flicker (i.e., change in brightness). At increasing substitution rates the two lights eventually "fuse" completely; that is, the disk appears to be a single,

unflickering color. Two lights are defined as having equal luminance when, at the minimum substitution rate, they have completely fused.[15] This definition of luminance also works well for describing the relative brightness, or contrast, of small targets.[16]

As already noted, however, (photopic) luminance will not describe our brightness perceptions below about 3 cd m². More interesting, perhaps, even above this level luminance does not adequately describe our general impressions of brightness for large colored objects. Deeply saturated (highly colored) lights can look up to six times brighter than faintly colored or white lights of the same luminance.[17,18] Another example of the inadequacies of luminance in characterizing brightness can be observed by placing a slightly yellow filter over the eye while a scene illuminated by a "white" light source is viewed. Naturally the yellow filter reduces the amount of light reaching the retina (i.e., luminance is reduced). Nevertheless, the scene can, depending on the density of the filter, appear brighter with the filter than without it.† Therefore, while luminance is very useful it does not completely describe brightness perceptions. Here again, then, problems may occur in practice when one tries to specify the brightness of colored objects like signs or signals. Researchers are presently working toward a more complete specification of brightness perception of colored objects.[11,19,20]

Color

Another obvious limitation of luminance is its inability to describe human color perception. A detailed understanding of color perception has emerged in the last 50 years; most of it is outside the scope of this discussion.[15] For this chapter, however, two important color phenomena must be differentiated: color matching and color appearance.

Color matching is an area of study that describes those combinations of wavelengths that will be indistinguishable for a given (usually "standard") observer.[11] Color matching can be understood

---

*The shift between the photopic and scotopic spectral sensitivity functions was first described by Purkinje in the last century. He observed a change in the relative brightnesses of red and blue objects as light level changed. A red sign was brighter than a blue sign in the daytime but the reverse was true in the late evening. This change in relative brightness with absolute level is called the *Purkinje shift* and is a natural manifestation of the different relative weightings of the short and the long wavelength regions of the spectrum by rods and cones.

---

†This phenomenon is readily apparent with commercially available yellow shooting glasses intended for marksmen.

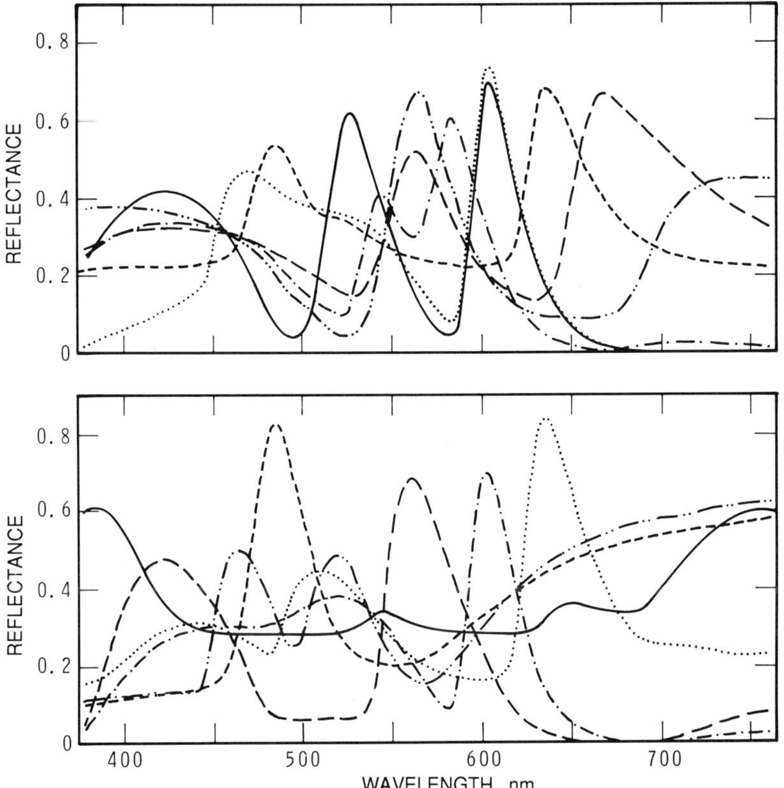

FIGURE 11.4. Twelve spectral reflectance curves for targets that would appear metameric to the Commission Internationale de l'Eclairage (CIE) 1931 standard observer under CIE standard illuminant *C*. (Curves from Figure 7 [3.8.2] of Wyszecki and Stiles.[11] A thorough explanation of them can be found in that publication. Copyright 1982, John Wiley & Sons, Inc.)

largely in terms of the linear combinations of the three cone spectral response functions (although under some circumstances rods may also play a role in color perception[11]). Essentially, when the neural outputs from the three cone types in the retina are the same, lights will be indistinguishable even though their spectral compositions might differ radically. Such lights are known as *metamers*.[21] All that matters for color matching, then, is that the outputs from the three cone types are identical; there is an infinite number of possible wavelength combinations that will produce equal cone outputs (Fig. 11.4).

Color appearance is much more complex. Although clearly the appearance of colors must depend fundamentally on the three cone types, the cones are not directly responsible for the hue perceived. Color is created by neural interactions at levels higher than the photoreceptors. Essentially, all per-

ceived colors are combinations of three pairs of primary, or complementary, colors: red or green, yellow or blue, and black or white. Each pair of primaries is associated with one "color channel" in the visual system. Thus we see, for example, dark reddish yellows (browns) or bright reddish yellows (oranges), but we never see reddish greens or yellowish blues.[22] As implied in these examples, color appearance also depends on the absolute level of stimulation. The same combination of wavelengths that gives rise to brown can also produce orange if the radiance is increased. To varying degrees this change in appearance occurs with all lights of changing radiant energy and is known as the *Bezold-Brücke effect*.[23] At low photopic levels all hues are dominated by red and green; at high levels they are dominated by blue and yellow.

Another difficulty in explaining color appearance is that the context in which colors are perceived must also be defined. For example, juxtaposed colors will influence each others' appearances. Thus, a blue patch adjacent to a white patch will make the white patch slightly yellow (the opposite of blue) and the white patch will make the blue patch darker (the opposite of white). Similar effects occur temporally; after one looks through a dark green filter a scene will appear whitish red, or pink (again, the opposite of dark green), when the filter is removed.

Essentially, color appearance depends on the ratios of stimulation to the three color channels; yellow-blue, red-green, and black-white. When the two color channels responsible for hue (yellow-blue and red-green) are perfectly balanced we see white, gray, or black. If the balance changes in only *one* of the channels responsible for hue, one of the "unique" hues is seen (red, green, yellow, or blue). If the balance changes in both hue channels, other colors are created. When the channels produce red and blue outputs we see purple or violet; green and blue outputs make cyan; red and yellow make orange; green and yellow make chartreuse.

It should be noted, however, that, just as it adapts to different absolute levels of stimulation, the visual system also adapts to moderate shifts in spectral composition. After a scene is viewed through a lightly tinted filter (e.g., sunglasses) for a time, the scene will look "normal" even though the spectral compositions of the scene on the retina differ with and without the filter. This phenomenon occurs through neural "rebalancing" of the color channels to provide the same relative output from all channels.

The significance of different light sources for color perception depends on the application, that is, whether one is concerned with color matching, color appearance, or luminous efficiency. One source, for example, may be more efficient in producing light than another (i.e., in terms of light per watt of electricity), but it may *appear* dimmer than another source because brightness perception is not always correlated perfectly with the physical quantity luminance. As noted in the previous paragraph too, different spectral compositions may have no effect on the appearance of colored objects as long as the color channels can "readapt." Thus, in many cases the apparent colors of some objects will not be affected significantly when they are illuminated with different light sources. Occasion-

ally, however, the spectral reflectance of an object is such that, when it is illuminated by light sources of different spectral composition, noticeably different hues will appear. Conversely, objects with completely different spectral reflectances appear to have the same hue under one (or more) light source. As already noted, different spectral compositions that produce the same hue are termed metamers.[21] Metamerism is quite important to the automotive industry, for example, which produces colored products from different materials. The appearance of metal and plastic objects must match in both daylight and electric light. If objects do not have the same spectral reflectance, care is taken to make them metameric for all the different light sources under which they will be seen.

Spectral composition and its effects on human perception are complex and multifaceted. Certainly many of the important issues have not been covered here. The most important point to be realized, however, is that physical definitions of light and the ways it is currently measured may not always characterize human brightness and color perception adequately.

Contrast

Contrast can be defined in terms of luminous differences with respect to some absolute level of stimulation. Formal definitions of contrast depend on the spatial or temporal characteristics of the visual stimulus. For spatially or temporally periodic stimuli (e.g., stripes, sinusoidal patterns, or flicker):

$$\text{Contrast} = \frac{(L_{max} - L_{min})}{(L_{max} + L_{min})} \qquad (11.1)$$

where L_{max} is maximum luminance and L_{min} is minimum luminance.

For small luminous decrements or increments on a large background (e.g., print on a page):

$$\text{Contrast} = \frac{(L_b - L_t)}{L_b}$$

$$= 1 - \frac{L_t}{L_b} \qquad (11.2)$$

where L_b is luminance of the background and L_t is luminance of the target.

Sometimes, for small luminous increments on a large dark background (e.g., characters on a visual display terminal):

$$\text{Contrast} = \frac{L_i}{L_b} \qquad (11.3)$$

where L_i is luminance of the increment.

Contrast is perhaps the most important variable for vision; without sufficient contrast in the visual scene there can be no stimulus for vision. The visual system is incapable of detecting very small luminous differences; only after contrast has reached some threshold level (i.e., the transition from non-detection to detection) can vision take place. Many studies have been conducted measuring contrast threshold that is affected by the spatial, temporal, and chromatic characteristics of the stimulus as well as the absolute level of stimulation. Figure 11.5 shows the results of a recent study of contrast threshold for squares of different sizes and contrasts flashed on backgrounds of different luminance.[24] In this study the probability of a subject's detecting these flashed squares of different sizes on different background luminances was determined and, by convention, the 50% probability of detection was taken as the contrast threshold for those stimulus conditions (Fig. 11.6).

Contrast perception is generally concerned with luminance differences that exceed threshold, that is, suprathreshold contrast. Interestingly, different visual responses can be produced from the same suprathreshold target. Cannon[25] has shown that subjective judgment of contrast, using magnitude estimations,[26] increases essentially linearly from threshold to higher contrasts (Fig. 11.7). Rea and his colleagues,[8,27,28] however, have shown that the speed and accuracy of response to variations in suprathreshold contrast are highly nonlinear; there is a rapid initial rise from threshold contrast followed by an extended region of response saturation (Fig. 11.8). Thus, for the same stimulus it was possible to show that appearance and response time follow completely different functions (Fig. 11.9). Analogously, Kaplan and Shapley[29] have recently recorded responses from two separate layers of the lateral geniculate cortex of monkey and obtained two different response functions to the same type of stimulus (Fig. 11.10). The similarity between the curves in Figures 11.9 and 11.10 is remarkable. Although completely speculative, the two psychophysical functions shown in Figure 11.9 may arise from the two separate visual channels exam-

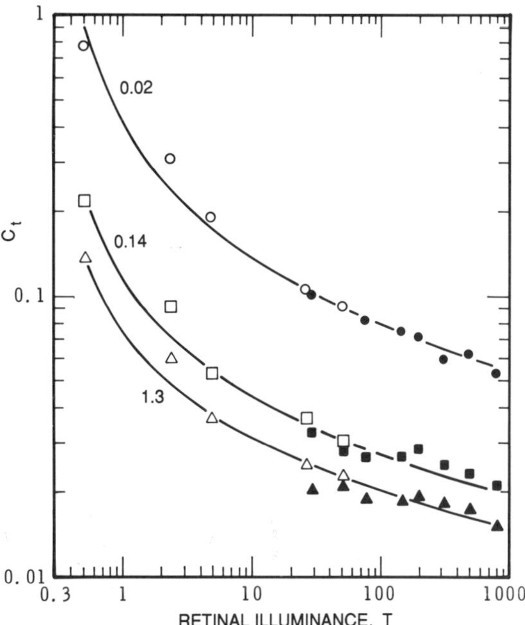

FIGURE 11.5. Contrast threshold (C_t) as a function of background brightness level, measured in trolands (T), for three target areas, 0.02, 0.14, and 1.3 microsteradians. Open symbols are for targets brighter than the background (increments) and closed symbols are for targets darker than the background (decrements). Every point represents the contrast needed for the 50% probability of the target being detected when flashed on a steady background. (Data and curves from Figure 6 of Rea and Ouellette.[24])

ined by Kaplan and Shapley[29] and discussed more extensively by Livingstone and Hubel.[30]

These various contrast response functions may also have different forms in combination with other variables important to vision. Magnitude estimations of contrast do not appear to depend on size,[25] but reaction times to targets of different size (having the same contrast) can be very different.[24] It is not clear whether subjective judgments of contrast depend on the absolute level of stimulation, but reaction times certainly do.[24,31] In general, with speed (or accuracy) used as the dependent variable, the contrast response function to large targets at high background luminance levels will be steplike in appearance. As target size becomes smaller and background luminance lower, however, the contrast response function becomes less steplike and the response level lower. The contrast

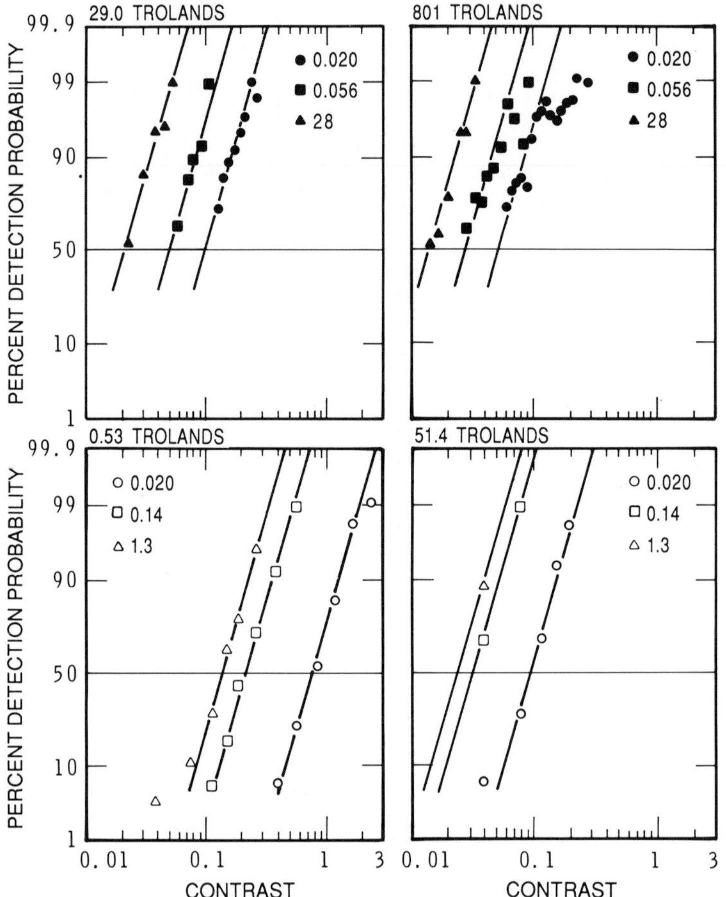

FIGURE 11.6. Probability of detection data under various experimental conditions. Subjects viewed a computer screen through an artificial pupil 2 mm in diameter. Square targets, either brighter than their background (increments; open symbols) or darker than the background (decrements; closed symbols) were flashed on the screen. Subjects were obliged to press a button as soon as the square was detected. Every panel relates the probability of detection of a square to the contrast of that square. Each panel shows data collected at a different adaptation luminance (0.53, 29.0, 51.4, and 801 trolands). Within each panel are sets of detection data for squares of different areas (0.020, 0.056, 0.14, 1.3, and 28 microsteradians). Each set of data is characterized by heavy straight lines of the same slope. The detection threshold for each set of data is determined by the intersection of the line designating the 50% probability of detection (the conventional threshold criterion) and the heavy line characterizing that data set. (Data and curves from Figures 3 and 5 of Rea and Ouellette.[24])

response function using response speed will also depend on the absolute level of stimulation.[24,28,31,32] Figure 11.11 shows results for targets of different sizes, contrasts, and background luminances with response time used as the dependent variable.

Lighting can affect the apparent contrast of objects in two general ways. First, the physical contrast of a task can be affected by changing the lighting-task-eye geometry.[33] Veiling reflections can reduce the contrast of the task by adding a luminous veil to the target and the background (e.g., light reflected from a visual display terminal reduces text contrast). Such a veil can, in some cases, enhance contrast if the directional reflection characteristics of the target and the background are markedly different (e.g., light reflected from a steel ruler can enhance the contrast of lines and numerals marked on its surface). Second, the con-

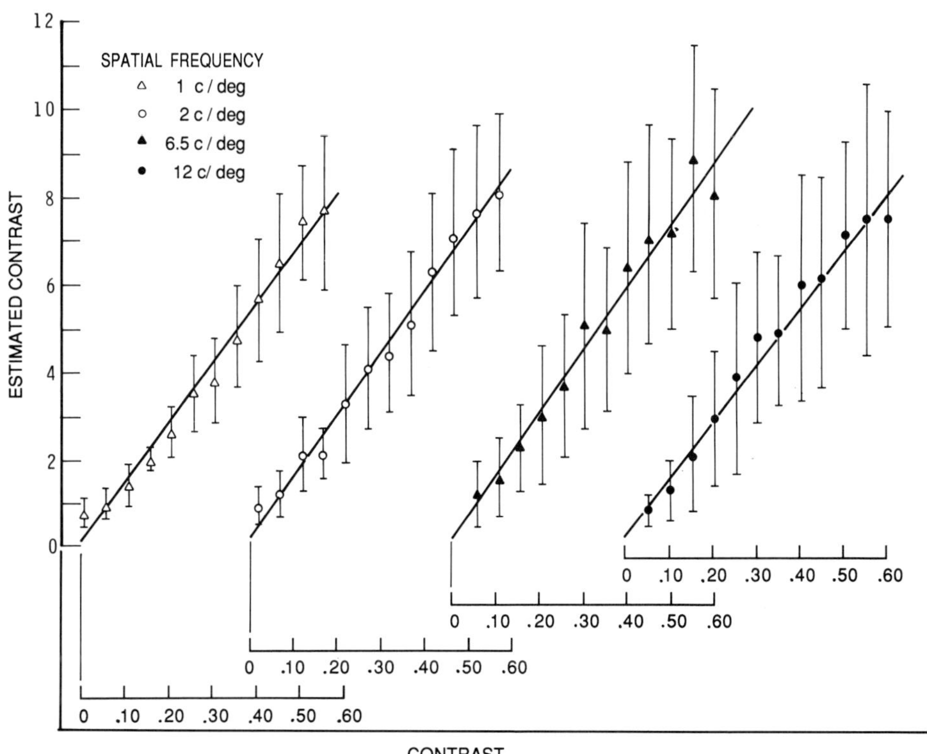

FIGURE 11.7. Contrast response functions using subjective scaling. Subjects gave magnitude estimations of target contrast to targets of different size, or spatial frequency measured in cycles per visual degree (c/deg). Vertical lines represent the standard deviations about the plotted geometric means. (Data and curves from Figure 4 of Cannon.[25] Reprinted with permission, copyright 1979, Pergamon Press PLC.)

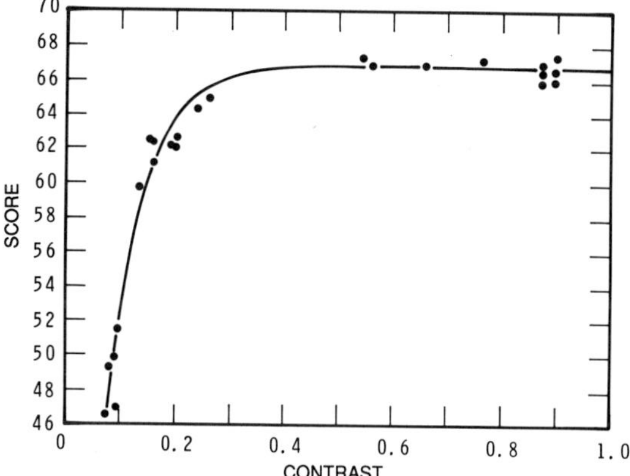

FIGURE 11.8. Contrast response function using time and errors. Subjects were required to compare two number lists of different contrasts as quickly and accurately as possible. Score is a composite of their speed and accuracy. (Data and curve from Figure 7 of Rea.[27])

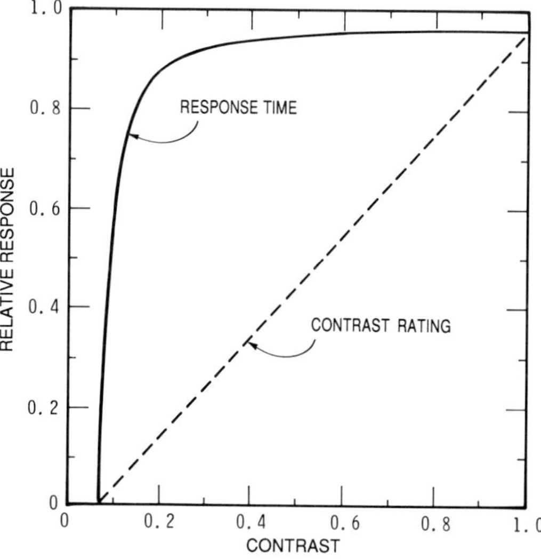

FIGURE 11.9. Two contrast response functions to the same stimuli — printed five-digit numbers of various contrasts — using different response measures. The solid line is based on the reciprocal of response time,[8] and the dashed line is based on unpublished data using magnitude estimations. Background luminance was 20 cd m^{-2} for both.

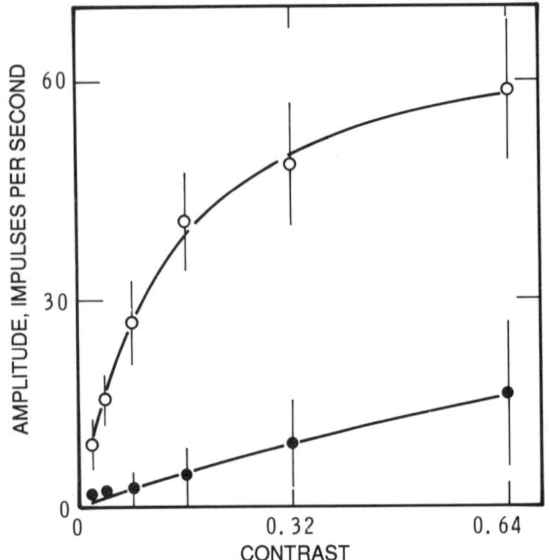

FIGURE 11.10. Contrast response functions from two layers of the lateral geniculate cortex of rhesus monkey. The rates of neural response from neurons in the different layers are plotted as a function of the contrast of a sinusoidal grating that evokes the best response from the cells in those two layers. (Data and curves from Figure 2 of Kaplan and Shapley.[29])

trast of a task can also be reduced by light scattering within the eye. This so-called direct glare is most important when the light source is bright and close to the line of sight to the task.[34] Old people are most seriously affected by direct glare because of age-dependent imperfections in the ocular media.[35]

For both of these cases, contrast losses are most important when the stimulus contrast is close to threshold. Relatively small losses in contrast near threshold may make the difference between seeing and not seeing an object on the roadway, for example. In terms of visual speed and accuracy, contrast variations near threshold will have a very large impact on the magnitude of the suprathreshold visual response. As contrast becomes higher, however, entoptic scatter and luminous veils are much less important (unless, for the latter case, conflicting cues for accommodation and convergence are created). Large losses in the contrast of dark print on white paper can occur without the speed and accuracy of reading being seriously altered, for example.[27] In terms of appearance,

glare will make both colored and achromatic targets less vivid. Any losses in "vividness" are proportionally equal for any suprathreshold contrast, since the contrast response function for appearance is approximately linear.[25] As will be discussed in a subsequent section, however, glare and veiling reflections can often be overcome when people move themselves, the light source, or the task to positions where there is little or no contrast reduction.[36,37]

Size

Visibility depends on the apparent size of a target, or more generally on its spatial frequency content. Targets can be made small enough to become undetectable; such targets are below the *acuity limit*. Generally, acuity is taken to be the reciprocal of the smallest visual angle, in minutes of arc, that can be resolved. Thus

$$\text{Visual acuity} = \frac{1}{\theta} \qquad (11.4)$$

where θ is the minimum resolvable angle in minutes of arc. A person with a visual acuity of 1.0, a value usually considered "normal," can resolve details 1 minute of arc or larger in size. A person who can barely see a target 4 3/16 in. (10.6 cm) in size at 20 ft (6 m), the standard viewing distance, has a visual acuity of 1.0. According to the Snellen convention for characterizing acuity, this person would have a visual acuity of 20/20 (or 6/6). The first number is the standard viewing distance and the second number is the distance a normal person would stand to have the same visual acuity. If a person has a visual acuity of 20/200 (or 0.1 from Eq. 11.4), he or she could resolve details at 20 ft (6 m) that a normal person could resolve at 200 ft (60 m). Young adults with good ocular health and with the proper optical refraction may have visual acuities as high as 2.0, or 20/10 (6/3), under high-adaptation luminances (i.e., they will be able to resolve a visual detail 0.5 minute of arc in size).

Acuity will depend on the contrast, temporal characteristics, and spatial extent of the target as well as on the absolute luminance of the target background. Generally, acuity improves as the

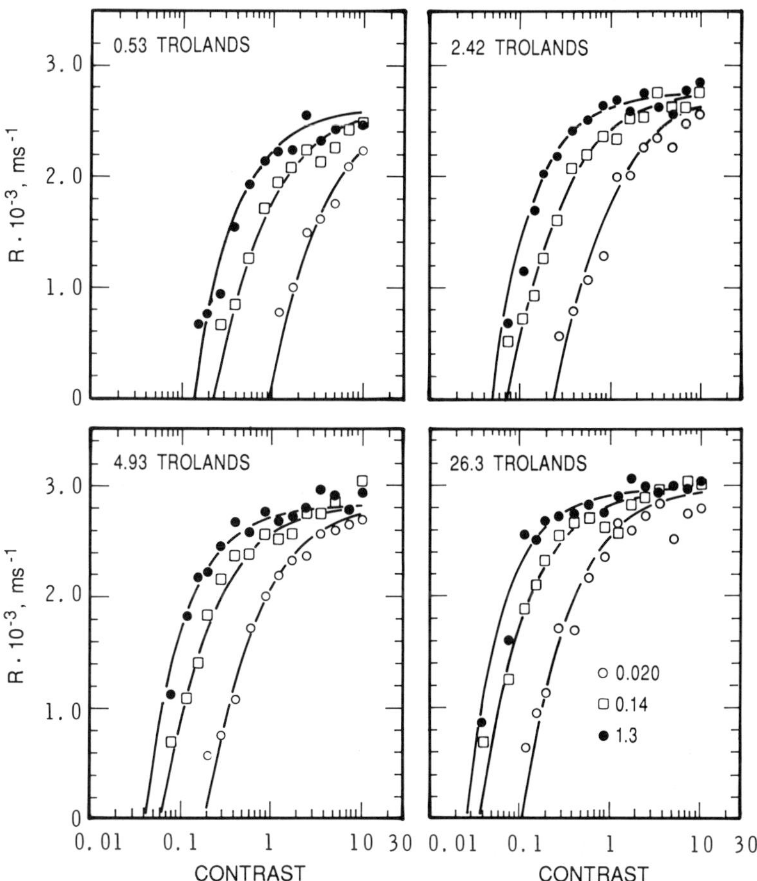

FIGURE 11.11. Contrast response functions using reaction times under various experimental conditions. Subjects viewed a computer screen through an artificial pupil .2 mm in diameter. Square targets brighter than their background were flashed on the screen. Subjects were obliged to press a button as soon as the square was detected. Every panel relates the reciprocal of reaction time, $R \times 10^{-3}$, to the contrast of the squares. Each panel shows data collected at a different adaptation luminance (0.53, 2.42, 4.93, and 26.3 trolands). Within each panel are sets of detection data for squares of different areas (0.020, 0.14, and 1.3 microsteradians). (Data and curves from Figure 11 of Rea and Ouellette.[24])

contrast,[7] presentation time,[38,39] and spatial extent* of the target increases. Acuity will also improve if the luminance of the background on which the target is viewed increases.[6] Another interesting factor to consider is the spatial extent of the target background: Acuity increases as the area on which the target must be seen increases.[6] Given a large uniform background, acuity will continue to improve with luminance, at least up to 5000 cdm⁻², a value well in excess of the values found in electrically illuminated interiors (Fig. 11.12).

As the size of the target increases, visibility, in terms of speed and accuracy, rapidly improves, until after about 20 to 30 minutes of visual arc further increases in size produce little if any improvement in performance.[24,40,41] A more detailed view of this effect can be seen in Figure 11.13.

Lighting can indirectly affect the apparent size of targets. If light levels are reduced, people will either move themselves or the task closer to the

---

*Lines are easier to resolve than points; this is known as *hyperacuity*.

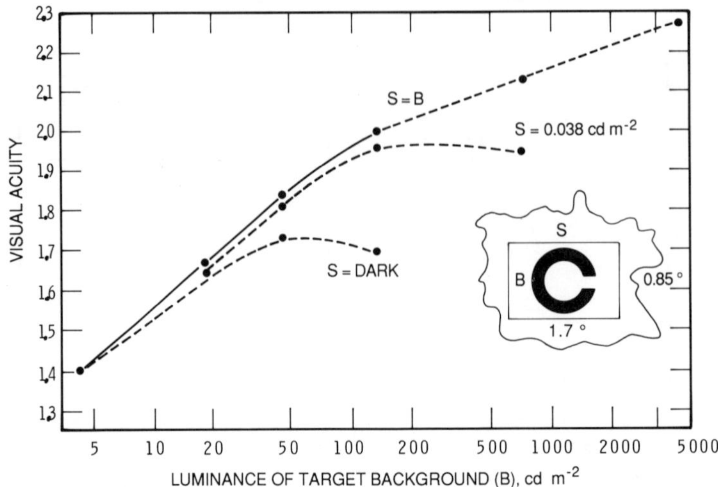

FIGURE 11.12. Effect of surround luminance (S) on visual acuity. Visual acuity is plotted as a function of the luminance of the background (B) for a high-contrast (0.98) Landolt ring acuity target. The Landolt ring and its immediate background are seen through a rectangular aperture 1.7 by 0.85 degrees of arc. The impact on acuity of the brightness of the area forming the aperture (i.e., the surround luminance, S) was determined at three values: S = dark, S = 0.038 cd m⁻², and S = B. Acuity continues to improve with background luminance as long as the surround luminance is equal to the background luminance. (Data and curves from Figure 10 of Lythgoe.[6])

eyes.[37] Presumably this occurs to overcome the coarser "grain" in the retinal mosaic produced by the lower adaptation luminances and creating reduced acuity.[42]

Temporal Modulation and Movement

Much like variations in spatial contrast, the luminance or brightness of objects can vary with time; this is called *temporal contrast*. As with spatial contrast, there is a threshold for temporal contrast. Very small variations in luminance over time cannot be noticed. Perception of temporal contrast will also depend on the frequency of luminance variation. Under the best conditions the eye will be unable to perceive variations greater than about 65 Hz.[43] This value is known as the *critical flicker frequency*.

Sensitivity to these temporal modulations, created either by modulating the output of a light or moving an image from one area of the retina to another, will depend on the other key aspects of the stimulus. For example, the size of a flickering light interacts with its flicker rate.[44] It is generally true that one is more sensitive to large flickering fields than to small ones; however, the reverse is true under certain circumstances (Fig. 11.14). Similarly, the mean brightness of the stimulus will affect the target threshold visibility. Typically, as brightness increases sensitivity increases.[45] Even suprathreshold modulations interact with other key aspects of the stimulus. For example, perceived flicker rate decreases with the size of the stimulus.[46] The apparent rate of motion interacts in a complex way with contrast; a reduction in contrast for rapidly moving stimuli increases apparent velocity, but the opposite is true for slowly moving stimuli.[47]

Most electric lights are supplied with alternating current, and therefore they flicker to some extent. In North America, where alternating current is supplied at 60 Hz, light source flicker (at 120 Hz) will typically be imperceptible. Depending on the characteristics of light source, however, visual problems can still occur. Objects moving under some types of electrical illumination appear to move in discrete steps rather than in a smooth continuous manner. This phenomenon is known as the *stroboscopic effect*[48] and must be considered seriously in many lighting applications. The strobo-

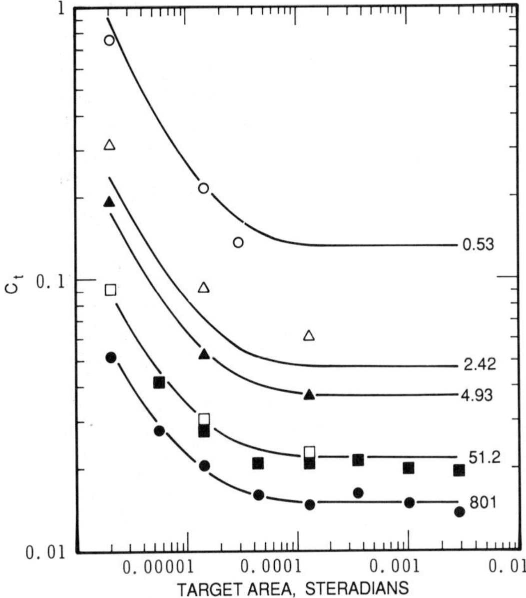

FIGURE 11.13. Contrast threshold (C_t) plotted as a function of target area, in steradians, for five background brightness levels (0.53, 2.42, 4.93, 51.2 and 801 trolands). Open symbols are for targets brighter than the background (increments); closed symbols are for targets darker than the background (decrements). Every point represents the contrast needed for the 50% probability of the target being detected when flashed on a steady background. (Data and curves from Figure 7 of Rea and Ouellette.[24])

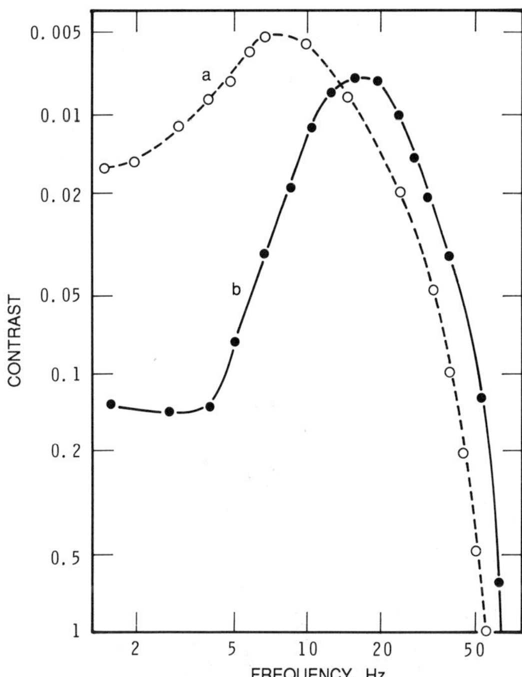

FIGURE 11.14. Flicker sensitivity to targets of different sizes. Curve a shows the contrast necessary to just detect a 2° flickering field in a 60° steady field of the same mean luminance at different temporal frequencies. Curve b illustrates the contrast necessary to detect a 65° flickering field at different temporal frequencies. (From Kelly DH: Effects of sharp edges in a flickering field. *J Opt Soc Am* **49**(7):730–732, 1959.)

scopic effect is important when the temporal contrast is high and the object traverses a large visual angle.[49] Rotating objects under flickering illumination (e.g., a lathe) may appear to stop altogether (as with a timing light used with an automobile engine), which creates a safety hazard—the operator cannot see whether the object is rotating or not. Use of light sources with very little flicker or on three-phase current can prevent annoyance and improve safety.[33]

Finally, recent evidence suggests that flicker above the critical flicker frequency (i.e., imperceptible flicker) may adversely affect certain individuals. Wilkins et al.[50] reported that the incidence of headache and eyestrain was reduced when high-frequency ballasts (32 kHz) were used instead of conventional (British) ballasts (producing 100-Hz flicker). Although these results should be considered tentative, they may point to future insight

about the causes of complaints about fluorescent lamps.

Field Applications

Illuminance and Luminance Meters

Despite relatively detailed understanding of how the visual system responds to key aspects of the visual environment, it has been difficult to translate this understanding into practice. Particularly troublesome to the illuminating engineer, much of this information cannot be applied in the field because of the limited range of necessary tools. Typically, an illuminance meter is the only instrument an illuminating engineer will have for assessing the lighting conditions in a working environment. An illuminance meter simply measures the amount of light falling on a surface. It is impossible

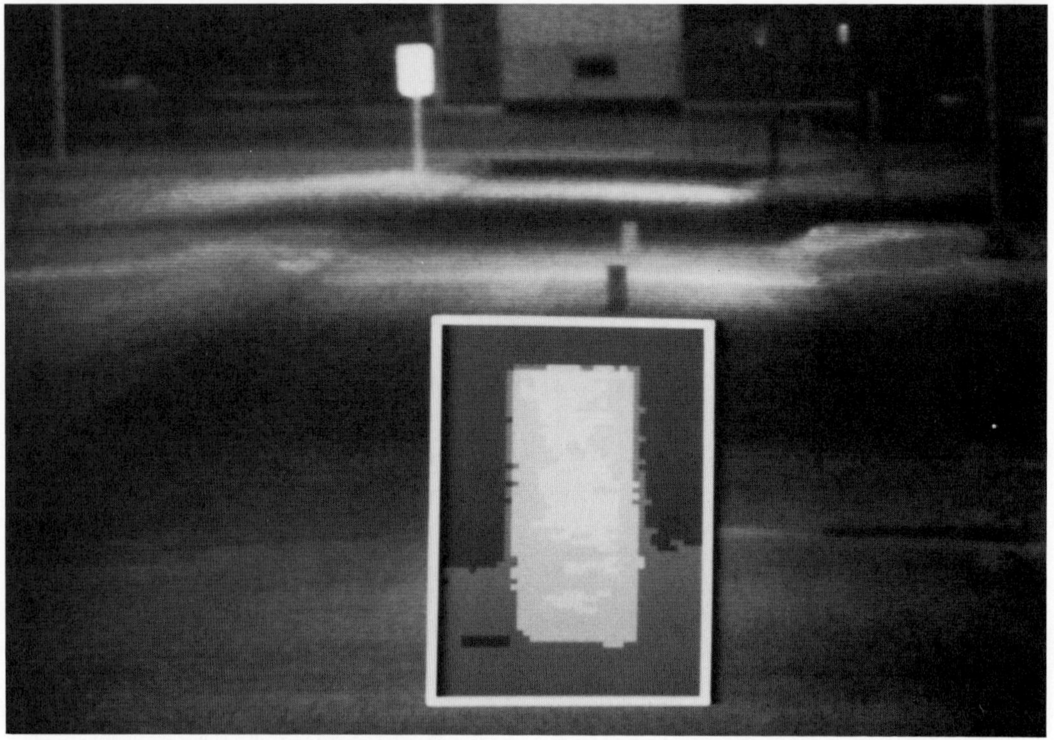

FIGURE 11.15. Digitized image of a roadway generated by the CapCalc (*cap*ture and *calc*ulate) imaging system. Several cement blocks were placed on the roadway at various distances from the driver. After the image was captured and stored in the computer, an area of the image including one cement block was enlarged through software for closer inspection by the system operator. (From Rea MS: National Research Council of Canada.)

to predict visual response without also measuring such important factors as target size and contrast.

Some illuminating engineers use luminance photometers to measure the brightness of objects. In principle, luminance photometers can be used to assess brightness levels throughout a visual scene as well as the contrast of targets against their background. In practice, however, this is almost never done because of the labor-intensive nature of measuring and recording the necessary data and then calculating the impact of those data on visual response. Without practical tools for making measurements of the relevant stimulus conditions, illuminating engineering is hampered in its mission of ensuring adequate seeing conditions in the workplace.

Visibility Meters

Many years ago Luckiesh and Moss[51] recognized the importance of including all of the key aspects of the visual stimulus in assessing lighting quality and quantity. They devised an instrument for assessing the relative visibility of actual tasks in the workplace.[52] The device comprised two filters (one for each eye) continuously varying in density. A person viewed the task through these filters and adjusted them until the task was "just visible." The filters changed both the absolute level and the apparent contrast of the task, but the technique was conceptually important as a starting point for field evaluations of lighting quality and quantity in terms of key aspects of the visual stimulus.

Similar devices, which came to be known as *visibility meters*, were developed to achieve the same goal, namely, to have a field instrument capable of assessing the key aspects of the visual stimulus. Subsequent visibility meters were typically based on the concept of contrast reduction rather than light attenuation as in the Luckiesh-Moss visibility meter.[53-55] All visibility meters have met with limited success for a variety of reasons.[56] Both practical and theoretical problems are inherent with these devices (e.g., stability of calibration, variability in operators, extrapolation of visibility at threshold to suprathreshold levels), but the approach has successfully drawn attention to the importance of measuring the key aspects of the visual stimulus when assessing the lighting conditions.

Imaging Photometry and Analysis System

Recent work at the National Research Council Canada (NRCC) has overcome many of the limitations inherent in visibility meters and produced an imaging photometric system that can rapidly acquire much of the information about the lighted environment that is important to the visual system.[57] It can also quickly compute the impact of certain key aspects of the visual stimulus on visual response. The system is called CapCalc (for *cap*ture and *calc*ulate) and is a fully calibrated luminance photometer linked with a personal computer. CapCalc consists of a solid-state video camera with photopic spectral sensitivity and a personal computer with image-processing board. Approximately 250,000 luminance measurements and their spatial distribution are recorded in a fraction of a second.

After the spatial luminance data have been acquired, it is possible to process those data according to any one of a number of algorithms based on visual science. Figure 11.15 shows an image captured and analyzed with the CapCalc system. From the spatial luminance data in this image, vision algorithms embodied in the computer software can determine, for example, the amount of glare produced by each luminaire[34,58] or the visibility of the objects in the roadway in terms of reaction time.[24] CapCalc and similar devices will probably revolutionize the field of illuminating engineering because, for the first time, it will be practical to make field measurements of the key aspects of the visual stimulus.

Although the CapCalc system allows the illuminating engineer more quickly and more adequately to specify the stimulus for vision and then calculate the impact of that stimulus on a "typical" individual, it is sometimes necessary to evaluate more precisely the impact of a particular lighted environment on a specific person.

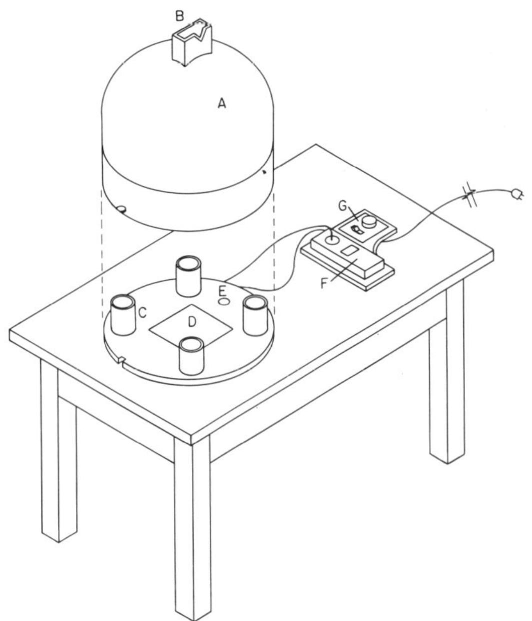

FIGURE 11.16. Components of the VALiD (vision and lighting diagnostic) kit used for diagnosing visibility problems in a working environment. The VALiD kit assesses the quality of the lighting conditions, the difficulty of the visual task, and the visual capabilities of the worker. (From Rea MS: National Research Council of Canada.)

Field Diagnostic Kit

There are three potential sources of problems for seeing in the working environment: The lighting may be inadequate, the task may be inherently difficult to see, or the individual may have impaired vision. Each of these sources can lead to complaints or poor performance by workers, yet it has been difficult to diagnose the problem in the field with currently available techniques.

Recent research at the NRCC has produced a vision and lighting diagnostic (VALiD) kit, which can assist illuminating engineers in analyzing visual problems in the workplace.[59] The kit comprises a standard reference task, an internally illuminated hemisphere, and an illuminance meter (Fig. 11.16). The standard task is an array of Landolt rings of different orientations, sizes, and contrasts. Using the standard task under the reference lighting conditions produced in the hemisphere, it is possible to compare a particular person's performance with that of a large population (approximately 2000 individuals).* From such data it is possible to determine whether the source of the problem likely lies with inferior visual capabilities. Of course the VALiD kit does not analyze all of the potential visual problems (e.g., sensitivity to discomfort glare) and is not a substitute for a clinical examination. It does, however, go well beyond other techniques that have been used in the field to analyze a person's visual capacity.

The kit can also be used to diagnose potential problems with lighting. With the standard task placed at the actual workstation, it is possible to compare performance on the standard task under the hemisphere with that at the workstation. Inferior performance on the standard task when positioned at the workstation would indicate that lighting is likely to be the problem. Using the illuminance meter supplied with the kit, it is also possible to determine whether the illuminance level at the workstation meets that recommended for the task being performed,[33] recognizing of course that illuminance is incomplete in describing the stimulus for vision.

Finally, certain kinds of tasks are inherently difficult to see. The relative difficulty of many visual tasks can be assessed by placing them in the hemisphere and adjusting the illuminance on the task to make it "just visible" or "just readable." From these two illuminance level settings it is possible for the illuminating engineer to assess the relative difficulty of a specific task. (In principle, this technique is similar to that used originally by Luckiesh and Moss.)

By analyzing the task, the lighting, and the eyesight of the worker, the illuminating engineer now has a more precise guide in solving potential problems in the workplace. Without such tools the illuminating engineer is hampered in meeting his or her professional obligation for providing appropriate conditions for seeing in the workplace.

Conclusions

As clinicians and illuminating engineers, our professional responsibility to the public cannot be fulfilled completely without an understanding of visual science. Of equal importance, such understanding can have little impact if we do not have the tools to implement our knowledge.

As professionals, then, we are first obliged to seek a deeper understanding of visual science and to foster that understanding through continued research. Development of new instruments, both for the clinic and for the field, must also be undertaken. We can only crudely analyze many problems facing office workers and highway drivers, even with the latest technology. Sometimes the problem lies with the person's eyesight, but often difficulties are created by the lighting or by the task itself. Without a deeper understanding of visual science and a proper set of tools for the field and clinic, "blame" can be wrongly ascribed to the clinician or the illuminating engineer. With ever-increasing litigation directed toward professionals concerned with seeing, the science and application of visibility is of growing importance.

Acknowledgments. I gratefully acknowledge the time granted me to complete this chapter while I was on staff at the National Research Council Canada, as well as the kind assistance of the following NRCC staff members: S. G. Brault, M. J. Ouellette, A. R. Robertson, J. D. Scott, and D. K. Tiller. Segments of this chapter were developed at the request of the National Electrical Manufacturers Association in Washington, D.C.

References

1. Illuminating Engineering Society of North America (IES): *IES Lighting Handbook* (1st ed). New York, The Waverly Press, 1947.
2. Weston HC: Visual fatigue. *Illumin Eng* **49**:63–75, 1954.
3. deGroot SG, Gebhard JW: Pupil size as determined by adapting luminance. *J Opt Soc North Am* **42**(7):492–495, 1952.
4. Brindley GS: *Physiology of the Retina and Visual Pathway.* London, Edward Arnold, 1970.
5. Dowling JE: The site of visual adaptation. *Science* **155**(3760):273–279, January 1967.
6. Lythgoe RJ: X. *The Measurement of Visual Acuity.* London, His Majesty's Stationery Office, Medical Research Council, Report No. 173, 1932.
7. Richards OW: Effects of luminance and contrast on visual acuity, ages 16 to 90 years. *Am J Psychol* **54**(3):178–184, 1977.

---

*Comparisons are based on the number of Landolt ring gap orientations correctly identified from a set of 156 under two illumination levels (110 lux and 1000 lux).

8. Rea MS: Toward a model of visual performance: Foundations and data. *J Illumin Eng Soc* **15**(2): 41–58, 1986.

9. Lit A: The magnitude of the Pulfrich stereo-phenomenon as a function of binocular differences of intensity at various levels of illumination. *Am J Psychol* **62**:159–181, 1949.

10. McCann JJ, Hall JA: Effect of average-luminance surrounds on the visibility of sinewave gratings. *J Opt Soc Am* **70**(2):212–219, 1980.

11. Wyszecki G, Stiles WS: *Color Science: Concepts and Methods, Quantitative Data and Formulae* (2nd ed). New York, John Wiley, 1982.

12. Alpern M, Ohba N: The effect of bleaching and backgrounds on pupil size. *Vis Res* **12**:943–951, 1972.

13. Kokoschka S: Untersuchungen zur mesopischen Strahlungsbewertung. *Farbe* **21**:39–112, 1972.

14. Sagawa K, Takeichi K: Spectral luminous efficiency functions in the mesopic range. *J Opt Soc Am* **3**(1): 71–75, 1986.

15. Boynton RM: *Human Color Vision.* New York, Holt, Rinehart and Winston, 1979.

16. Ingling CR, Martinez-Urieagas E: The spatio-temporal properties of the R-G cell channel. *Vis Res* **25**(1):33–38, 1985.

17. Alman DH: Errors of the standard photometric system when measuring the brightness of general illumination light sources. *J Illumin Eng Soc* **7**(1): 55–62, 1977.

18. Alman DH, Breton ME, Barbour J: New results on the brightness matching of heterochromatic stimuli. *J Illumin Eng Soc* **12**(4):268–274, 1983.

19. Commission Internationale de l'Eclairage (CIE): *Light as a True Visual Quantity: Principles of Measurement.* Paris, CIE Publication No. 41, 1978.

20. Kaiser PK: Models of heterochromatic brightness matching. *CIE J* **5**(2):57–59, 1986.

21. Robertson AR: Critical review of definitions of metamerism. *Color Res Appli* **8**(3):189–191, 1983.

22. Hurvich LM, Jameson D: Some quantitative aspects of an opponent-colors theory. II. Brightness, saturation, and hue in normal and dichromatic vision. *J Opt Soc Am* **45**:602, 1955.

23. Purdy D: Spectral hue as a function of intensity. *Am J Psychol* **43**:541–559, 1931.

24. Rea MS, Ouellette MJ: Visual performance using reaction-times. *Light Res Technol* **20**(4):139–153, 1988.

25. Cannon MW: Contrast sensitivity: A linear function of stimulus contrast. *Vis Res* **19**:1045–1052, 1979.

26. Stevens SS: *Psychophysics.* New York, John Wiley, 1975.

27. Rea MS: Visual performance with realistic methods of changing contrast. *J Illumin Eng Soc* **10**(3):164–177, 1981.

28. Rea MS, Boyce PR, Ouellette MJ: On time to see. *Light Res Technol* **19**(4):101–103, 1987.

29. Kaplan E, Shapley RM: The primate retina contains two types of ganglion cells, with high and low contrast sensitivity. *Proc Nat'l Acad Sci (USA)* **83**: 2755–2757, 1986.

30. Livingstone MS, Hubel DH: Psychophysical evidence for separate channels for the perception of form, color, movement, and depth. *J Neurosc* **7**(11): 3416–3468, 1987.

31. Vicars WM, Lit A: Reaction time to incremental and decremental target luminance changes at various photopic background levels. *Vis Res* **18**:1579–1586, 1975.

32. Burkhardt DA, Gottesman J, Keenan RM: Sensory latency and reaction time: Dependence on contrast polarity and early linearity in human vision. *J Opt Soc Am* **4**(3):530–539, 1987.

33. Kaufman JE, Christensen JF (Eds): *IES Lighting Handbook, Reference Volume.* New York, Illuminating Engineering Society of North America (IES), 1984.

34. Fisher AJ, Christie AW: A note on disability glare. *Vis Res* **5**:565–571, 1965.

35. Vos JJ: Disability glare—a state of the art report. *CIE J* **3**(2):39–53, 1984.

36. Rea MS: Behavioral responses to a flexible desk luminaire. *J Illumin Eng Soc* **13**(1):174–190, 1983.

37. Rea MS, Ouellette MJ, Kennedy ME: Lighting and task parameters affecting posture, performance and subjective ratings. *J Illumin Eng Soc* **15**(1):231–238, 1985.

38. Riggs LA: Visual acuity. In Graham CH (Ed), *Vision and Visual Perception.* New York, John Wiley, 1965, Chap 11.

39. Burg A: Visual acuity as measured by dynamic and static tests: A comparative evaluation. *J Appl Psychol* **50**(6):460–466, 1966.

40. Legge GE, Pelli DG, Rubin GS, et al: Psychophysics of reading. I. Normal vision. *Vis Res* **25**(2):239–252, 1985.

41. Bradley A, Ohzawa I: A comparison of contrast detection and discrimination. *Vis Res* **26**(6):991–996, 1986.

42. Patel AS: Spatial resolution by the human visual system: The effect of mean retinal illuminance. *J Opt Soc Am* **56**(5):689–694, 1966.

43. Brown JL: Flicker and intermittent stimulation. In Graham CH (Ed), *Vision and Visual Perception.* New York, John Wiley, 1965, Chap 10.

44. Kelly DH: Flicker. In *The Handbook of Sensory Physiology, Visual Psychophysics (VII).* New York, Springer-Verlag, 1972, Chap 11.

45. Kelly DH: Visual contrast sensitivity, *Opt Acta* **24**(2):107–129, 1977.

46. Bowker DO: Perceived flicker rate of suprathreshold stimuli: Influence of spatial-frequency content and modulation amplitude. *J Opt Soc Am* **72**(12):1652–1659, 1982.

47. Thompson P: Perceived rate of movement depends on contrast. *Vis Res* **22**(2):377–380, 1982.

48. Frier JP, Henderson AJ: Stroboscopic effect of high intensity discharge lamps. *J Illumin Eng Soc*, October 1973, pp 83–86.

49. Rea MS, Ouellette MJ: Table-tennis under high intensity discharge (HID) lighting. *J Illumin Eng Soc* **17**(1):29–35, 1988.

50. Wilkins AJ, Nimmo-Smith I, Slater AI, Bedocs L: Fluorescent lighting, headaches and eye-strain. *Proceedings of the CIBSE National Lighting Conference*, Cambridge, England, March 1988, pp 188–196.

51. Luckiesh M: *The Science of Seeing*. New York, D. Van Nostrand, 1937.

52. Luckiesh M, Moss FK: A visual thresholdometer. *J Opt Soc Am* **24**:305–307, 1934.

53. Eastman AA: A new contrast threshold visibility meter. *Illumin Eng* **63**:37–40, 1968.

54. Blackwell HR: Development of procedures and instruments for visual task evaluation. *Illumin Eng* **65**:267–291, 1970.

55. Slater AI: A simple contrast reducing visibility meter. *Light Res Technol* **7**(1):52–55, 1975.

56. Rea MS, Ouellette MJ: *An Assessment of the Blackwell Visual Task Evaluator, Model 3X*. Ottawa, National Research Council Canada, Division of Building Research, NRCC 22960, 1984.

57. Rea MS, Jeffrey IG: CapCalc: *A New Luminance and Image Analysis System for Lighting and Vision*. Ottawa, National Research Council, Institute for Research in Construction, Report No. 565, 1988.

58. Hopkinson RG: Evaluation of glare. *Illumin Eng* **52**:305–316, 1957.

59. Rea MS: *Population Data on Near Field Visual Acuity for Use with the Vision and Lighting Diagnostic (VALiD) Kit*. Ottawa, National Research Council Canada, Institute for Research in Construction, Report No. CR5544.3, March, 1988.

12
Contrast in Photography

Daan Zwick

Introduction

"I don't know what it is, but I know it when I see it," could be a characteristic response of most casual photographers when asked about contrast. A closer study of photographic contrast reveals that it can be as complex as any other visual sensation. It is thus useful to commence the topic with definitions of the pertinent terms. The following arrangement results from long discussions with the late C.J. Bartleson, my colleague at the Kodak Research Laboratories, and owes much to his orderly mind.

Definitions

Contrast is the perception of differences among stimuli or stimulus elements of an array. This perception is formed from several aspects of our visual sensation and also from our experience. As a result, there are several kinds of specific contrast.

Two that may first come to mind are *color contrast* and *brightness* (or *lightness*) *contrast*, which are the perception of differences in color and brightness (or lightness), respectively, among stimuli or stimulus elements. Although the terms *brightness* and *lightness* when used with precision refer to self-luminous and illuminated surfaces, respectively, brightness contrast is often used generically, and is probably the concept that comes most readily to the mind of the layperson in this connection. However, the effect on contrast of chromatic differences can be just as great as that of luminance differences.

Less obvious is *border contrast*, the enhanced difference in perceived color and brightness between juxtaposed stimuli or stimulus elements, at their points of contiguity. *Surface contrast* is the enhanced difference in perceived color, brightness, and texture between two surfaces, usually juxtaposed ones. The visibility of surface differences is strongly influenced by the geometry of the lighting of these surfaces. *Simultaneous contrast* is that induced on simultaneous presentation of stimuli, for example, one stimulus presented against a background of another stimulus, or two different stimuli in the same field. Simultaneous contrast is a significant perceptual effect during the viewing of any complex array, such as a scene or a picture. Related to this is *binocular contrast*, which refers to contrast effects resulting from differential sensitivity or stimulation of the two eyes.

Besides these spatial effects, there can be the temporal sensation of *successive contrast*, the contrast induced on successive presentation of stimuli. This effect can be particularly strong if the first stimulus has been presented long enough for brightness or color adaptation to occur.

These several effects can combine to affect *image contrast*, which is the integrated impression of differences in color (using the broad meaning of color, which includes brightness and lightness) among elements of a spatially complex stimulus array *viewed under a specified set of conditions*. The generic image contrast is called *photographic contrast* when the images in question are produced by photographic means.

Attributes of Photographic Contrast

From the preceding discussion it should not be unexpected that photographic contrast is the result of complex cognitive perceptions involving not only direct visual experiences (perception), but also past or learned experiences (apperceptions), which are brought to bear to form an integrated impression of a complex optical image. For example, a particular picture may be perceived as having low contrast if the viewer expects that it was photographed under harsh sunlight, but can be perceived as having higher contrast if the expectation is that it was photographed under "flat" or diffuse lighting.

Because of this personal involvement, image or photographic contrast may consist of a number of specific attributes. One, *subject contrast*, refers to the perception of differences among elements of the reproduction of a scene that are cognitively ascribed to the relative radiances (or brightnesses) of those elements in the original scene. A difference in lightness of the skin of two people in a picture may be ascribed by the viewer to apparent racial differences between the subjects. *Lightning contrast* refers to the perception of differences among image elements that are recognized as variations in the uniformity of illumination of the original scene. In the example just cited, the viewer noticing that one of the two people was in sunshine and the other in shade might have reached the conclusion that the differences in skin lightness were not in the subjects but in their lighting.

When the differences among the elements of a scene are believed by the viewer to be distorted by flare, haze, or other veiling illumination, this perception can be called *veiling contrast*. This perception, of course, can be affected greatly by the degree of clarity or flare in the viewer's optics, or in the optics of the cameras and projectors used in obtaining and presenting the image.

Attributes of the Imaging System

(Imaging) system contrast is that perception of differences among elements of the image of a scene that are ascribed by the experienced viewer to characteristics of the imaging system itself. An observer having familiarity with imaging systems may be able to isolate specific aspects of the system contrast, which are given names such as *highlight contrast* (perceived differences among image elements that correspond to the brightest areas, i.e., highlights of the image of a scene), *shadow contrast* (perceived differences among image elements that correspond to the darkest areas, i.e., shadows), *mid-tone contrast* (perception of differences among the important image elements that are neither highlights nor shadows), and finally *highlight-to-shadow contrast* (perception of differences between the brightest and darkest areas of the image).

Without striving for this detailed analysis, even the naive observer sees an *overall contrast*, which is the perception resulting from an integrated response to all of the foregoing specific attributes of image contrast (viz., highlight contrast, shadow contrast, mid-tone contrast, highlight-to-shadow contrast, subject contrast, lighting contrast, veiling contrast, and system contrast).

Viewing Conditions

Some of these separate factors are most directly related to the scene and its lighting, some are properties of the imaging system itself, and all are affected by the experience and expectations of the viewer. Another important factor determining our perception of contrast is the conditions under which we view the photograph or other image. The level of illumination on the print or through the transparency, and the level of ambient illumination in which the picture is seen, are critical to the perception of contrast. Thus the definition of image contrast must have the qualifier, "for a given set of viewing conditions."

Hunt, Pitt, and Ward,[1] have quantified the effect of ambient illumination. Figure 12.1 shows how the level of ambient illumination, which sets the adaptation level of the observer, affects perceived contrast. The adaptation levels shown correspond with three methods commonly used to present photographs: darkness in which transparencies may be projected; full illumination in which reflection prints may be viewed; and a low level of illumination, in which large transparencies or radiographs may be examined by transillumination, or in which television screens may be viewed.

A practical consequence of this effect is the requirement that photographic transparencies

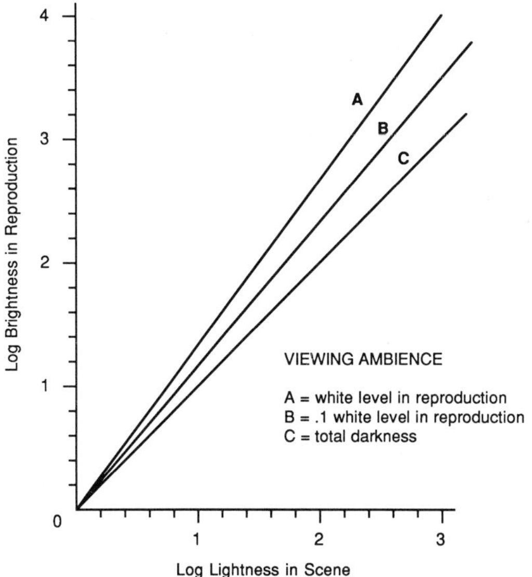

FIGURE 12.1. Appearance of scene elements in reproduction (brightness) versus their scene lightness, as a function of ambient illumination during viewing.

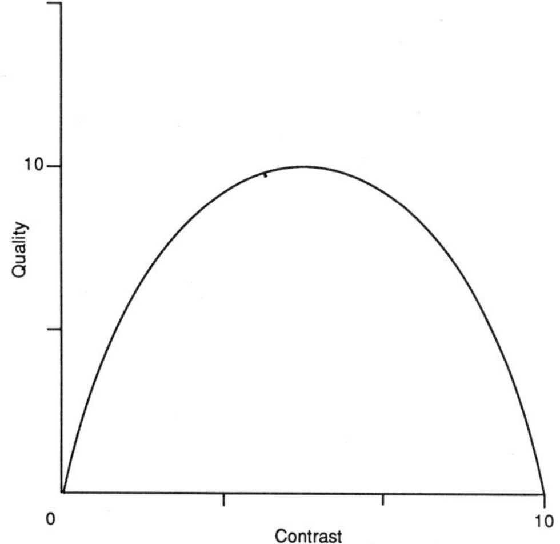

FIGURE 12.2. Picture quality as a function of picture contrast. (Scales are arbitrary, from very low, to very high.)

designed to be projected in a darkened theater be prepared on higher gradient materials than transparencies that are viewed on a large illuminator. Photographic prints, viewed at higher levels of ambient illumination, will require a photographic system of still lower gradient.

Image Quality

Image contrast can be *relative* in the sense that the viewer assesses the degree to which overall contrast matches or resembles that of some tangible reference (e.g., another image), or it can be *absolute* in the sense that its overall contrast is compared with some intangible reference that represents a condition of optimum contrast.

The existence of the concept of an optimum level of contrast brings up questions of the goodness, or *quality*, of the image. Image contrast influences image quality according to the degree to which the overall contrast matches an observer's expectations or desires for the image. Observers with disparate experiences or different expectations for an image can arrive at different concepts of what is optimum contrast for that image. Some photographic systems allow for this by providing means for the photographer to manipulate the image (system) contrast, for example, the provision of several "contrast" grades of printing paper in black-and-white photography.

Some perceptual aspects of photographs, such as graininess or sharpness, are monotonically related to picture quality. That is, the lower the graininess, or the greater the sharpness, the better the picture. However, for contrast the relationship takes the form shown in Figure 12.2. Picture quality is low or nonexistent when contrast is very low. It is also low or nonexistent when contrast is extremely high. A change in contrast from either of these two extremes can produce a rapid increase in quality until maximum quality (limited by factors other than contrast) is approached.

For some scenes or picture uses, maximum quality may be achieved over a relatively wide range of contrasts; for other scenes or uses, the correct contrast may be critical to maximum picture quality. For example, a scene in which the subject lightness differences are very high, such as that of a bride in a white gown next to a groom in a dark tuxedo, will require very careful control of contrast to produce the expected lightness relationships in the

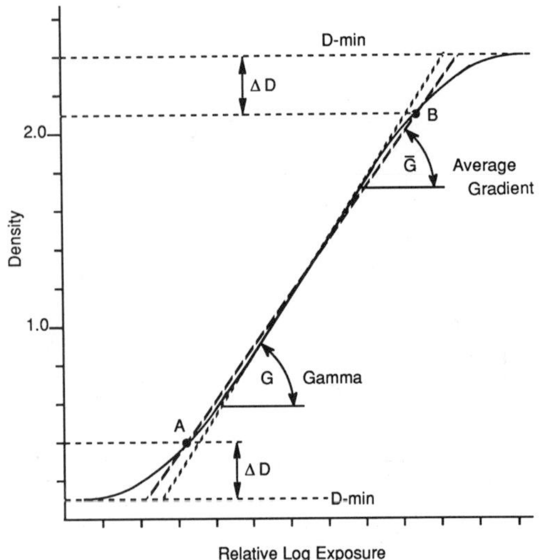

FIGURE 12.3. Average gradient ($\bar{G}$) determined from a density versus log-exposure curve. A standardized method would include criteria for selection of points A and B.

reproduction. Conversely, the observer of a reproduction of an unfamiliar landscape may tolerate a wide range of contrasts on the assumption, for example, that the lighting contrast of the scene was "hard" or "soft."

Similarly, some observers may be more or less tolerant of differences in contrast on the basis of their experience or intended use of the picture information. A viewer of a snapshot who is thinking, "This *is* my daughter" (not "This is a *photograph* of my daughter"), may be quite unaware of such a photographic attribute, and may be very tolerant of variations in contrast provided the picture of the child is flattering. On the other hand, a person producing a textbook or catalog will be very sensitive to the contrast in the illustrations.

A high contrast that enhances differences among the elements of a scene may be desirable for a photointerpreter who is counting aircraft in an aerial photograph of an airfield. Similarly, such contrast may aid a doctor in analyzing a radiograph of a fractured bone. Legibility of alphanumeric characters is also enhanced by high contrast. However, high contrast can cause a loss of information (and thus, a loss in quality) when the photographic material does not have sufficient exposure or density range to record or display the full range of lightnesses that need to be recorded. For example, the radiographer who needs simultaneous information about abnormalities in soft tissue and in bone must accept a compromise lower contrast system.

A photographic system such as Kodak Ektachrome transparency films may have its characteristics optimized for some "normal" amateur photographic use such as "snapping" landscapes on a holiday. The photographer will recognize a higher contrast picture as one taken on a clear, sunny day, and a lower contrast picture as one portraying a harbor in a mist, and feel that the two pictures both have optimum contrast. A pilot using the same system to take pictures from an airplane at high altitude will probably feel that all of those pictures are too low in contrast, for even on a bright sunny day the normal scattering by particles in the atmosphere will reduce the subject contrast greatly. The pilot may know this, but may still have expectations of a more satisfying contrast on the basis of experience at ground level.

Physical Indices of Contrast

I have used the word *contrast* thus far consistently to refer to a subjective perception. However, the word is frequently used also in the objective sense of a physical measurement, or index. An *index of contrast* is a numerical specification, calculated from one or more physical measurements of image characteristics, that is intended to be highly correlated with the subjective image contrast. In this sense, a physical index can be used as a predictor of the subjective sensation.

Relatively few physical indices of contrast have been proposed, probably because many of the factors that influence perceived contrast have not been studied systematically. Studies that have been conducted imply that many physical factors affect perceived contrast. In one study, Bartleson, Jenneiahn, and Woodbury[2] showed that image contrast was related to density range, average gradient, and spatial frequency response of images. A later study by Bartleson (private communication, May, 1987) of the factors that influence image contrast showed that acutance, granularity, average gradient, physical tone reproduction characteristics, printing exposure, lighting (physical) contrast, object haze, image exposure, subject (physical) contrast, and distribution of relative radiances in the scene all influence contrast.

The effects of most of these interrelated factors have been clearly demonstrated in a series of illustrated lectures by Ralph Evans, and many of these are summarized, with illustrations, in his books.[3,4] Evans discusses the interrelationships of the perceptual factors and relates them to physical phenomena.

Two commonly used physical indices of contrast are *gamma* and *average gradient*, although these simple indices are only rough approximations to something as complex as image contrast. Gamma (symbolized G) is measured as the slope of the linear portion of the transfer function relating density to log exposure (Fig. 12.3). Since this is, therefore, the exponent of the power function of the *transmittance* or *reflectance* versus *exposure* curve ($T = -\log D$) over the range that may be characterized by a simple power function, gamma should (strictly) be specified only when such conditions exist. Average gradient (symbolized $<G>$ or sometimes $\overline{G}$ [bar Gamma]) is the slope of a line connecting two coordinate points of density, log exposure that are selected by criteria relating to density or log exposure relationships. An example is shown in Figure 12.3. American National Standards (ANSI) and international standards (ISO) define the measurement of average gradients for different types of photographic products.*[5]

Optimum Gradient

What is the relationship between optimum contrast, the perceptual attribute of a picture, and optimum gradient, a physical descriptor of the photographic system? Earlier we defined optimum contrast according to the degree to which the appearance of the contrast of the reproduction matched the expectations of the viewer, expectations based on experience with the scene or similar subject matter. A photographic material with a gradient of 1.0 (one in which double the exposure results in double the transmission or reflection of illumination to the viewer of the reproduction) will

seldom achieve this desired result. We almost never view a photograph in the same ambience as we viewed the scene, even with "instant" photography. Cameras, projectors, and screens all affect image gradient differently from the way our visual system affects our perception of the scene, due to light-scattering properties. If the sharpness of a picture is at all degraded, as it frequently is, this reduced sharpness produces the appearance of lower contrast, which demands a compensating increase in gradient. And if color saturation in the reproduction is reduced, that, too, will reduce perceived contrast.

It is possible to calculate quantitatively the compensations in gradient required by flare components. This is done in the "tone reproduction" diagrams originated by Jones.[6] However, information does not exist that allows such calculations to compensate for degradations in color or sharpness.

Flare

Photographic exposure due to *flare* can be defined as that component of the total exposure arriving at a particular area in the film plane that does not originate directly from the object that is being imaged in that area. It occurs because energy from objects other than that intended to be imaged is scattered or reflected by components of the imaging system into that area. Flare can have many sources. A considerable volume of atmosphere with many scattering particles between the scene and the camera, as there is in aerial photography or in photography of distant scenery, will induce flare. The lenses used to image the object can introduce varying amounts of flare even if clean, and of course any dust or smudges on the glass will increase flare. The multiple reflections that can occur at the glass-air interfaces between the elements of lenses can be a significant cause. Modern multielement lenses use an antireflection coating on all surfaces to reduce this degradation. However, the many surfaces in some telephoto lenses can induce measurable flare effects.

Behind the lens there can be other sources of flare. A carelessly designed lens mount can leave shiny retaining rings to reflect stray light toward the film. Multiple reflections can occur, at extreme angles, from blackened lens barrels. The surface of the film itself may reflect and scatter light that can

---

*American National Standard PH2.2-1966 and subsequent revisions. American National Standards Institute, 1430 Broadway, New York, NY 10018 can also supply copies of the standards generated by the International Organization for Standardization (ISO).

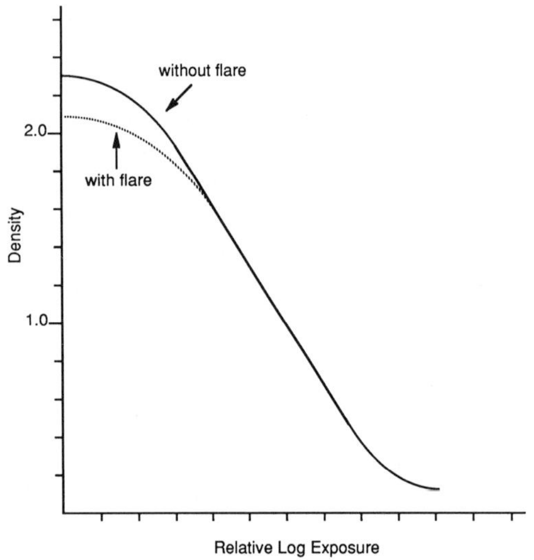

FIGURE 12.4. The effect of veiling flare on the photographic density versus log-exposure relationship. The level of flare shown could result from a dirty multielement lens.

then be rereflected by the inner surfaces of the lens and camera body. A peculiar reflection, called *halation*, can occur inside the film itself, when light scattered by the sensitive silver halide crystals encounters the interface between the smooth surface of the plastic film support and the air, which have different optical indices of refraction. At this optical interface, rays exiting at less than the critical angle will pass through, but rays reaching the interface at the critical angle or greater will be reflected. This phenomenon was given the name halation because it was first described by astronomers, who saw it as a circular halo around images of stars. A small object such as a star will produce a recognizable halo; with larger objects the potential halo from each point merges with those from other points to produce a general flare exposure. Most modern films use some sort of filter or layer beneath the sensitive layers to reduce this internal reflection.

Some components of the flare energy exist uniformly over the film plane, but often much of that energy is in localized areas surrounding sources of high exposure in the scene. Because of the density-log-exposure relationship, the energy in the flare component has greatest effect in areas of low image exposure. In a positive transparency, flare reduces the density of large dark or shadow areas that had little or no image exposure, and thus reduces con-

trast. It also reduces the density in small dark images, affecting both sharpness and contrast. The effect of flare in bright areas of the image may not be noticeable, because the flare exposure is a negligible part of the total exposure of those areas. These effects are illustrated in Figure 12.4; density is plotted versus log exposure with and without the addition of a uniform flare exposure.

Conclusion

The phenomena just described inherent in photographic flare are, in general, no different from flare phenomena occurring in visual systems. Because the responding element, the photographic image, is accessible to measuring instrumentation, we find it relatively easy to quantify the direct results of flare on the physical index of contrast, photographic gradient. However, this chapter has pointed out the complex relations among the sensations of sharpness, graininess, color and lightness contrast, subject contrast, and lightning contrast, as well as flare, that determine the overall perception of contrast in a photographic image. Faced with this multitude of affective elements, we do not yet have enough knowledge to predict the sensation of contrast generated in the mind of the viewer of something so complicated as a picture, from physical measurements of that image.

Knowing this, the intelligent investigator of visual effects avoids these problems by designing simpler geometric or alphanumeric test patterns more appropriate to the type of information being sought.

References

1. Hunt RWG, Pitt IT, Ward PC: The tone reproduction of colour photographic materials, *J Phot Sci* **17**:198, 1969.
2. Bartleson CJ, Jenneiahn RH, Woodbury WW: Visual contrast in photographic prints, *J Phot Sci* **11**:35–41, 1963.
3. Evans R: *An Introduction to Color.* New York, John Wiley, 1948.
4. Evans R: *Eye, Film, and Camera in Color Photography.* New York, John Wiley, 1959.
5. *SPSE Handbook of Photographic Science and Engineering.* New York, Wiley-Interscience, 1973, pp 817–822.
6. Jones LA: On the theory of tone reproduction, with a graphic method for the solution of problems. *J Franklin Inst* **198**:39, 1920.

Index